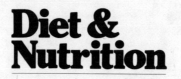

Diet & Nutrition

Diet & Nutrition

a holistic approach

Rudolph Ballentine, M.D.

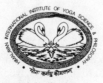

Published by
The Himalayan International Institute
Honesdale, Pennsylvania

Library of Congress Catalog Card Number: 78-110274
ISBN 0-89389-022-7
ISBN 0-89389-048-0 pbk.

Copyright 1978

Himalayan International Institute
of Yoga Science and Philosophy
Honesdale, Pennsylvania

Second Printing, 1978
Third Printing, 1979

Publisher's Note

Proper diet and good nutrition have become an increasingly and realistic concern in recent years. The Himalayan Institute is pleased to present this unique work which provides an integrated and holistic approach to a field too often fragmented by controversy.

Diet and Nutrition demonstrates how modern science and traditional wisdom can come together to provide practical answers to the issues that surround nutrition so that one is brought into greater harmony with the environment and into closer touch with the inner Self.

Acknowledgements

The author was privileged to be assisted in the preparation of this book by an unusually talented and dedicated staff. Special appreciation is due to the staff physicians of the Himalayan Institute, who worked tirelessly in researching and verifying detailed areas of the book: David Anderson, M.D., Greg Manteuffel, M.D. and especially Matthew Monsein, M.D., who labored alongside me through long days and late into the night on many occasions. Special thanks also go to Mrs. Betty James who unselfishly gave a year of her time to collect and index information; also to Arpita and my mother who devoted many months to editing and organizing the manuscript; to Randy Black and Bala for illustration and design, John Miller who did the indexing, and last but not least, to Theresa O'Brien who carefully and painstakingly typeset the many, often technical, pages of this book.

Many others contributed information, suggestions, and help of all sorts. I also owe a debt of gratitude to those students and patients whose thoughtful questions, whose clippings and reprints, and whose very real needs prompted and stimulated the writing of *Diet and Nutrition*.

Contents

Preface

This book is not intended to be an encyclopedia of nutrition. It is quite clear that no one book can even begin to encompass the wealth of data available today on the various aspects of nutrition. The valuable literature on trace elements alone would easily fill several volumes. The accumulated research on vitamins is even more massive. To orient the student properly to only one vitamin, its history, its meaning in nutrition, and the essence of its use would require at least a small book.

Nor is this book intended to popularize a "new diet" or new twist to nutrition. Rather it is offered as an overview. It is an attempt to put the field of nutrition into some coherent perspective. One who begins to develop awareness of diet and is interested in further understanding finds himself confused and frustrated by the disparate and apparently irreconcilable differences in attitudes and theories about nutrition.

This book then is an attempt to provide a holistic and comprehensive overview of the field that is designed to orient the serious student whether he is lay or professional. While no one area is dealt with in the detail that might be possible, it is hoped that a single volume integrating the major approaches used in nutritional research and practice might reduce somewhat the feeling of fragmentation and contradiction that confronts those who are beginning to explore the subject. If the reader comes away from this book with the feeling that nutrition can be productively approached from a number of angles but that each approach has its limitations as well as advantages and that, moreover, they can all be fit together to form a complex and yet coherent science, then this work will have served its purpose.

In keeping with this intent, copious footnotes and references are provided so that the student who wishes to delve into an area in more depth may be able to do so without the frustrating and time-consuming work that is ordinarily needed to get at solid and reliable information. An attempt has been made to provide references to the best and most current information on the subject, but because of the rapidity with which knowledge is being accumulated in the field of nutrition, it should be understood that such efforts may at times be only partially successful. Clive McCay, one of the outstanding nutritionists of this century, writing in the 1930's, estimated that in order to keep up with the published literature on nutrition, one would have had to read one article every three minutes during his entire working day of eight hours. Even so, he would have been behind since he would have only covered the chemical aspects of nutrition, ignoring the medical literature. And that was nearly a half century ago. In the meantime, the *Index Medicus*, which simply lists research articles on medical and related sciences, has grown from one small volume a year to more than a half dozen huge ones, and research published in the field of chemistry has increased proportionately. Clearly, no one person can be even vaguely aware of such a mass of information. In any event, the intent of the present author is not to have the last word on the subject but rather to suggest some models for thinking about diet and nutrition and to establish an approach which might serve in the coming years to integrate the rising flood of data which is becoming so overwhelming.

Many of the most fascinating areas in nutrition are controversial. Perhaps no field of scientific endeavor today is so filled with contradictions. It has not been the purpose of this book to take sides. Rather there has been a serious and sincere attempt to outline various positions to show the truth in each and to attempt to provide a perspective that permits as much as possible an integration of the most valid points of all. The greatest challenge here was the effort to cope with the disparity between traditional Eastern and modern Western ideas about nutrition. One of the major goals of this book is to bring together some of the insights of the East with the scientific research of the West. While contemporary laboratory research has been very productive in providing great quantities of information, it seems increasingly likely that we will have to look beyond it for the insights and perspectives that will enable us to assimilate and organize this data. It is the opinion of the author that the more experientially-oriented concepts about diet and nutrition that come from the ancient traditions of the East will be very useful in this respect. It is hoped that this book will explore that possibility in a practical and understandable way.

Rudolph M. Ballentine, Jr. M.D.
Honesdale, Pennsylvania
February 17, 1978

I

The Ecology of Nutrition

The complex interplay of animate and inanimate systems on the surface of the earth—soil, air, water, plants and animals—has come only recently to be appreciated as a delicate but fundamental factor in the welfare of the planet. We have just begun to realize that our unthinking interaction with these systems—air, soil and water—multiplied by families and groups and cities and crowds can burden them and shift them from a state of equilibrium, the thrust of which can recoil, damaging us, our food supply and our health in turn.

The movement of certain minerals and plant-made compounds into the body of the human, a phenomenon we call "nutrition" is but one small aspect of the overall ecological whole. Though it is our purpose to examine this aspect in detail, in order to do so properly we must have a clear understanding of how it fits into the larger picture. We must understand the nature of the human cell and the nature of the plant cell which provided the nourishment around which animals and man evolved; we must grasp the relationship between the quality of cellular life and the quality of the soil from which it springs, and we must become aware of what impact social, tribal and economic influences have on the eating patterns and food habits of man.

Eating Patterns—
Ancient and Modern

1

Cookbooks outsell all others in most bookstores today, and interest in nutrition is constantly growing. While in many cultures eating habits are established by tradition and the principles of nutrition are assumed rather than discussed, in this country there is much confusion about exactly what a healthy diet really is. People are concerned, and legitimately so. There have been serious trends away from wholesome foods, and many people sense the negative effects of such changes. Our major purpose in this book is to understand how we can evolve for ourselves a diet of high nutritional quality despite unhealthy social trends.

CURRENT EATING HABITS

First, however, we need some perspective on changing food patterns. It is important to understand what the general public is eating and why they are eating it. It is now estimated that food-away-from-home expenditures account for about 36% of the total food dollar,[1] and they are expected to be half again as much by 1985. This trend is both a cause of and a result of a change in family structure. The family meal, once a sacred institution, is being gradually eroded. What was once a major focus of family life is gradually shifting outside the home. The "limited menu restaurants," which include most fast food chains, are growing rapidly, their sales increasing almost fifteen percent each year.[2] Hamburger, hot dog, and roast beef restaurants are the most prevalent of these fast food chains with pizza, chicken, taco, seafood, and pancake outlets following. Last year, over 15 billion hot dogs were eaten in America.[3] If these were lined up end to end, they would extend to the moon and back four times. The most frequently purchased foods, comprising

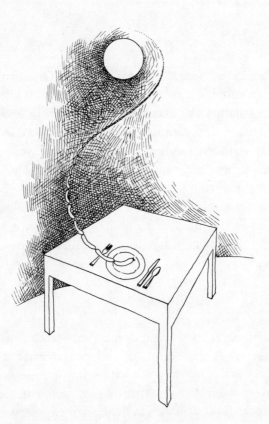

the most popular American meal, are hamburgers, french fries, a small salad, coffee and soft drinks.[4] The nutritional content of such a meal is questionable. However, the consumption of foods that are even less nutritious than these, such as "snack foods" and "junk foods," is of even more concern from a nutritional point of view. Since World War II, the consumption of soft drinks, for example, has gone up about 80%. These drinks are essentially sugar unless they are "diet pop," in which case they are merely a solution of chemicals. In the same time period, the consumption of pastries has gone up 70% while that of potato chips has gone up 85%.[5] Meanwhile, the consumption of dairy products has gone down 21%, that of vegetables has decreased by 23%, and fruits by 25%.[6] This is a steady, definite and important change.

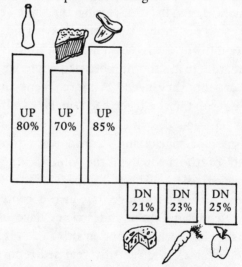

Changes in Eating Habits since World War II

The major ingredients of most poor-quality foods are fats and sugars. Fat constitutes about 45% of the calories that most people take, and sugar accounts for about another 20%. Therefore, the diet of the average person is between 60% and 70% fat and sugar. Such a diet does not provide room for other needed nutrients.   Moreover, snacks and ready-prepared foods that are high in fats and sugars require the addition of flavorings, colorings, and conditioners to give them appeal and preservatives to retard deterioration so they can remain on the shelf until used.   There are about 2,000 such additives used by the food industry today, and the average person eats between an estimated three[7] and five [8] pounds of these chemicals a year.

DIET AND HEALTH

The government regularly does a nutritional survey in which families are randomly sampled in ten selected states to try to assess how much of different nutrients the average American gets.   In 1955, the survey estimated that 60% of the people had an adequate diet.   In 1965, using the same criteria, it was down to 50%.[9]   This shows that within a period of ten years there was a significant decrease in what is considered, by conservative standards, to be the number of people who are getting all the vital nutrients they need.   A more recent survey has been made, but the results haven't yet been analyzed.   If the 1955 to '65 trend has continued, which seems likely considering the increases in sales of snacks and "convenience foods," by now well over half of the people in the United States are eating definitely deficient diets.   The full impact of this on the health of the people is difficult to judge, but in this century a number of carefully researched books and articles have documented a close relationship between diet and health.[10, 11] "Nutritional Goals for the United States," the recently released report of a Senate Select Committee, attempts to summarize current trends in eating and to see if there is any correlation between these and trends in health.   The committee decided that there was indeed a relationship and that, in fact, the most common diseases today are related at least in part to diet.   This seemed particularly true in the case of heart disease and cancer, which are the two major causes of death at present.   There is conclusive evidence that diet plays some role in both of these diseases, and for many people that role is highly significant.[12]

Besides the suffering that results from such diseases, their cost is monumental not only in terms of loss of work time, but also in terms of medical care. From 1960 to 1976, the total cost of medical care increased from 27 billion dollars to over 137 billion dollars per year,[13] the bulk of it being used for the treatment of such diseases as cancer, arteriosclerosis and diabetes. That is an increase of over 500 percent in sixteen years.* Moreover, costs have been climbing with increasing rapidity in the last five years so that the outlook is bleak unless major steps can be taken to prevent the most widespread diseases. From all evidence, this could be accomplished most simply and directly through changes in dietary habits.

The cost of the food itself has also increased, in part because of the more elaborate and sophisticated processing that goes into the preparation of snack and ready-prepared foods. Current agricultural practices are more expensive too, despite the reduction in manpower they have made possible. Fertilizers, pesticides and herbicides have all added to the cost and energy consumption involved in farming. Whereas at the turn of the century one calorie of food value was produced by the input of less than a calorie of energy so that there was actually a "gain," today ten calories of energy are used to produce the same one calorie of food value.[15]

The problems of modern nutrition extend from the soil and farmer to the processing plant and advertisers, to the grocery store and consumer and, sadly, often to the doctor's office. Despite the disheartening situation that exists, there are many things that we can do to extricate ourselves from it. In order to accomplish this, however, we must understand the nature of the

___

* Though part of this is due to inflation, much of it is real. In the decade from 1965 to 1975 the cost of medical care increased from 5.9% to 8.3% of the gross national product.[14]

cell we are trying to nourish, of the food we are consuming, and of the soil from which it comes. We must also have some perspective on the origin of man's eating habits and what happens when he breaks with traditions of sound nutrition that were evolved over many generations.

TOTAL HEALTH EXPENDITURES

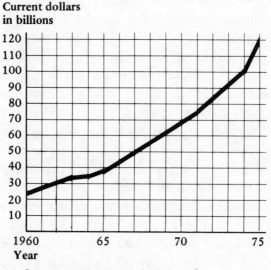

Current dollars in billions

Source: Mueller, M.S. and Gibson, R.:
National Health Expenditures. 1929-75.
Social Security Bulletin 39:3-20 February 1976.

ORIGINS OF FOOD PATTERNS

When man abandoned the forest and began to form villages, his food habits changed. No longer was he roaming about eating what was available, shifting his home to correspond to the changing seasons, the coming and going of various fruits and leaves, or the migrations and movements of game animals. Instead he began to live permanently in a confined space. His food was no longer a matter of what could be plucked from the trees or gathered wild from the fields, but rather what could be cultivated, what could be stored, and what could provide the most food for the most people. The first agricultural communities were organized around what could be grown in their area, and this was supplemented in some cases by what animal food could be killed nearby and brought back to the home base.

Food collectors were able to accumulate a rich lore based on experience with the wild plants and animals of their locale. They knew their habitat so well that they gradually learned to domesticate the plants and animals they had previously been collecting and hunting. This was a very natural process, and it seems that the first step was an unintentional breeding of the kind of food source needed. As wild grain was harvested, for example, one would necessarily reap those plants with tough spikes and intact heads because the grain of other varieties would have already fallen to the earth. When he finally came to sow seeds, he would naturally have on hand a large proportion of grains from plants which retain their seeds longer—exactly the kind he needed for farming. He then apparently found it advantageous to move these grains down from their natural mountain habitat to land which was flatter and closer to water. It was probably then that domesticated grain, having adapted itself to the new environment, lost its ability to disperse its seeds and became totally dependent on man. Man in turn, became dependent on his plants. Cultivation of such grains led to the development of small farming communities.[16]

The eventual emergence of cities and urban civilization was therefore based on the development of agricultural skills. Only if a consistent supply of food could be grown in the surrounding area, and only if a sufficient amount could be stored to last through famines and off-seasons could the village or town evolve. Survival was dependent on the food supply. If it was adequate, the town could flourish. If it became scarce, health and stamina declined until the people were forced to desert their settlement to seek new land or else remain eventually to face disease and conquest. Archaeological digs tell the story of this cycle time and again.

This process apparently occurred many times in many different locales over the earth's surface. The details are clearest perhaps, in the Middle East where archaeologists have studied the emerging civilizations in the greatest detail. Early cities located in Mesopotamia consisted of small communities scattered along natural waterways. Cultivation was confined to narrow enclaves of irrigated plots along swamp margins and stream banks. The farming villages of the pre-urban era covered at most only a few acres. When the course of the river shifted, when the climate changed, when the limited pasturage declined, or when a roving band of nomads destroyed the settlement, the town vanished.[17]

CIVILIZATION AND AGRICULTURE

Yet, while man's newly domesticated food supply was often his limitation, in many senses it was also his liberation, for the evolution of a stable, storable, and accessible source of nutrition freed him from the necessity of being constantly preoccupied with food. No longer was it necessary for him to spend his time stomping through the forests or chasing after animals in an attempt to get enough to eat. No longer did his life need to be organized around the search for food. No longer was he forced to pass his day and night engaged in survival struggles and hunting, exposed to the dangers of the open forest. Now he could turn his time and energy to other pursuits. Agriculture brought the potential for peace and stability. Now a smaller percentage of the population was involved in the hunting, growing and preparation of food.[18] More and more people could devote themselves to exploring man's potential for creativity, discovery and understanding. Oral traditions became more elaborate, and a continuity of thought and learning was established. The stage was set for the emergence of highly developed art, philosophy and techniques for the cultivation of personal growth.

But there were definite pitfalls during the development of agricultural settlements. Farming practices often involved continual repetition of the same crop, resulting in gradual depletion of the soil. This, plus the disruption of the soil's natural balance that occurs when the soil is turned, frequently opened the way for erosion. As the soil became exhausted, the quality of the food declined, and ultimately the crops failed. Where man's ingenuity triumphed, where methods of crop rotation and composting were developed, and where the art of restoring and preserving soil fertility was learned, an enduring culture was established. By contrast, where these lessons were not learned, settlers were forced to move on. The result, during the early stages of the development of agriculture, was one wave of migration after another, sweeping across Asia north and west through Europe or Northeast to China[19] leaving only islands of more firmly rooted communities where the earth and its nurturance had come to be regarded with respect.

The records of man's struggle with his food supply are left buried with the remains of villages and often etched by disease in the bones and teeth of the men who inhabited them.

NUTRITION AND DENTAL PROBLEMS

Of the various kinds of tissue breakdown and disease processes that can result from dietary deficiencies, that which involves the teeth is perhaps the most accessible to objective evaluation and statistical analysis. Nutritional studies based on dental disease can be extended into past generations and sometimes even prehistoric times, since the teeth and jaws remain intact longer than the rest of the body and are frequently identifiable in anthropological explorations.

In the early part of the 20th century, Dr. Weston Price, who was a dentist, became interested in the relationship between nutrition and tooth decay. It had long been said that sweets caused dental decay, or that a poor diet resulted in bad teeth, but he determined to establish to his satisfaction whether, in fact, there was such a relationship and if so, exactly how important it was. In the 1920's and 30's, it was still possible to find areas where modern industrial civilization and its more processed diet was just beginning to make inroads into traditional food habits. So, Dr. Price set out on a series of expeditions, traveling around the world to compare various population groups in their native setting where their traditional diet continued unaltered, with the same tribes or ethnic groups where the refined foods that were brought in by modern civilization had become a major part of the diet.

In 1931 and 1932, for example, Dr. Price compared traditional areas of Switzerland with more "modernized" ones. One community he studied was that of the Loetschental valley where the agricultural practices and the way of life were completely self-sufficient and had been for centuries. Life was simple but stable, and cultural and spiritual values were highly prized. The valley, enclosed on three sides, was very isolated, containing a community of only 2,000 people. These valley dwellers had neither physician nor dentist because they had little need for them, nor had they policemen or jail because they had no need for them either. Dr. Price found that it had been the "achievement of the valley to build some of the finest physiques in all of Europe." In fact, a surprisingly large percentage of the Swiss guard had been customarily recruited from this tiny valley.

The bulk of the diet of these valley people consisted of bread made from their own home-grown rye which was taken with the fresh milk of their own goats or cows, or the cheese they made from it. Dr. Price had samples of this food sent to him twice a month throughout the year and, using the laboratory technology then available, he tested them for their mineral and vitamin contents. "The samples were found to be high in vitamins and much higher than the average samples of commercial dairy products in America and Europe and in the lower areas of Switzerland." Dr. Price also observed that the hay on which the cows were fed throughout the winter proved, upon chemical analysis performed in his laboratory, "to be far above the average in quality for pasturage and storage grasses."[20] In the summer, he noted, the cows "seek the higher pasturage lands and follow the retreating snow." During this time "they have a period of high and rich productivity of milk." It seems likely that the melting glacial snows played an important part in keeping the soil rich in minerals so that it was fertile and could produce good pasturage, good hay and good rye for bread. As we shall see, life-giving food springs from healthy, fertile soil.

Dr. Price's dental survey of this valley's inhabitants revealed that among the children between seven and sixteen years of age, the number of cavities per person was 0.3. On the average, in other words, it was necessary to examine three children to find one cavity. Two out of three had absolutely perfect teeth! A complete absence of all dental caries and fillings is, of course, something seen very rarely in Europe and America today. But in a neighboring valley, Dr. Price found that the incidence of tooth decay was dramatically higher. Here there were 20.2 cavities per hundred teeth. That is, virtually every child had cavities, with an average of about six or seven decayed teeth each. Though the way of life and surroundings of these two valleys were very similar, in the second valley a roadway had been brought in some years before and modern foods such as refined flour and sugar had become available.

In an intermediate area located between the other two, Dr. Price found an incidence of 2.3 cavities per hundred teeth, a little less than one per person. This was more than seen in the Loetschental valley where teeth were so often perfect, but less than that seen in the second valley. Food habits were intermediate too. The use of bought foods was not uncommon, but it was less frequent than in the valley where tooth decay had run rampant. Curiously, however, he found evidence of previous,

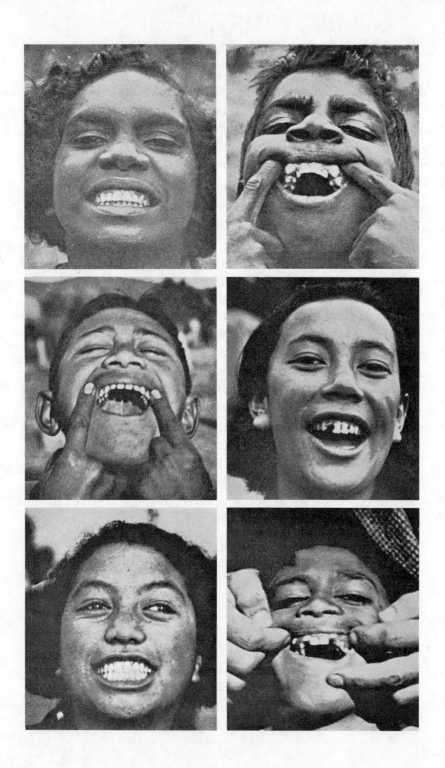

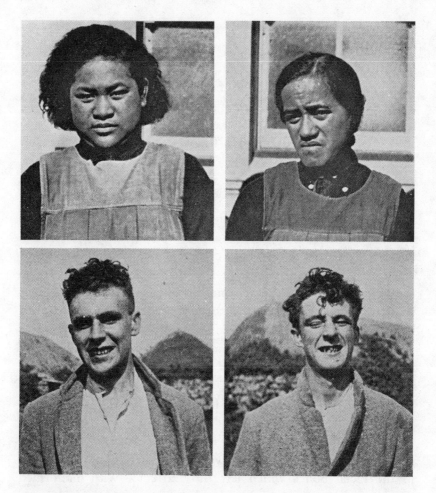

The photos on the left side of each page are of native peoples who lived on their traditional diets. Those in the right hand column of each page are persons of the same race, culture and living habits who had adopted a "modern" diet. Note the overall differences: the wide sturdy dental arches of those on natural diets compared with the malformation and decay of those on industrialized food. The first pair are Australian aborigines whose traditional diet is fish, game, roots, stems, leaves, berries, grains and peas. The woman on the left had adhered to this while the young man on the right had been raised on canned food, white flour, sugar, etc. The bottom two pairs on the page at left and the sisters above are Maori of New Zealand. Their native diet is primarily such foods as shell fish and fern root. Of each pair, however, the person on the right had subsisted on industrialized foods and showed decayed teeth, narrowing of the dental arches, and, in more severe cases, deformity of the facial bones with narrowing of air passages. The same principles apply to the brothers above who are from the Isle of Harris off the coast of Scotland. The traditional diet there is largely oatmeal, oatcakes and seafoods. Yet it can sustain excellent health as exemplified by the brother on the left. Only one in a hundred teeth were decayed among these people. The brother at right, however, (surprisingly, the younger of the two) had used modern white bread, jams, marmalades and canned foods for some time.

Photos reprinted with permission from *Nutrition and Physical Degeneration*, Weston A. Price, Price-Pottenger Nutrition Foundation, Inc. PO Box 2614, La Mesa, CA 92041.

more extensive tooth decay in some adults. On questioning such people, he usually found they had been away a year or two, living with relatives in an urban setting and eating other than the traditional diet of locally grown food.

Comparable results were found in other areas of Switzerland. Over many years, Dr. Price made similar extensive studies among the Gaelics in the outer and inner Hebrides; the Eskimos in Alaska; the American Indians in the western and northwestern United States, in Florida and in central Canada; the Malanesians and Polynesians on eight different archipelagos of the Southern Pacific; tribes in eastern and central Africa; the aborigines of Australia; Malayan tribes on the islands north of Australia; the Maoris of New Zealand; and ancient civilizations and their descendents along the coast, in the mountains and in the Amazon basin of Peru. The results were invariably the same: there was an obvious and direct relationship between the incidence of tooth decay and the adoption of a "modern diet."

FROM DECAY OF TEETH TO DECAY OF HEALTH

However, Dr. Price made other observations which he did not expect at all. Besides decayed teeth, there were deformities in the facial bones which left those affected with malformed dental arches and crowding of the teeth. Moreover, this deformity of the dental arch and the malformations of the bones of the face and head were correlated with lower IQ's, with personality disturbances and with a dramatically higher incidence of degenerative diseases such as tuberculosis. The incidence of birth defects was dramatically higher among families in which the parents had adopted the "new diet" before the birth of their children. No such defects were seen among brothers and sisters who were born before the "new diet" was adopted. They did not seem to be "hereditary" in the usual sense of the word.

But what was the shortcoming in this "modern diet" which Dr. Price so frequently found associated with degenerating

health? First of all, he noted an increase in "processed foods"—
those which are not used as they are found in nature. In some
cases this involved preserving, for example canning foods, a trend
which, as the graph shows, has continued.

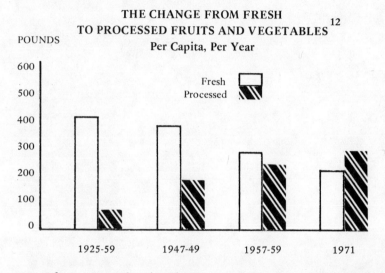

THE CHANGE FROM FRESH
TO PROCESSED FRUITS AND VEGETABLES [12]
Per Capita, Per Year

POUNDS

Fresh
Processed

600
500
400
300
200
100
0

1925-59   1947-49   1957-59   1971

Often processing involves removing some of the nutrients.
It is only relatively recently, in the last few hundred years, that
man has had the technological ability to break the food down
from its natural intact state into its separate components and to
consume these one at a time. The valley dwellers of Switzerland,
for example, who ate whole rye bread seemed invariably to be
less susceptible to tooth decay than those who ate white bread
made from refined flour.

We cannot assume, however, that the differences in health
are due simply to the refining of rye and wheat. We must also
consider the quality of the grain, be it whole or refined. Grain
from the isolated valley watered by glacial snows where, Dr.
Price emphasizes, the soil is painstakingly tilled by hand, varied
significantly from that of the plains where it is cultivated under
increasingly "modern" conditions, plowed on a large scale, and
fertilized artificially.

Nutrition and the Soil

2

From dust we came and to dust we return. Man's body is made from earth which has been transmuted by plants. Over the long course of evolution it was plant matter which provided the food around which animals, and eventually man, developed. The plants in turn derived their nourishment from the soil. The soil was populated by one-celled plants, bacteria, and other microbes that made it rich and fertile. Thus the dead stone of the earth's crust was brought to life.

The quality of that life has remained to a great extent, dependent on the quality of the interaction between dust, plant matter and the microorganisms of the soil. The soil itself is living and it is from it that more evolved forms of life take their origin. When man learned to drop seeds and cultivate crops, he discovered, in effect, how to exploit the life-giving potential of the soil. With this discovery came both power for good and the risk of abuse. Unfortunately, over the millenia soils in many areas have been depleted and destroyed leaving great wastelands and deserts as monuments to our mistakes.[1] But with more understanding of the nature of the soil, and how its delicate balance can be maintained and strengthened, we open the possibility of a new era of enlightened land use and more vibrantly living and life-giving foods.

MOVING WEST

In the 1940's when the transportation of foodstuffs in the United States was still rather limited, what most people ate was grown in the region where they lived. For this reason, one could still study the relationship between tooth decay, for example, and the condition of the soil. Statistics on dental health collected during the induction of personnel for service in the military during World War II showed an interesting correlation with the condition of the soil in their home regions:

> The East coast, from Florida through the rural South to the urban Northeast and Maine, showed an average of 17.55 caries per mouth. The next North/South strip from Alabama and Mississippi to Ohio and Wisconsin, where soils have been farmed for fewer years, showed an average of 14.9 cavities. The prairie states from the Dakotas and Minnesota down to Texas and Louisiana showed 12.1 cavities per person. Further West, where the soils were poor and underdeveloped, the incidence mounted again.[2]

Incidence of Dental Cavities in Regions of Varying Soil Conditions

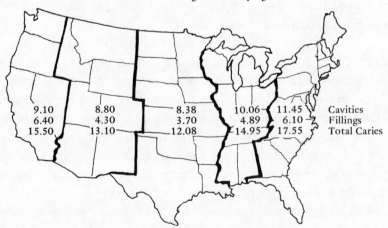

9.10	8.80	8.38	10.06	11.45	Cavities
6.40	4.30	3.70	4.89	6.10	Fillings
15.50	13.10	12.08	14.95	17.55	Total Caries

Dr. William Albrecht, the soil scientist who brought these facts to the attention of the scientific community, observed that our movement in this country has been consistently westward. The advice to "Go west young man" was given for a reason. The opportunity that lay westward often had to do with the fertility of the soil.

In the early nineteenth century, an American of English descent named Nichols cleared hundreds of acres of rich virgin land in South Carolina, on which he grew crops of cotton, tobacco and corn so abundant that with the revenue he built a big house and educated a large family. Not once in his lifetime did he add anything to the soil. When it became depleted and his crops dwindled, he cleared more land and continued his exploitation. When there was no more land to be cleared the family fortunes declined.

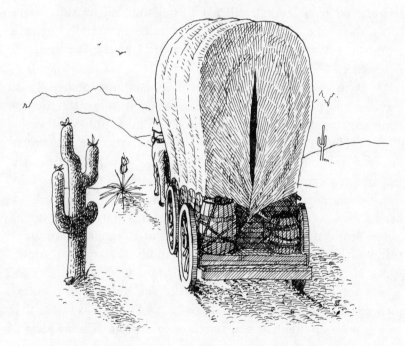

Nichols' son, grown to manhood, looked at the poverty-stricken acreage and moved west to Tennessee, where he cleared two thousand acres of virgin land; like his father he planted cotton, corn and tobacco. When his own son was grown to manhood, the land was once more so depleted that he moved on to Alabama, there to purchase another two thousand acres of fertile soil and raise a family of twelve children on the proceeds; the town became Nicholsville; Nichols became the owner of a sawmill, a general store and a gristmill. This man's son also grew up to see devastation where his father had grown rich. He decided to move further west and settled in Parkdale, Arkansas, where he bought one thousand acres of good land on the bayou.

Four moves in four generations. Multiplied by thousands, this is the story of how Americans raised food on a continent which was there for the taking.[3]

As the land has been exhausted we have moved on, clearing new land and benefitting from its fertility. This westward tendency in America is, however, only a reflection of the same trend that has existed over several millenia throughout the world. Migrations from the East brought the "Indo-European" linguistic groups into Western Europe and later brought the Europeans to America.

With the arrival of the multi-racial immigrant peoples to the east coast of North America and their movement across the continent to the Pacific, the circle of migration was almost closed. The Pacific theater of World War II and the subsequent "bush wars" in Korea and Indo-China are of epochal significance. Expansion westward has reached its ultimate limit, and westward moving America has now encountered the Orient. The result has been a new sobriety, a re-examination of our materialistic values, a new sense of ecological perspective, and a reappraisal of man's place in the universe. Instead of the spoils of war, many American soldiers brought home with them a nearly vegetarian diet and a new respect for the quiet wisdom of the Orient. In the East, man has long since learned to live with his limitations rather than to move on looking for new territory to exploit. The meeting of Western analytic nutrition based on the concepts of chemistry with the Eastern reverence for basic natural foods as the link that ties man to the soil and to the overall ecological system promises to bring a new perspective to nutritional science.

THE NATURE OF SOIL

It is only recently that our research technology has become sophisticated enough to allow us to probe the mysteries of the soil and to understand nature's complex methods of feeding plants.   In the wild there is a natural cycle involving plants and soil.   The plant, after reaching maturity, drops its leaves or dies, the remains returning to the earth where it decomposes.   The organic matter left plays an important role in the natural movement of nutrients from soil to root, for it provides the food which is consumed by the microbes growing in the soil.

A complex mixture of bacteria and fungi inhabit the soil in areas where it has not been tampered with. These microbes play extremely important roles in the biochemistry of the soil. First of all, they break down the plant matter. It is customary to think that the leaves "rot" and that this provides an opportune place for such microorganisms to grow. In fact, however, this "rotting" involves very active and energetic work on the part of the bacteria which convert the cellulose and other plant materials into a series of simpler compounds.[4] If the conditions in the soil are right, then these simple compounds recombine to form complex substances called humic acids. Humic acids make up nearly 50% of the weight of the organic material or "humus" which makes natural soil rich, dark and spongy. The other major constituent of the soil is clay, which, because of its composition, is able to hold water molecules between its layers, swelling to accommodate increasing amounts from rain or irrigation. This clay, or *Montmorillonite*, as it is technically called, is able, when appropriate, to release the stored water, shrinking its mass again. This is dramatized by the cracked surface of a sunbaked field where the soil is depleted of humus and is too clayey. In moderate amounts, clay is valuable, however. It's ability to hold moisture is very convenient for the plants which need water in a gradual, consistent way rather than in huge amounts all at once and then none at all.[5]

It has recently been discovered that the humic acids play much the same role with regard to minerals as does clay with water. The complex organic molecules of humic acids are able to hold the trace elements and other minerals of the soil in reserve, releasing them to the plant as they are needed.[6] Experiments have shown that when plants are rooted in a soil that is rich in humic acids the concentrations of trace elements may vary tremendously without either producing deficiency or toxic effects in the plants. Humic acids apparently serve then as a sort of buffer, though actually the technical term is "chelator."

Chelation has been studied by medical researchers who use chelating agents to remove toxic minerals such as lead from the body. A chelating agent is a large molecule which locks around a mineral, holding it and carrying it along. The word "chelation" comes from the Greek *chela* which means "claw." It derives from the ability of the molecule to hold a mineral much as a crab would hold a morsel of food between its pincers. Recent research on trace elements such as zinc, copper and manganese stimulated the study of chelation which is important not only in the soil but in animals and man as well. It has been shown in some cases that chelated minerals are better absorbed from the digestive tract than are simple mineral salts.*

The chelation of minerals by the humic acids of the soil means that they are "in reserve" so that they can be picked up as they are needed.[7] This means then that plants are able to flourish in a wide variety of soils where mineral content may vary tremendously. This explains in part, at least, why it is that some farms, where production has been very low, have suddenly become much more fruitful when the amount of humus in the soil is increased. Minerals which are naturally in excess in the soil

---

* See Chapter 8, Minerals.

can be held in abeyance until they are needed and therefore do not crowd into the plant displacing others. At the same time, those which are in minimal supply are also available on demand, so that minerals present in small quantities in the soil are not so likely to lead to deficiencies in the plant.[8]   While man's nutrients are fats, protein, carbohydrate, vitamins and minerals, the nutritional requirements of the plant are simpler. It makes its own carbohydrate, protein and fat. The only nutrients it needs from the soil are minerals. That the plant can get these when it needs them and keep them out when it doesn't is a crucial issue in the production of healthy, nutritious plants.

Humic acids also form insoluble complexes with calcium which help to hold the soil in place.[9]   If all the plants are harvested from the soil leaving little organic matter to form humus, the soil is more easily washed away. This tends to remove the fine particles of clay, so that the soil becomes coarse and sandy. In the absence of clay, water is not held in reserve and the plants grow with more difficulty, reducing the amounts of organic material further. Besides, without their roots to help hold the soil in place, gullies soon form and more minerals and clay are washed away. The result is a vicious circle. On most of our farmland, little or no organic matter is put back in the soil, and erosion takes an average of twelve tons of topsoil per acre per year. Since only about a ton and a half is formed during that time, there is a large net loss of soil, usually the part that is richest in minerals.[10]   The sandy soil doesn't have the capacity to retain water like the clay-humus mixtures, and plants growing in it are easily damaged by droughts. In 1974 when rainfall was scant and the average yield for dry land corn in Nebraska was twenty-nine bushels per acre, three organic farms in the area which made a practice of adding large amounts of organic matter to the soil produced about 100 bushels an acre, more than triple the amount produced by their neighbors.[11]

The combining of minerals with humic acids is only one aspect of the complex biochemistry of the soil and plant interaction.

There is at least one other important link in the chain of events which brings the mineral into the plant. In natural soils the roots of many trees[12] and other plants are found to be surrounded by extremely tiny filaments of fungi, called "mycorrhiza." Fungi are known to make and release a series of chelating agents.[13] It may be these which pick up the minerals from the humus reserves and "package them" in such a way that they are acceptable to the plant root. Research has shown that seedlings whose rootlets are coated with mycorrhiza are better able to absorb a number of minerals from the soil than those whose rootlets are "bare."[14] The chelating agents produced by fungi are often toxic to bacteria. They are, in fact, one way the fungi hold the bacteria, with whom they are competing for living space in the soil, at bay. Penicillin is one such antibacterial or "antibiotic" chelating substance which is secreted by a fungus to destroy nearby bacteria. Such antibiotics enter the plant and may serve many other functions as well—perhaps helping to make the plant resistant to infection.[15]

In turn for their services to the plant, the mycorrhiza are permitted to derive nourishment from the plant itself. However, the soil is not suitable for the growth of a particular plant, for example, when an alkaline soil is needed but the soil is highly acidic, the plant will not be healthy and vigorous. The mycorrhizal fungi then become invasive, or "pathogenic" in the botanists' terms, helping nature to destroy the weak plant so as to make way for others that are more robust. For this reason it was long mistakenly thought that most of these fungi were "disease causing" when in fact their role in the nourishment of the plant may well be strategic.[16]

When plants are cultivated in a soil which is balanced, healthy, rich in humus and alive with the best varieties of microbes, they are of excellent quality, like the rye and the hay grown in the Swiss valley visited by Dr. Price. But a vibrantly healthy soil is rare. Though there is an interesting awareness that how a food is grown has a great deal to do with its quality and though one hears much of "organic foods" these days, it is seldom possible to know what kind of soil they were grown on or even what, in fact, is being meant by the term.

WHY BUY "ORGANIC"?

Historically, organic chemistry was the study of the complex molecular structures found in plant and animal matter. This was in contradistinction to the inorganic or simple compounds that were found in non-living rocks, stones and other mineral substances. The organic branch of chemistry was concerned with the large carbon-based molecules that are characteristic of living protoplasm and included such substances as petroleum, which is plant matter that was deposited in the earth eons ago and is partly decomposed.

As the technology of chemistry improved, scientists became increasingly capable of synthesizing in the laboratory many of the compounds which they had formerly been able to obtain only by extracting them from plants and animals. Thus it happened that many "organic chemicals" were actually synthetic. Modifications of these produced others which did not even exist in a natural form. Nevertheless, since they were related compounds of a similar structure, they were included in the category of "organic." In the field of agriculture, the use of these terms has taken a different turn. Soils which were rich in decomposed plant material (humus) and derived their fertility from this were said to be rich in "organic materials." This stood in contrast to farmland where fertility came from the application of simple chemical compounds such as potash, nitrates and phosphates. These latter chemical fertilizers are "inorganic." They dissolve in water and are absorbed directly into the plant roots, without going through the intricate complexing with humic acids, clay and so forth. For this reason they are independent of the microbes and are able to nourish the plants even when the soil is not healthy. At the same time, their concentrations must be carefully adjusted, since the buffering action of the living soil is by-passed.*

To contrast them with those produced through the use of inorganic phosphates, nitrates and potassium compounds, vegetables and fruits grown on the humus-rich soil came to be spoken of as "organically grown." The term did not remain so clearly defined, however. Plants grown on chemically fertilized soil were not as robust and resistant to attack by insects or competition from weeds as those grown on healthy, humus-rich soils, so insecticides and herbicides were used to protect them. Soon foods came to be called "organic" simply because they had not had heavy applications of chemical pesticides, or even because they had not been dyed or coated with wax or exposed to chemical ripeners after harvesting. Though free of chemicals, they were not necessarily grown on a soil that was properly balanced or particularly rich in organic material. Therefore, even though they may have been less contaminated, they could still be deficient in certain minerals.

At present there are still no clear-cut standards for officially designating one food "organic" and another not, though some states are beginning to take action in the direction of setting up guidelines for this. Even though the shopper may not be able to know with any certainty what is meant when a food is labeled organic, there are still definite clues that can help him in shopping. The first and most important is the condition of the food. For instance, vegetables whose stalks are split or skins cracked are most likely deficient in some mineral. Those whose coloring is "too green" might be suspect of having had large quantities of nitrogen-based fertilizer dumped on them. Where leaves are yellowed, there is often a lack of iron.[18] Besides these characteristics, there is also the "taste test."

---

* There is some suggestion that inorganic fertilizers may destroy the mycorrhizae, disrupting the natural system of mineral chelation and absorption[17] forcing the plant to rely entirely on water soluble fertilizers. This would mean that once the use of such fertilizers is begun, a "dependency" on them develops.

It is a common belief in every culture that the fruits and vegetables which have the most flavor are nutritionally superior. It is logical that our tastes would have evolved to lead us to the most valuable foods.   Whether taste reflects the quality and quantity of vitamins, minerals and protein, or whether it is an index of other as yet undiscovered nutrients or properties of foods, has not been verified in the laboratory. Nevertheless, as a working hypothesis, it is probably safe to assume that produce which looks pretty but has no taste is less desirable in the diet.[19] There are some clearly negative effects from tasteless fruits and vegetables.   For example, if experiences with mealy, bland fruit causes a child to turn away from it, then he may lose his natural impulse to eat fresh food. His sense of taste may become diverted and, in a futile attempt to satisfy his body's needs, he may turn increasingly to artificially flavored and seasoned snack foods and sweets.

The cultivation of a healthy soil through the addition of organic matter may also be an economic boon. Not only does it help to dispose of animal manure which is a problem in America, but by increasing the humus in the soil, erosion is diminished and this in turn slows the silting of waterways which increases liability to floods. It also eliminates the need for expensive fertilizers and pesticides.

Research in Europe and in America has shown that farms using no chemical fertilizers, pesticides or herbicides have consistently turned out yields as good as their conventional counterparts and in many cases at less expense.[20] During the droughts of early 1976, one agriculturalist's examination of numerous fields verified that humus-rich soils produce crops in even dry years, whereas chemicalized soils don't.[21]

AGRICULTURE OF THE FUTURE

Eliminating chemicals is only one technique that has great potential for improving food production. Another is the use of minimum tillage techniques. "Minimum tillage" is a fancy name for the reversion to one of the most primitive and perhaps soundest of all agricultural practices. It means that the earth is disturbed as little as possible in the process of its cultivation. Nowadays this may mean that strips of grass are left between the rows so that only a portion of the earth is actually turned. This, of course, can be very helpful in retarding erosion, both from water and from wind, since the strips of land provide a a kind of windbreak. Not only is this practice based on sound ecological principles, but it is also attractive to the average farmer because it is cheaper and easier. Authorities feel that among all the soil conservation measures that have been proposed in the last half century and promoted with billions of dollars* this particular one may have a chance of being widely adopted and of serving its purpose. One expert notes that in Nebraska soil erosion averaged only 3.4 tons per acre using minimum tillage as compared with losses of 10.7 tons for the conventional "plow disc planting system."[23] Of course, even a 3.4 ton loss is more than twice the 1.5 ton of topsoil that is formed by natural weathering process on the average acre of land. Something more is needed if we are to stop the progressive loss of soil rather than only slow it.

Close on the heels of the realization that minimum tillage makes sense comes the idea that *no tillage* may be an even better answer. In experiments in Ohio, soil erosion rates for no tillage corn were less than a hundredth of that for conventional corn.[24] With such an approach, not only could we stop soil loss we could even gradually (though very slowly) restore some of what is already gone. Unfortunately, in the context of large-scale agriculture where there is a heavy reliance on artificial fertilizers and the natural health of the soil has not been maintained, the no-tillage technique has resulted in increased problems with

---

* $15 billion has been appropriated by the government for this purpose since 1935.[22]

insects and even more with weeds. Therefore, farmers in America using the no-tillage approach have greatly increased their use of pesticides and herbicides.[25] No-tillage methods are being promoted by the chemical industry which calculates that this will boost sales immensely.

By contrast, small-scale experiments using year-round cultivation with overlapping crops have reported extremely good yields without any cultivation and without either the use of chemicals or difficulty with weeds or insects. In Japan, one such farm adopting the no-tillage system was reportedly able to grow, on the same plot, barley, rice, buckwheat, soybeans and garden beans. Rice was sown in the early summer before buckwheat was harvested so that the cutting of the buckwheat would allow the already germinated rice to show through. Before rice was harvested, barley was sown, and so forth. This method is said to have produced per acre per year 6,400 pounds *each* of rice and barley from the same plot.[26] Yields of buckwheat and soybeans were also good from that same field. This is "beyond organic farming" and might be called "natural agriculture." Once a healthy condition is established in the soil, this process might go on indefinitely.

ECOLOGICAL STABILITY AND FOOD PRODUCTION

Throughout the world there remain a few pockets of civilization that have found ways to maintain their stability and continuity for hundreds or even thousands of years. Among these are the Incas of Peru and certain communities in the Himalayan Mountains, as well as some in China. In China, for example, a study of the agricultural practices has revealed that composting was a highly developed art. Every fragment of material that came from the land was returned to it. This included not only the animal manure, but also the plant wastes and even the silt that escaped into the rivers and irrigation canals. All of these components were carefully mixed into heaps which would encourage the growth of desirable bacteria and fungi, and the finished material was then returned to the land. In this way the Chinese have escaped what would otherwise have been certain annihilation due to complete exhaustion of their farmlands.

The mountain communities which have maintained their stability have done so by virtue of elaborate terrace farming. Some of these "megalithic people" have cultures that date back further than anthropologists have been able to determine. The hill terraces are built of huge stones which apparently were put in place thousands of years ago. Their careful construction shows high development of civilization even at that time. The result is an effective system for holding the soil and preventing erosion. Again, everything taken from the soil is returned to it, and in addition, the terraces are irrigated with a constant supply of melted ice and snow. These glacial waters are brought by aquaduct over the mountains to the fields. They seem to keep the soil rich and fertile probably in part because such waters are extremely high in the minerals that come from a constant grinding by the glacier against stone.

Dr. Price in his study of the Swiss valley peoples found that those who lived in the mountains and maintained the most vibrant state of health placed particular value on the mountain waters. It was when the cows were grazed at the edge of the melting snow in the summer that milk productivity increased, and it was from this milk that the women made and stored cheese for the winter. "This cheese contains the natural butter-fat and minerals of the splendid milk, and is a virtual storehouse of life for the coming winter." The people of the valley had a special reverence for the butter and cheese "made when the cows eat the grass near the snow line."[27]

Ecological health depends on keeping the surface of the earth rich in humus and minerals so that it can provide a foundation for healthy plant and animal life. The situation is disrupted if the soil loses these raw materials or if great quantities of contaminants are introduced into it. When man goes beneath the surface of the earth and drags out minerals or other compounds that did not evolve as part of this system, then problems follow. The mining of lead and cadmium* are examples of this. Petroleum is also a substance that has been dug out of the bowels of the earth and introduced into the surface ecology by man. Though it is formed from plant matter, the highly reduced carbon compounds that result are often toxic to living protoplasm. In some cases this is true of even very tiny amounts, as in the case of "polychlorinated biphenyls" (PCB's), a petroleum product which can cause cancer. Because they are not easily broken down by plants and animals, these compounds accumulate in the environment. They are also concentrated by animals so that fish, for example, may contain twenty thousand times as much as the water in which they are caught.[28] Public concern was aroused when dangerous levels of PCB's were found in the milk of nursing mothers.[29]

Ecological stability leads to cultural stability. The Swiss mentioned earlier, who Dr. Price found to have sound agricultural practices, had essentially no crime and no disease. The same is true of mountain cultures in the Himalayas, where a constant supply of wholesome food and a stable, well-maintained soil has served as a foundation on which a healthy and sophisticated culture could evolve. The enduring traditions that resulted have given rise to some of the highest accomplishments, both physically and spiritually, known to man.

It would seem that a return to careful maintenance of the soil through such techniques as well-engineered composting, minimal or no-tillage, and the closer regulation of our chemicalized technology, could provide the foundation for restoring ecological harmony to America and the West. In the meantime, many available foods may be less than ideal. Fortunately, as we shall see in later chapters, there are techniques of food selection

* See Chapter 8, Minerals.

and preparation that can work around these difficulties and maximize the nutritional value of the food that is available.

An understanding of nutrition and diet can provide the nidus from which a new ecological harmony can be created. The food that one eats is his own personal contact, day in and day out, with the ecological system in which he is embedded. Consciousness of food then becomes ultimately a consciousness of the overall ecological matrix. An appreciation of the purity and of the vibrant, health-giving properties of the food that we eat will lead us gradually to realize that our own clarity of mind and well-being is inextricably linked with the clarity and well-being of the universe of which we are but a small part.

Nutrition and the Cell

3

Pushed by the necessity of understanding his diseases and bolstered by his leisure time and insatiable curiosity, Western man has used the tools of modern science to probe the mysteries of living matter. Over the last century, medical science has come increasingly to focus on the basic structure of protoplasm. The human body has been examined in increasing detail even exploring the inside of what had been considered the smallest unit of life, the cell. Recently our understanding of the events inside the cell has become more and more detailed. The electron microscope has revealed for us the inner structure of the cell's substance and has helped us to explore its tiniest components.

A JOURNEY THROUGH THE CELL

Any effort toward good nutrition must start with and be organized around an awareness of the cell and its central importance in human nutrition. The clearer the picture we have of cellular function, the better we can provide for its nourishment. The busy world that exists there is as fascinating as it is complex.

When we look inside the cell, we see embedded in its substance compact little units like tiny rooms where a great deal of activity is going on and from which heat emanates. These mini-power-houses are called "mitochondria." Outside, a continuous line of medium-sized molecules of fat and sugar wait to get in. Inside, they are broken down, and a continuous line of the by-products exits. The energy released is transferred to energy-carrying phosphate molecules (ATP). Highly charged streams of these issue from the mitochondrian, like electricity flowing from a generator. They serve as one of the chief sources of the energy that keeps the cell active.

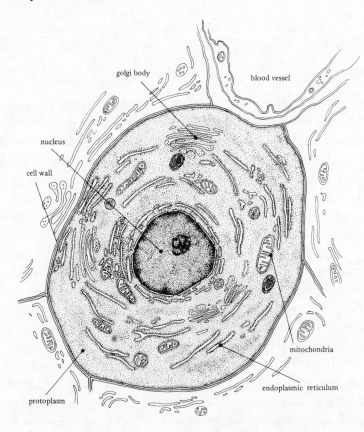

There is a trend in the movement of other molecules as well. Various molecules filter in through the outer covering of the cell (the cell membrane). They are of several types: first are the glucose, fructose and other sugars which will be burned inside the mitochondria, producing carbon dioxide, water and energy. Another rather frequent arrival is the protein molecule, sometimes coming in large chains (some too large to get through the rather small openings in the wall) and other times in little detached segments which are called amino acids and which pass through readily, only to be reassembled again into protein chains inside the cell.

The influx of sugars and amino acids is a routine matter in the cell, but occasionally a special molecule arrives which creates a flurry of unusual activity in the cell. It is called a hormone and plays a very strategic role in regulating the chemical processes going on in the cell. Thyroid hormones, for example, speed up the overall tempo of cellular metabolism while adrenalin molecules accelerate the conversion of stored carbohydrate into a usable form, gearing the cells for emergency operations. Upon their arrival in certain areas of the cell, the whole course of activity shifts.

Other entering molecules that seem to play a strategic role in making metabolism possible are the vitamins. They are of many sizes and participate in many biochemical processes, but the one thing they are said to have in common is that the cell is generally unable to manufacture them, so they must come "ready-made" with the diet. Minerals can also be seen to enter the cell from outside. They vary in character but are generally smaller and even less frequent than the vitamins, though perhaps of equal or even greater importance. Calcium ions are among the more common of the minerals, whereas some of the others are so rare as to be called "trace elements." Zinc, copper, cobalt and manganese are some of these. Technically, the ever-present potassium ions also are "minerals," but they are involved with water molecules and are distributed throughout the cellular protoplasm as is sodium, though it is more concentrated in the fluid outside, that surrounds the cell.

CHROMOSOMES AND GENES

In most cells, one will find a great deal of traffic coming and going from a central compartment, the nucleus. Small "messengers" enter and leave, carrying orders that are issued from here. The nucleus serves as a sort of central computer bank where plans for the cell's functioning are more or less encoded on long chains or coils of a protein-like substance called DNA. These chain-like coils are called chromosomes, and each spot that carries a bit of information is a "gene." Periodically, an assembly of special units called nucleic acids are brought to the nucleus to line up in order against a portion of the DNA chain, forming its mirror image, and these are joined together by a special molecule called an enzyme. After this process has been repeated a predetermined number of times, this new chain separates and moves out of the nucleus to another part of the cell, where the process is repeated. The end result is that a protein chain is synthesized. The order in which the units line up is extremely important, and it is the enzyme which helps them to interact in such a way that they are joined together with very little energy input.*

Throughout most of the cells, it is the enzymes that do the bulk of the work. For each biochemical reaction that occurs, there is a special enzyme, and the reaction can proceed only in its presence. Some enzymes break down old molecules while others reassemble new ones. Other enzymes make sure that oxygen combines with sugar for its combustion, while still

---

* Because of the complexity of the subject matter and space limitation, this description has been intentionally over simplified. For those interested in more detail they should consult the excellent *The Molecular Biology of the Gene* by James D. Watson, W.A. Benjamin, Inc., New York, 1970.

others break down fat chains.

While enzymes help build protein chains, actually they are themselves proteins. It is their special shape that endows them with the capacity for grasping, holding and bringing together other molecules. Many of them also depend in some way on a mineral (or "trace element") for their mysterious ability to create and destroy. In fact, the regulation of the cell's overall performance is carried out through altering the activity of the enzymes. As the enzymes go, so goes the entire metabolism. In many cases, molecules of a foreign substance, a contaminant, or a medicinal compound, for example, shapes the course of events in the cell by affecting the enzymatic activity.

NUTRITION FOR THE INTRACELLULAR WORLD

Studying the inner workings of the cell confronts us with a confusing maze of molecules. Our confusion is due in part to the fact that the molecules vary so much in size—some are huge, coiled, knotted up giants, while others are tiny by comparison. Gradually we realize, however, that there is actually a definite order to the apparent chaos. Careful scrutiny reveals a sort of lattice work made up of protein molecules that extends in every direction, creating a three-dimensional frame within which the rest of the cellular components are moving. These beam-like structures form a sort of huge "jungle gym" that both preserves the shape of the cell as well as maintaining each of the components in place. The chains of protein which make up this interior skeleton also seem to serve as sort of "assembly lines" along which the various molecules move, being altered at each juncture. What seems at first like random motion in the cell protoplasm is really very orderly, only it is so complex that the order is not at first apparent. In the spaces lying between the protein beams, the other molecules are separated by water molecules which serve as a sort of "fluid cement" holding them apart, and yet securing them in place, as the positive and negative poles of the water molecules shift and swing like swarms of tiny tugboats moving huge ships.

The intricate inner workings of the cell require certain molecules at each position and function well only if their components can be supplied. If "imported" material is not available, then some of the cell's processes may stop altogether while others are slowed. Though there are many alternate paths and much flexibility, repeated shortages or "deficiencies" result in malfunctioning of the cell and even, if they continue, in its death.

For tissue integrity to be maintained, the cells must have a ready supply of carbohydrate and fats which are used as the fuel for metabolism, a supply of protein for building materials and a supply of the many miscellaneous components of biochemical reactions such as vitamins and minerals which the cell does not itself manufacture. These raw materials which the cell needs from outside are called "nutrients," and our primary source of them is another cell—that of the plant. Here we find all the needed nutrients combined in ideal proportions and neatly packaged for our use.

Whether man takes his food directly from plants or indirectly from animals, it is the plant cell which is ultimately the source of the substances he needs. It is the nature of the plant cell to take energy from the sun and, using water and carbon dioxide along with the minerals it draws from the soil, to create the protein, the carbohydrate and the many other nutrients on which the animal cell relies.

The Biochemistry of Nutrition

When man first began the chemical study of nutrition, he became aware of the need for those nutrients which were used in the largest quantities. These were the carbohydrates such as sugar and starch which provide the fuel on which the body runs, and which comprise the largest bulk of what we eat. Although the body can burn fats or proteins, it does not do so as efficiently as it burns carbohydrate, so for smooth physiological functioning, substantial quantities of carbohydrate are constantly used.

The body can convert excess carbohydrate into fat which is essentially a storage form of fuel. This can later be burned when there is no ready source of carbohydrate. Other animals besides man, of course, also make and store fat in the same way, and when animal foods (meat, fish, fowl, etc.) are eaten, then fat becomes a significant part of the diet. Plants make some fats too, the majority of which tend to have a low melting point and are therefore normally encountered in a liquid form which we call "oil." Certain of these oils, which are much more plentiful in plants than in animal food, cannot be manufactured by the body and must be taken in the diet in small amounts. Otherwise fat in the diet is taken less out of necessity than out of preference. While fats are ordinarily taken in lesser quantities than carbohydrates, protein is usually taken in still smaller amounts.

Protein is the basic building block of the body and makes up the framework of its more rigid structures such as the cell walls, skin, bones, solid organs, blood vessels, etc. It is the framework of protein molecules inside the cells which serves as the inner skeleton that helps the cell to maintain its integrity. In most cases, protein structures are relatively stable, and there is not a rapid turnover of protein in the body. During times of growth, more protein is needed, but during adulthood there is a decreasing requirement. If more protein is taken in than is needed and if the intake of carbohydrate is low, the body will tend to burn the extra protein as fuel, which may as we shall see, cause problems.

These three basic nutrients—carbohydrate, fat and protein— stand quite apart from other requirements of the body such as vitamins and minerals since they are needed in comparatively larger quantities. If they are the fuel and the building materials which are used in bulk, the vitamins and minerals are, by contrast, analogous to the screws and bolts necessary for the construction and operation of the body. More precisely, if we think in chemical terms of the carbohydrate, fat and protein as the basic compounds out of which the body is composed, then the vitamins and minerals are the catalysts which prompt these compounds to interact. While daily requirements of vitamins and minerals are recorded in amounts that can be measured in milligrams or even micrograms, protein, fat and carbohydrate intakes are expressed in grams, which is to say they are needed in amounts one thousand to a million times as great.

Most whole natural foods (with the exception of meat, which contains no carbohydrate) contain a balance of the three major nutrients as well as appropriate amounts of vitamins and minerals. Only with the coming of modern technology has man been able to cheaply and easily separate out the basic nutrients, yielding relatively pure fat or carbohydrate, for example, and creating the "refined" foods, mineral tablets and vitamin pills that are increasingly available today. This provides both the possibility of quickly supplying that which is deficient as well as the danger of taking excessive amounts of one of these nutrients. It also presents the hazard of disrupting the balanced food that nature offers us, thereby destroying the equilibrium of natural diet. To understand how to restore and maintain this natural balance, we must probe a bit deeper into the composition and the sources of carbohydrates, fats, proteins, vitamins and minerals, as well as their relationship to one another and to the maintenance of good health.

Carbohydrate: Our Source of Energy

Carbohydrate is probably the oldest subject in Western nutrition. It is the fuel on which body functions are based, and in the 1800's the study of nutrition was considered to be the study of this fuel. Nutritional value was judged largely on the number of calories that a food could provide, so that foods like tomatoes, which are low in calories were considered to be of "little nutritional value."

Though many other nutrients have since been discovered, in terms of sheer quantity, carbohydrate remains the most important. If one leaves out the water and fiber content of food, it is carbohydrate which makes up the bulk of the diet. The average person eats ten ounces of carbohydrate for every ounce of protein. This huge amount of carbohydrate is used by the animal body for energy, and through its oxidation or "burning," energy is produced. It is on this energy that all of metabolism depends. Without the burning or "internal combustion" of carbohydrate, the body's primary source of energy would be missing. Just as the automobile runs on gasoline, so the body runs on carbohydrate. In fact, the principle is not very different.

Gasoline is a hydrocarbon, that is, a carbon to which hydrogen has been added, and it is the combination of oxygen with this hydrocarbon which produces the energy on which the automobile functions. The carbohydrate, by contrast, on which the animal cell functions, is so called because it is a form of carbon to which water has been added. Plants take carbon dioxide from the atmosphere and water from the soil and, using the energy of sunlight to force the two together, combine them to form the series of complex chains called sugars and starches. These hydrated carbon chains, or carbohydrates, are then eaten. So the plant does the crucial work while man takes the carbohydrate and burns it with the oxygen he breathes, producing carbon dioxide and water and releasing the original energy derived from sunlight.

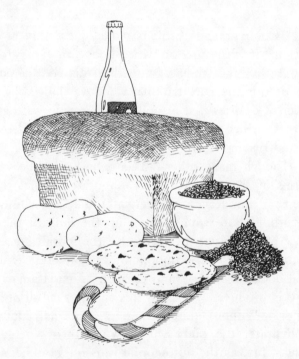

In this way, the body is able to maintain within itself an internal source of energy which acts as a "little sun." It is perhaps no accident that the area of the body where food is primarily broken down, assimilated or burned is traditionally called the "solar plexus" and in many of the ancient writings is symbolized by a flame.

The combustion of carbohydrates by the animal cell breaks the carbohydrate molecule back down to its original components: carbon dioxide and water. The water is vaporized in the breath and excreted in the urine; the carbon dioxide is exhaled and returned to the atmosphere. There, plants once more take it up and combine it with water, producing, when they are exposed to sunlight, more carbohydrates. In this light-dependent reaction, called photosynthesis, the combination of the water and carbon dioxide releases oxygen which is returned to the atmosphere from the plant for use again by the animal.

In the animal cell the oxygen is used to burn carbohydrate. Thus there is a constantly recurring cycle; carbohydrate being formed by the plant with the release of oxygen and the entrapment of the sun's energy; carbohydrate being oxidized by the animal with the throwing off of carbon dioxide and water, and the recovery of that energy derived from the sun. The plant reaction takes up energy; the animal reaction releases it.

While the plant has the advantage of a certain kind of independence, of being able to synthesize its own nutrients from light, air and soil, it must remain stationary with its roots thrust deep into the earth and its leaves turned up toward the sun. Therefore, the nature of its vegetative existence is a sort of rigidity and immobility. The animal, by contrast, has gained mobility and freedom, but he lacks the ability to synthesize his own food. He remains utterly dependent on the patient, stolid plant which alone has the capacity to capture energy from the sun and "package it" as carbohydrate. This provides the animal with the fuel he needs to create his own internal source of energy. He has sacrificed self-sufficiency for mobility.

From a practical point of view, it is as though it is necessary to fuel up periodically with plants which are burned little by little to supply the energy required. Despite the dependency on the plant that it implies, this capacity permits movement from place to place, and it has provided the opportunity for evolution in the animal kingdom to reach the great heights of agility and consciousness that characterize man.

The carbohydrate molecule, then, is a fairly simple structure. It contains only carbon, hydrogen and oxygen plus the energy from the sun that was trapped during their combination. The smallest unit or molecule of carbohydrate produced by the plant is called a "sugar." There are various types of sugar molecules. A few contain five carbon atoms, but most contain six.

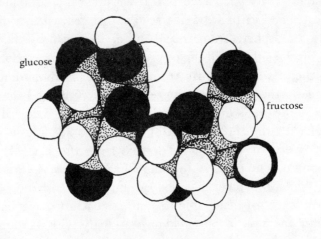

Sucrose Molecule

Attached to each of these carbon atoms are either hydrogen, oxygen or a combination of the two. The sequence of these elements is what makes fructose, the most commonly occurring sugar in fruits, different from glucose, which is the primary sugar in the blood. Other sugars are made up of pairs of such simpler molecules. When fructose and glucose are coupled together, for example, the result is sucrose or "table sugar."

THE SUGAR STORY

Most of the sugar in the diet of primitive man was found in fruits. Whereas a seed, a nut or a grain is a dormant or embryonic plant awaiting the opportunity to sprout and grow, the substance of a fruit is something different. A seed may be contained within the fruit, but the fruit itself is not necessary to the nourishment of the seed during the early stages of its growth. In fact, the sweet part of the fruit seems to be a rather clever innovation on the part of the plant designed primarily to tempt a man or animal. Nature has known for a long time that the way to get the cooperation of the animal world is to offer it something sweet, and this is especially true of man. The sweetness of the fruit entices him to eat it, carrying with him the seed to deposit elsewhere and propagate the growth and spread of the plant species. The delicious and seductive sweetness of fruit is a matter of legend, and the ancient poets tell the story of Hercules who tromped about the earth searching for the golden apple, or of Adam and Eve who, unable to resist the temptation of the fruit's sweetness, learned the lessons of Good and Evil. By concentrating sugars around their seeds, the fruit-bearing plants are able to please the palate and successfully compete for attention.

No doubt man's natural affinity for sweets stems, at least in part, from the relationship of sugar to the appetite mechanism in the body. When blood sugar begins to drop, one usually develops a feeling of hunger. When the blood sugar is elevated, the feeling disappears. In natural circumstances this mechanism worked well. Normally the foods that early man ate contained only small or moderate amounts of sugar, and as these were absorbed from the stomach and intestines, his appetite disappeared. The reduction in the hunger drive would occur as sugar reached the bloodstream. Some of this would be the sugars contained in the food, but most of it would come from the breakdown of starch. Starch is a complex chain made up of sugar units which are broken off one at a time by the digestive enzymes so that they reach the bloodstream over a period of time. As one digests starch he also digests and absorbs the numerous other nutrients which he needs, such as protein, fat, vitamins and minerals. These would also be present since most whole, natural foods contain not only sugars and/or starch, but a balanced complement of the other necessary nutrients as well. As the carbohydrate in the food is burned to supply energy, the blood sugar gradually begins to sink, and once more one experiences an appetite and is prompted to look for food. Carbohydrate absorption, then, serves as a sort of signal, letting one know when he has enough food or when he needs more. One might wonder why carbohydrate should be the nutrient that's used for this purpose, but its "choice" is logical since it is the nutrient one needs in the greatest quantity and is the fuel on which the body operates. It is also what one needs most urgently in the case of an emergency since carbohydrates are "energy foods." If one could choose only one gauge to appear on the dash of his car, he'd probably pick the gasoline gauge. Oil, water, etc., can be checked periodically, but gasoline is of more urgent concern.

Inevitably, man gravitated toward the cultivation of plants such as sugar cane that contain extraordinarily high concentrations of sugar. Eventually, he even discovered how to extract the sugar from the food where it is normally found, throwing the rest of the food package away. He could then eat the sugar, delight the taste buds, kill the hunger and not bother with all the rest. In fact, his body wouldn't even have to break down the starch into small sugar units. He could put the individual sugar units into his belly and they would be immediately absorbed and the hunger would disappear. This had—and still has—a great attraction for him. But when such concentrated sweets are taken alone, their sudden absorption results in an immediate rise in blood sugar. One may experience an immediate but short-lived burst of energy. This rush of energy and euphoria may be followed, however, by a period of letdown, exhaustion, weakness and tremulousness. The weakness that follows this exhilaration leads, of course, to craving for another dose of sugar and perpetuates the cycle. So there is an important difference between taking sugar and taking starch. Whereas sugar is absorbed immediately and may give a sudden burst of energy and then a drop, starch is gradually broken down into sugar units, giving little bits of useable carbohydrate spread out over a longer period of time so that the blood sugar doesn't drop as fast or as low. The difference between eating a piece of pastry that has refined sugar in it and eating a piece of bread or a bowl of rice is obvious. The reaction which follows, called the hypoglycemic effect, is not as pronounced with the complex carbohydrate.

NATURAL SUGAR

The major concentrated source of sucrose is in sugar cane and sugar beets. Up until the last hundred years or so, the process of extracting sugar from its natural sources was expensive and impractical. In the 13th and 14th centuries in Europe, a pound of sugar cost more than a week's wages for a servant. It was a rare delicacy, available only on the tables of royalty. As the process of refining sugar and extracting it from sugar cane and beets became industrialized, however, it became more widely available and its cost decreased.

When purified white sugar is made from the piece of sugar cane, everything is taken out except the sucrose. While sucrose is the only completely purified sugar commonly used in the diet, there are other sweetening agents which are produced by the process of refining sugar cane, each having different properties and different effects. Molasses is one of these by-products and consists of all the miscellaneous material remaining when sucrose is removed from sugar cane juice. Molasses varies in its composition. So-called sweet molasses has a fair amount of sugar left in, while "blackstrap" molasses has less sugar but a correspondingly stronger and more unpleasant taste. Since it is a concentrated residue, molasses contains significant quantities of minerals such as iron, a fair amount of calcium and generous quantities of trace elements such as zinc, copper and chromium.[1] Of course, other substances will be concentrated in the molasses too: environmental pollutants like lead, chemicals incident to the cultivation of the cane such as pesticides, or substances involved in its processing, for instance, sulfur. So-called unsulphured molasses is prepared with these considerations in mind, but it is usually difficult to know exactly what by-products of the refining process a given lot of molasses might contain since such information is not mentioned on the label. Even when carefully prepared, blackstrap molasses is the final residue of the sugar cane and in the traditions of the East is considered inferior, the least wholesome of the products extracted from that plant.

Sorghum and cane syrup are a step closer than sugar to a whole food since they are the boiled down juice of the sorghum or sugar cane plant without anything removed except water. Sorghum cane syrup is prepared from the juice of sorghum, which is a member of the millet family, and has a richer and heartier taste than sugar cane syrup. Pure sugar cane syrup, of course, contains most of the nutrients that are in molasses though in lower concentrations and subjected to less processing. However, it is usually difficult to find a pure cane syrup since its shelf life is fairly short. For this reason many additives such as refined sugar, corn syrup, etc. are often used to help preserve it.

Genuine raw sugar is made by simply evaporating the water from sugar cane juice and allowing it to solidify and granulate. In years past, such sugar was readily available and inexpensive since relatively little work was required for its preparation. In such areas of the world as India where much of the processing of sugar cane is done by hand on a small scale, this raw sugar, called *gur* in Hindi, is still common. Its flavor is rich, and it contains all the nutrients which are found in sugar cane since it is essentially the same as sugar cane except that the fiber and water are removed. By contrast, the modern industrialized processing of sugar is geared to the total purification of sucrose, and crystalline table sugar is thus one of the purest chemicals regularly produced in large quantities.[2]   In fact, government regulations in the U.S. require that sugar be purified at least to some extent.

Sugar in this country is made in a two-step process. The sugar cane is crushed at the mill, pressed and the juice is treated to remove some impurities, then boiled down until it begins to crystallize. The liquid is separated by centrifuging, leaving a "raw sugar," which is shipped to the refinery. Though this raw sugar is 96-97% sucrose, it contains a number of contaminants such as soil, molds, yeasts, bacteria and waxes and cannot be sold until it is washed with steam. This is marketed as "turbinado sugar" but is not very different from white sugar—since it is more than 99% sucrose. It may contain traces of minerals like chromium, however, which gives it a slight edge over refined sugar.

Brown sugar is prepared by pouring a small amount of molasses over pure granulated white sugar. While this returns some nutrients to the sugar, the desirability of brown sugar will depend to some extent on the methods used for sugar refining and the quality of the molasses that results.

In the old-fashioned home methods of processing sugar cane, the juice was allowed to crystallize slowly, and when large sugar crystals had formed, the mixture was poured into burlap bags and piled up so that the remaining liquid could drip into a container below. This produced a pure home-made molasses, leaving large chunks of highly purified sugar which was crushed for table use or eaten as "rock candy." This method is still used in certain rural areas of India today.

Though it is now clearly established that there is a definite relationship between sugar consumption and tooth decay, it is surprising that people who chew sugar cane don't suffer from an increase in cavities. As a matter of fact, cane workers in South Africa who chewed four stalks of sugar cane a day had better than average teeth.[3]   In the laboratory experiments have yielded similar results. Sugar cane juice was mixed with saliva in one container, and sugar was mixed in the same proportions with saliva in another. Teeth which had been removed, but had no cavities, were placed in each. Weeks later, the teeth in the sugar cane juice had not decalcified at all while about half of those in the sugar had.[4] There is apparently something (perhaps molyb-denum,[5] it has been hypothesized) in cane juice which has a protective   effect that is lost when pure white sugar is made.

Among the Zulu and Pando cane cutters in Natal who chew a great deal of sugar cane, diabetes is virtually unknown. By contrast, very high correlations have been found between deaths from diabetes and consumption of refined sugar.[6] In the 1920's in Panama, construction workers in the Canal Zone who came from the Dominican Republic and had consumed quantities of sugar cane from early childhood had no trace of diabetes although over 5,000 were examined. Wealthy Spaniards living in the same area, however, who used large quantities of refined sugar had a high incidence of the disease.[7] Apparently, large amounts of cane sugar cause little difficulty as long as one is taking it as part of the natural cane juice. Separating and refining it seems to change its effects on the body.

REFINED SUGAR

At present in the industrialized West most foods are grown on specialized farms in huge quantities and are often shipped halfway across the continent; the major factor in their cost comes from transportation and storage. Because of the availability of modern technology, the process of refinement has become so streamlined as to be relatively cheap. Meanwhile the refrigeration and special handling that is necessary for a food which will spoil is much more expensive. Refined sugar is, of course, very stable and like most other purified chemicals will keep indefinitely.   It has therefore gone from an extremely costly commodity to one which is quite cheap.   This has brought sugar from a rare delicacy to one of the least expensive of all sources of carbohydrate.   As a result, the use of sugar has increased from about 15 pounds per person per year in 1815 to about 120 pounds per person at present,* an eight-fold increase in 150 years.[8]   In other words, the majority of people eat their weight in sugar each year.   This comes out to more than a teaspoonful every hour, day and night.

NUTRIENT DEBTS

A large percentage of this sugar is "hidden."   A cursory examination of labels in packaged and canned foods in a modern supermarket turns up sugar as an ingredient in the most unlikely places.   Even meat products contain nearly 3% by weight of added sugar, while more than 13% of processed vegetables is added sucrose.[10]   When sugar is taken into the body, one's need for carbohydrate is satisfied.   At the same time his hunger is eliminated. The very real need for other nutrients, however, goes unmet as sugar contains no protein, no vitamins, no minerals and no fat or fiber. It is a stripped carbohydrate and consists essentially of "empty" calories. We might say that, nutritionally speaking, when one eats sugar he has incurred a "debt." Though he has met the need for carbohydrate, he owes himself a corresponding quantity of vitamins, minerals, fat, protein and fiber.

The metabolism of sugar will proceed only through the use of all the accessory nutrients which are involved in its combustion.   Vitamins, minerals and even some protein and fat molecules are all necessary. These "incidentals" are not replaced by

___

* It is sometimes stated that sugar consumption has not increased in the last fifty years. This is essentially true if present figures are compared with exactly fifty years ago, since that happened to be a period of unusually high sugar consumption for that era.   However, the overall trend over the past 150 years has been one of increase.[9]

the "meal" of refined sugar. Therefore, as sugar eating becomes a habit, the supply of vitamins, minerals, fats and protein gradually becomes depleted, and such nutrients must be pulled from tissues somewhere in the body in order to continue support of the metabolic activities fueled by the sugar. Even though weight is gained when large quantities of sugar are eaten, the continued consumption of refined sugar can result in the body becoming increasingly deficient in important nutrients. In some cases only a limited amount of the sugar is burned since one feels too tired to be very active. Without the proper vitamins and minerals to facilitate the metabolism of carbohydrate and create a desire for exercise, much of the sugar is stored away as fat. The result is a bloated or pasty sort of obesity that has come to characterize those who regularly indulge in soft drinks, candy, etc., incurring nutrient "debts" which they never pay off. It is important to realize that with "modern" refined foods, especially those containing large amounts of sugar, obesity and malnutrition may occur together. Under a mountain of fat, many obese people are starving to death because they're not getting what they need.

By contrast, on a diet comprised of whole foods in which one component has not been separated from another, weight gain will usually mean an increase in all nutrients, and is a sign of good health. Thus it is that among peasant folk the world over where whole, unaltered foods are taken, a hefty body is regarded with pride and pleasure. But in the context of an urban environment and an industrialized food supply, weight gain is anathema, and to "keep it off" is a constant struggle. In such a setting, obesity is recognized as an indication of serious health problems.

Other untoward effects of refined table sugar on health have also been documented. A heavy intake of table sugar has been shown, for example, to be associated with high levels of blood fats such as triglycerides and cholesterol.[11] Yet this does not mean that sugar itself is harmful. Used in small quantities in a diet otherwise rich in essential nutrients, it can be a useful adjunct. As long as it is used as a condiment rather than a food, it will cause no trouble. If it is taken as a major source of energy, however, replacing whole foods, problems will definitely follow.

OTHER SUGARS

While sweets like dried fruits and honey contain large amounts of sugar, this is not all in the form of sucrose (table sugar). Half or more may be, according to the fruit, but there is usually a large percentage of fructose too. Other sugars are also present, as in the example of grapes where the preponderant sugar is glucose (also known as dextrose). Whereas glucose requires insulin for its movement from the bloodstream into the cell, fructose does not.[12] It is also absorbed somewhat more slowly,[13] and for these reasons, fructose is thought to be less likely to trigger hypoglycemic attacks. In fact, this property has led to its popularization as a sweetener, and granulated fructose (sometimes called levulose) is now being marketed on a large scale as a replacement for ordinary table sugar.[14] Fructose is also probably less likely than sucrose to cause dental carries.[15] Though dried fruits, honey, etc. may not have all the undesirable effects of pure sucrose, they still may, if taken alone in quantity raise the blood sugar too far too fast, only to have it drop too rapidly thereafter. This results in the familiar "roller coaster" effect that follows eating large amounts of any kind of sweets, though it may be less severe than what occurs after table sugar.

HONEY

Honey is a very complex substance consisting mostly of fructose and glucose with a few minerals, very few vitamins, little or no protein or fat, and small amounts of sucrose.[16] Honey varies depending on where it comes from, what flower it is made from and how it is made. It contains not only the various sugars derived from the nectar of flowers, but also some "additives" from the digestive system of the bee. These substances serve as a preservative, allowing the honey to remain nutritious for a long time.

When used as a sweetener in the diet, honey has the advantage of being absorbed relatively slowly, probably because of its high fructose content. Because of the complexity of the carbohydrates and other substances in honey, it is delicate and easily damaged so that any heating should be avoided. Labels should read "raw" or "unheated." "Uncooked" honey may have been heated enough to extract them, and enough to ruin their flavor and quality. In the ancient writings in Ayurvedic medicine in India, heated honey is emphatically said to be harmful. The honey made from certain flowers is quite dark and has a strong taste, however, which many people find unpleasant. It is probably primarily to remove this strong flavor that much of that honey marketed in a large scale is cooked and filtered. This removes much of the color and taste but it produces an acid off-flavor that is quite different from that of raw honey. While millions of people are using the cooked, refined honey sold in most supermarkets, no laboratory research has been done to investigate its possible undesirable effects.

An increasing awareness that refined sugar can be harmful when taken in large quantities has led to an attempt to find a substitute. While many people who have had experience with honey insist on that which is raw, they often unthinkingly follow recipes that involve cooking it. According to traditional lore, however, honey is unsuitable for such foods unless it can be added after the cooking process.

While there are disadvantages to concentrated sugars of all kinds, even honey, there is clearly a need for carbohydrate in the diet. A certain amount of fuel must be burned each day, and if sufficient carbohydrate is not taken in the diet, the body must turn to the use of fats or proteins. However, neither of these burns well, especially in the absence of carbohydrates, and the residues they produce can cause problems. Therefore, a form of carbohydrate other than simple sugars is most ideal.

STARCH

Carbohydrate, or fuel, can be taken in one of two forms: simple or complex. Simple carbohydrates are sugars, which we have discussed. Complex carbohydrates are the large, branched chains formed by many sugar molecules linked together. This is called starch. While total carbohydrate consumption has decreased in the last 100 years, probably because increased mechanization has resulted in less physical work for the average person, the use of simple carbohydrates, like table sugar, has more than doubled. It is the amount of complex carbohydrate or starch, such as that found in grains or beans, that has decreased dramatically.

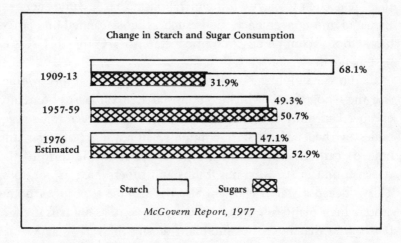

Change in Starch and Sugar Consumption

1909-13 68.1% 31.9%

1957-59 49.3% 50.7%

1976 Estimated 47.1% 52.9%

Starch □ Sugars ▨

McGovern Report, 1977

Nutritional surveys suggest that this is one of the most major changes in dietary habits in the last 100 years. Since it is during this period of time that arteriosclerosis became the major cause of death in the West, it has been suggested that this might be connected with such shifts in carbohydrate consumption.[17] As we have seen, there are a number of studies that show a connection, at least among some people, between increased consumption of refined carbohydrates and an increase in blood fats and arteriosclerosis. Moreover, there are also studies which have shown a *decrease* in blood fats and arteriosclerosis when diets are high in *complex* carbohydrates such as grains and dried beans and peas.* There are also a number of studies which show that whole grains containing their natural fiber lower blood fats and may help to protect against arteriosclerosis.[18, 19, 20]

In fact, it may be the whole grains and beans that are important rather than the starch itself. Starch alone, while it may release sugar molecules into the blood more slowly than sugar, since they have to be chopped off one by one, is still essentially a stripped carbohydrate. Purified starch like corn starch is "empty calories," failing, like sugar, to bring with it the necessary complement of vitamins, minerals and proteins that are needed to carry on the metabolism that it could energize. Prepared and convenience foods such as most canned and jarred baby foods containing "modified starch" are for this reason best avoided.

Fortunately, the refining of starch is a lot of trouble, and the whole foods which contain starch are at least potentially cheaper and more accessible. Though fruits and even some vegetables in their natural state contain small amounts of sugar, the bulk of carbohydrate occurring in nature is in the form of the starch found in seeds, grains, bulbs and tubers such as potatoes. This is because starch is essentially the storage form of carbohydrate which plants use in much the same way as animals use fat. It is starch that nourishes the plant during the early stages of its development before it establishes a root and leaf system for manufacturing its own nourishment. Therefore, it is "packaged" along with the other critical nutrients, vitamins, minerals and protein that will be needed during its growth. Though some carbohydrate is present in the leaves and stems of plants, man and many animals depend for the bulk of their fuel on certain seeds. Throughout the world, such seeds or "grains" are the

* See Chapter 6, Protein.

most highly valued source of starch.

GRAINS: FOOD FOR AN OVERPOPULATED WORLD

In the diet of modern man, grains are the most common source of starch and the cheapest source of calories in most parts of the world,* supplying the vast majority of fuel that is burned by human beings. Though some writers on nutrition believe that grains have been used by man too short a time for him to be adapted to them,[21] other authors disagree.[22] Actually, the history of grains is the history of civilization, and it was largely the storable, compact grain that made towns and cities feasible. Throughout the world, there is a wide variety of grains cultivated, and each climate and culture has its favorite, be it rice, wheat, rye, millet, corn, oats or barley. Basically, a grain is a seed and is made up of three parts: the *germ*, which will, upon germination and sprouting, give rise to the first tiny leaves and rootlets; the *endosperm* or starchy bulk of the grain which nourishes the seedling during its early growth before its leaves have begun photosynthesis; and the *bran* or tough outer covering that protects the grain. The germ contains vitamins, oils and proteins. It is an especially important source of vitamin E, and diets which use degerminated and refined flours are usually deficient in this important nutrient. The endosperm is made up of starch granules packed into tiny compartments, the walls of which are mostly protein. This protein is not an insignificant part of the diet. The bran is composed of several layers and contains minerals, fiber, significant amounts of protein, and also small amounts of certain vitamins.

As long as the grain or seed remains intact, it will live for some time in a dormant condition. When exposed to warmth and moisture, it will begin to wake up and sprout, reacting as

---

* As mentioned above, in industrialized areas white sugar has often come to be cheaper than grains calorie for calorie—though not nutrient for nutrient.

though spring had arrived and it were time to grow. On the other hand, if the integrity of the grain is disrupted by grinding, cracking, or rolling, it cannot remain alive. It dies, and decay will eventually begin. For this reason, any whole grain which is not in its natural state, such as whole grain flour, cracked wheat, corn meal, etc., will eventually spoil unless it is refrigerated. Even under cold storage, it will remain fresh only for a limited amount of time.

Longitudinal Section through a Grain of Wheat

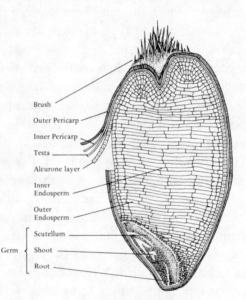

Brush
Outer Pericarp
Inner Pericarp
Testa
Aleurone layer
Inner Endosperm
Outer Endosperm
Germ { Scutellum
Shoot
Root

Wheat

Wheat is one of the oldest grains cultivated by man. There is evidence of wheat cultivation in the Middle East as early as 10,000 years ago. In the U.S. and Europe, wheat is the most widely consumed grain, and it has progressively edged out other grains in the rest of the world. There are now a billion people who use it regularly in their diets, and since the beginning of this century wheat production has more than doubled. Though wheat is seldom eaten as the sole item of the diet, a good quality wheat is remarkably well-balanced. It can be nearly one-fourth protein and is also rich in other nutrients. When taken with small quantities of other foods, such a good quality wheat can support vigorous health, even when it makes up three-fourths or more of the diet.[23]   Unfortunately, wheat varies more in nutrient content than any other cereal, and ranges in protein content from 8% to 24%.[24]   Other nutrients in the grain also vary widely depending on the health of the soil and the other conditions under which it is grown.

Basically, there are two kinds of wheat grown today. One is a hard wheat whose grain is flinty and contains a relatively high percentage of protein, and the other is softer and contains a higher proportion of starch. Hard wheat is generally used for the flour that goes into bread while that of the softer wheat is favored for pastries, cakes and so forth. It is the gluten in wheat* which makes up the majority of the protein, and gluten is also the substance which is responsible for making bread springy. As bread dough is kneaded, the gluten molecules join together, or polymerize, forming long chains that make it elastic. Flour which is low in gluten is difficult to develop into a springy mass and is not likely to produce a light bread. On the other hand, pastries and cakes depend for their flakiness and tenderness on the absence of the stretchy gluten. Pastry flours, then, are usually low in gluten, and good cooks know that pastry dough should not "be handled too much" because this will develop what gluten there is and make the pastry tough. There is a third variety of wheat that is particularly hard called durum wheat. Because of its high gluten content, it is especially suitable for making pasta such as macaroni and spaghetti. If these Italian delicacies are made with other kinds of wheat, they do not hold their shape as well and tend to come apart when cooked.

Gluten is the major source of protein in the diets of many people who live on a wheat-based diet. Some vegetarian cook-

---

* as well as several other grains including oats, rye and barley

books offer methods for isolating gluten from wheat flour to make a meat-like substance that can be sliced into cutlets, added to stews, or even stretched into lengths and roasted over a fire to make "barbecued ribs"![25] To prepare such gluten, the wheat flour is simply kneaded until it is stretchy, after which the kneading process is continued under water. As the starch in the flour is washed away, a rubbery mass of gluten is left. Gluten does not agree with everyone, however, Some digestive diseases for example, known to be aggravated by wheat, have been found to be based on an intolerance to gluten. Certain persons with schizophrenia also seem to react adversely to wheat, and research has demonstrated that there is often overall improvement by putting such patients on a wheat-free diet.[26] Again, it is suspected that gluten is the substance to which such people react, though other constituents of the wheat might also play a part.

In India, where it has been a major part of the diet for many thousands of years, the ancient medical traditions ascribe special and unique properties to wheat. It is said to be particularly prone to produce growth, thus being suitable as a food for children. It is also prescribed for convalescents, but traditional physicians are wary of its growth-producing tendency in adults and suspect it of aggravating the tendency to develop cysts and other benign growths and tumors in the body. Wheat is also especially good at helping put on extra pounds, even when they are not wanted, so dieters often substitute rye bread for wheat bread when they wish to lose weight.

Brown Bread or White?

The nutrients that are contained in the separate parts of the wheat grain are vastly different. Most of the starch and large amounts of the protein are concentrated in the center, that which we grind to make white flour. In the germ, the part which would grow to make leaves if the seed were allowed to sprout, there's a high concentration of protein, fat and certain vitamins, especially vitamin E. The covering layers or bran contain many minerals and B vitamins, as well as a significant amount of protein.

Actually, the various covering layers that are usually grouped together as "bran" are not uniform in their makeup. The outermost layer, for example, which is tough and flaky (called technically the epiderm or epicarp) was traditionally known to the miller as the "bee's wing" because it flaked off into pieces like fragments of the wing of a bee. It contains primarily cellulose and very little useful nutrients. The layers beneath that, however, (the endocarp, testa, hyaline and aleurone layers) contain progressively less cellulose and increasingly more protein and vitamins such as thiamin and niacin.[27]

During most of man's 10,000 years of wheat cultivation, he has used the grain as it is harvested, or ground the whole grain into flour, mixing it with water and cooking it to produce one of the many kinds of bread which are staples the world over. Though such whole wheat bread is of course the original and earliest form, man discovered thousands of years ago how to sift the flour through a finely woven silk fabric to remove part of the bran. This produced a lighter flour which was more delicate in taste and easier to digest. The light, delicate loaves that could be prepared from such sifted flour were the perogative of the privileged classes and were considered an enviable delicacy. To serve anything but white bread on a ceremonial occasion was considered an insult. Nevertheless, whole wheat bread was still the daily fare of most people who ate a wheat-based diet and was probably even a common food among those who could afford the whiter breads. As the refining of flour became more prevalent, however, the practice developed of adding the left-over bran to coarser grades of flour, often that of cheaper grains like barley, thereby providing an inexpensive product that was used mostly by the poor. Even whole wheat flour is whiter than the flour made from such grains, so that dark bread was less likely to be wheat bread.[28] This brown or "black bread" as it was often called was disdained by the wealthy and was generally regarded by knowledgeable physicians as being hard on the stomach. Medieval writers in England said, "Brown bread fills the stomach; white bread nourishes the body."

The Bran Question

It is obvious then that exactly which parts of the wheat are eaten is very important not only for the palate, but for the maintenance of good health too. Since certain bran layers are more nutritious than others, the question is not whether the bran is removed, but rather which part of it is removed. Modern steel mills, which are much more thorough than the silk sifters of hundreds of years ago, are geared to produce the kind of white flour that's used in commercial bread. They tend to extract all of the bran, not only the coarser outer layers which are of little food value, but also the more digestible inner layers which are rich in vitamins, minerals and protein. They also remove the germ, which can be a valuable source of both vitamin E and protein, and its adjacent structures (the "scutellum") which contain most of the thiamin. Current milling techniques tend to selectively remove the outer and inner layers of the grain where many of the nutrients are concentrated, while the middle, which is proportionately richer in starch, is left. Because the wheat germ is the part of the grain that decomposes most readily, omitting it from the flour greatly increases the shelf life of the product. White flour can remain in the grocery store at room temperature almost indefinitely without becoming rancid, whereas whole wheat flour cannot. The bran, although it is not subject to spoilage, is also removed from the flour because it makes bread heavy and dark and interferes with the light color and springy texture that are often desired. Because of the many nutrients it contains, it is used in animal feeds.

In the U.S., the familiar white flour which is the result of this modern refining process is "72% extraction."[29] This means that it has lost 28% of the bulk of the wheat, including half or more of many of the crucial nutrients. Reducing the extraction rate, that is, including a larger percentage of the whole grain, will improve the nutritional status of the flour, but this will occur at the expense of adding great amounts of cellulose. As we have seen, not only is the cellulose fraction largely indigestible, but it contains the majority of the phytic acid in the grain as well.

Phytic acid is a phosphorous compound found in most plant foods but in especially large amounts in whole grains, beans and peas. It has the property of combining with minerals, especially calcium, iron and zinc to form insoluble compounds which are carried out in the stool.[30] It was noted long ago that foods high in phytic acid can lead to rickets in dogs,[31] a disease which stunts the skeletal growth of children, causing deformities of the head, chest and limbs, or which can cause enough softening in the bones of adults that they break even during normal use. Bread with added bran, for example, has been associated with calcium deficiency and rickets in certain villages in Persia.[32] At one point, English researchers claimed that because of its phytic acid content, the Scotsman's traditional oatmeal was dangerous and unsuitable for human consumption, nearly provoking a civil war. But further research showed that the hearty Scotsmen who had lived for generations on oatmeal had acquired the ability to break down phytic acid in their intestines and thus prevent its robbing them of minerals.[33] Other research also shows an adaptive effect when man or other animals are fed on whole grain bread. It seems likely then that phytic acid is ordinarily a nutritional problem only during the time that one is adapting to whole grains, beans or peas recently added to the diet. There are, however, probably some people who do not readily acquire the ability to deal with excessive quantities of phytic acid as is suggested by such problems as rickets among the Persian villagers. It is also likely that the ability to develop a capacity for handling phytic acid in the food is related to overall health and nutrition.

"Bran breads" and "fiber breads" are currently marketed as an aid to weight loss with the idea that indigestible fiber can't cause weight gain. For people who are not accustomed to eating even whole wheat flour, bread with extra bran can be even more troublesome, producing gas and a bloated feeling. Some fiber bread, rather than having extra bran, actually has ground wood fiber added to it. As we shall see later, the human digestive system is not well designed for processing sawdust, though little is known about the long term effects in humans of eating wood fiber in quantity.

How Refined Should a Fine Flour Be?

The refining of flour can drastically change the content and proportions of other vitamins, minerals, protein and even in some cases, toxic contaminants. Zinc and cadmium, for example, are both found in wheat. While the zinc is essential, the cadmium is toxic and exerts its negative effects by replacing zinc in strategic enzymes which are thereby inactivated. Thus the ratio between zinc and cadmium in food is very important, but zinc is concentrated more in the outer layers of the grain while cadmium tends to be found in its center. Milling, then, selectively removes the zinc, while leaving the cadmium so that the zinc/cadmium ratio is reversed.[34]

Many other minerals are also lost in significant quantities in milling. For instance, white flour contains only 13% of the chromium, 9% of the manganese and 19% of the iron which is contained in whole wheat.[35] Also, many of the B vitamins are concentrated in the outer parts of the grain. For example, while the silk-bolted flour which was used until the colonial American era probably contained 60% of the thiamin[36] present in the whole wheat berry, the white flour of present day production contains 20% or less. There may also be other valuable nutrients or properties of the bran and germ which have not yet been clearly identified but which are nonetheless lost in significant quantities.

Because of this loss of nutrients during the milling and refining process, wheat flour in this country is required by law to be "enriched." This is a method of replacing some of the vitamins and minerals, namely thiamin, riboflavin, niacin and iron, which are lost. For this reason, one might think that the removal of these nutrients doesn't matter since they are eventually returned to bread anyway. However, only these vitamins and minerals are replaced, leaving the flour stripped of many other important nutrients. White flour contains, for example, less than one-third of the pyridoxine and folic acid contained in the whole wheat flour, and less than one-half the pantothenic acid; moreover, it contains as little as 14% of the vitamin E since bleaching destroys much of it.[37]   Besides the nutrients which are lost by discarding all but the starchy, white endosperm, some are lost in the modern process of grinding.

Despite these drawbacks, this does not mean that white flour is never useful. In fact, experiments have shown that about 95% of the calories and protein of white flour are fully utilized whereas only 85% of these nutrients are used in whole grain flour.[38]   If we remember that whole wheat flour contains a lower percentage of starch and protein than flour containing all of the bran, then it is easy to see that one whose digestion is weak might find white flour beneficial. It is, in fact, a time honored practice to use the more digestible refined flour for those who are ill, but in such cases, careful attention must be given to supplying adequate quantities of the other nutrients that have been lost in refining.

It is interesting to note that the traditional milling procedure in India, where wheat has been used perhaps as long as anywhere in the world, includes stone grinding with a subsequent sifting that removes 5-10% of the grain.[39]   What tends to flake off in the largest pieces and be most easily removed is the "bee's wing" which, happily, is that fraction of the grain which is primarily cellulose and devoid of most nutrients. The result is a 90-95% extraction rate flour which retains almost all the nutrients of the grain while simultaneously eliminating that part of the grain which is most indigestible and the most likely to cause trouble since it contains most of the phytic acid which could bind and carry away minerals such as calcium, zinc, iron and so forth.[40]   Therefore, while Indian-style flour is not technically "whole wheat," it may be superior to the usual whole grain flour that is produced by simply grinding everything to a fine powder. It has a more delicate flavor and produces a lighter bread, yet it remains a satisfying, high protein grain. In the West, the battle over whether white bread is better than brown has been fought since the days of classic Rome, and continues to the present with scientists entering the fray in the last century or so. As early as 1826, a French physiologist reported that a dog fed on white bread and water died within 50 days, while one fed on "the coarse bread of the military" thrived.[41] The death of the dog on white flour would be ascribed today to thiamin deficiency, and since modern white flour in the U.S. has thiamin added, such results should not be seen. Yet a few years ago, a similar experiment produced the same results. Rats fed a diet of only commercial "enriched" white bread showed stunted growth and two-thirds of them died of malnutrition within 90 days.[42]

More recently, however, it was found that when experimental animals were fed a variety of commercial or even "health food" whole wheat breads or white breads, there was no difference between the two. In fact, while the best results came from one carefully made whole grain loaf,* some of the white breads, especially ones made with milk, came out ahead of whole grain ones.[43]

So the age-old controversy rages on while the Indians continue, as they have for thousands of years, to quietly grind

---

* which has since been taken off the market—perhaps because it was too time-consuming or expensive to make

their flour with stone mills and sift out the coarsest 5%, producing a bread both wholesome and digestible. It seems likely that this process approaches the ideal, and there is no reason why modern steel roller mills could not be adapted to produce a similar product.

Rice

While wheat is the predominant grain of Western Europe and North America, rice is clearly the staple of most of the Far East. Rice may well be the most ancient of food grains, and next to wheat, it is the grain grown in largest quantity throughout the world today.   Over 200 million tons are grown annually, and most of this is consumed by Asians who eat an average of 200 pounds per person per year.[44]   In fact, the Chinese written character for "food" is the same as that for "rice."

Interestingly enough, though most people picture the typical Chinaman with a bowl of rice in one hand and a pair of chopsticks in the other, rice actually originated in India. It is said that Buddhism, when it spread from the Indian sub-continent to the Far East, brought with it the custom of eating rice. Alexander the Great, when he returned from India, brought rice back to Europe, and its cultivation and popularity spread throughout the Western world. During colonial American times, rice was an important crop along the southeastern seaboard, and Carolina rice became famous for its flavor and quality. In America today, rice is grown primarily in Louisiana, Arkansas and California, but rice culture has never attained the sophistication in the West that it enjoys in Asia. From India to Japan, there is a wide spectrum of climatic conditions, and literally hundreds of varieties of rice are grown, each being prized in its native locale for its particular nutritional value and flavor. There are sweet rices which are glutinous and are favored for dessert-making by the Chinese. There are long grain and short grain varieties with different tastes and textures. Some rices are brown before milling, others are red and some are simply white or cream-colored.

Whole grain rice, like whole grain wheat, retains all of the nutrients, including those which are concentrated in the outer layers. This has lead to the current emphasis on brown rice, which is based on a rationale similar to that for the whole wheat bread. Surprisingly, however, unlike wheat which is still most often taken with little refining except in the industrially developed countries, the bulk of rice eaten in the world is polished.

The first step in processing rice is to remove the coarse and rather loose husk. This is generally done by pounding the grain with a wooden pestle. The husk can then be separated by winnowing. What is left is the whole rice grain. If continued, home pounding can produce a "polished" rice by removing the outer layer or bran of the grain too. It is often said that rice is polished primarily to improve its appearance and taste appeal, but it seems unlikely that the millions of people who hand-pound rice for many hours to polish it, thereby sacrificing many of the vitamins and minerals that are contained in the outer coating, go to such trouble and expense for mere taste and color. In fact, research has shown that the proteins of polished rice are more available than those in unpolished rice, and test subjects maintained a better balance of protein on a polished rice diet.[45] This could be extremely important in countries where the diet is almost exclusively rice, as is the case in certain regions of China and India. It is crucially important for those who depend primarily on rice for their protein to have as much of that protein available as possible, since there is not enough present to provide a wide margin of safety. Polished rice also keeps better than brown rice,[46] and because of the decrease in bran is less likely to cause intestinal gas.

Unfortunately, polishing removes a large proportion of many minerals and vitamins, especially the B vitamins. Only about 60% of the riboflavin remains in the polished rice, only one-third of the niacin and less than one-half the pyridoxine.

The Preparation of Rice

Cooking rice properly is a true art developed only after much experience. Generally, however, the less done to it the better it is. The first step in preparing rice is to pick it carefully to be sure it is free from stones, dirt or spoiled grains. Then it should be rinsed in tepid water until the water is clear. Next, place the clean rice in a pot and add enough water to cover the middle finger to the middle of the second joint as the fingertip rests lightly on the top of the rice. For quantities of less than one half cup of uncooked rice, use two to three parts of water to one part of rice. If too much water is added, one can later remove some of it by placing a cloth over the pot and putting the lid over it. In this way, the steam can be captured and removed. If too little water is added, one can carefully pour in a small amount of hot boiling water, taking care not to disturb the rice. Using more water makes the rice lighter and easier to digest, but it should not be soggy.

Bring the rice to a boil, cover it, and turn it to the lowest heat, allowing it to simmer gently until all the water is absorbed. Do not stir it again, but listen to it boiling occasionally to determine how much of the water is left. It is very important not to stir the rice because as it cooks, little passageways are formed throughout which allow the steam to escape and the rice to cook properly and evenly. Disturbing this network causes the rice to lose its fluffy quality, and it becomes gummy and sticks together.

Different varieties of rice require different cooking times. Brown rice, for example, requires about forty-five minutes while parboiled white rice needs only about fifteen. If selecting brown rice, the organically grown short grain varieties from Arkansas and Louisiana are especially delicious. For variety, spices, onions and mushrooms stir-fried in ghee can be added to the rice before cooking it.* Leftover rice can be used within a day or two if it is kept refrigerated. In this case it can be dumped into a heated pot with a little ghee in the bottom. The rice is then fried in the ghee, stirring constantly until it is lightly coated and sizzling. Then it can be covered for a few moments so that it regains its tenderness.

* See *Himalayan Mountain Cookery* by Mrs. R. Ballentine, Sr., p. 73-86 for more information.

The situation is even worse with thiamin, or vitamin B_1, however. Only about 20% of it remains.[47] When thiamin is deficient in the diet for a prolonged period of time, certain people will develop heaviness and weakness of the legs, fluid accumulation and swelling in the limbs and face, degeneration of the nerves with a loss of sensation, and eventually death. This condition, which is not uncommonly seen in those who subsist almost exclusively on polished rice, is called beri-beri. One way of preventing it is to substitute unpolished rice for the polished. If this reduces the availability of the protein, however, it may not be a practical solution unless supplemental sources of protein in the diet like meat, milk, fish and beans are available.

In India where lightly polished rice is often used, the problem has been traditionally solved in a more ingenious way. The rice is steamed or boiled before husking. This not only loosens the husk, making it easier to remove, but it also drives many of the nutrients deep into the grain where they will not be ground away during the polishing. Since the enzyme in the bran that initiates spoilage is destroyed by heating,[48] this is probably also helpful in preventing the rancidity and unpleasant flavor that develop when raw, unpolished rice is stored.[49] This process, called parboiling, has been widely used throughout India, and beri-beri is essentially unknown on the Indian sub-continent. The only documented cases have occurred in a certain coastal region north of Madras, the one area in India where the rice is not parboiled before milling.[50]

Rice is a well balanced food, and while it does not contain an unusually high percentage of protein, it is of particularly good quality. Therapeutic diets based on rice have been very effective[51] for the treatment of some diseases like diabetes. Not only is complex carbohydrate in general helpful in normalizing blood sugar because of its gradual absorption, but rice is particularly useful here. Calorie for calorie, rice that was tested was found to require 50% less insulin than potato.[52] It thus serves as an ideal source of carbohydrate for diabetics. Unfortunately, it is difficult to be specific about the properties of rice in general, since one variety is said to be very different from another in both flavor and effects on the body.[53]

Corn

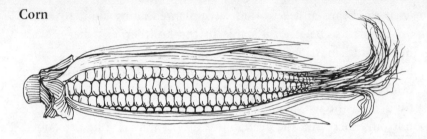

In medieval English, the word "corn" meant grain, and wheat, oats and rye were all corn, not to mention the barley corn, from which the Englishman's brew was made. When the English settlers came to the new world, their crops imported from home were less than successful, but they were quick to rely on the grain crop grown by the native Americans. The strange new grain which grew on large ears had been called maize by the Spanish explorers, but it became the English colonists' "corn." The American settlers learned how to use this new corn from the Indians, and many of their recipes such as hasty pudding* which were famous at the time of the Revolutionary War were adaptations of the traditional Indian dishes. Corn-based diets were found not only in the area colonized by the English and French, but were also widespread throughout Mexico, Central America and down into the Andes.

It was in the Southeast and Southwest of what is now the United States, however, where the Indian tribes did their most extensive farming, and their agriculture was based primarily on corn. The use of corn in the diet in New England and the middle

* so called perhaps because it was made by dropping handsful of corn meal into boiling water along with bits of nuts and dried fruit, meanwhile stirring hastily.

Atlantic States gradually faded out despite Thoreau's praise of hoecakes "of rye and Indian corn" cooked over an open fire. But in the Southern colonies, the settlers adopted the cuisine of the Indian farmers to a great extent, and corn, along with the beans and peas that were planted alongside it to climb on its stalks, became a staple in the Southerner's diet. Most of the Indian tribes used little corn until it was mature and had dried. Then it was pounded into meal, or what was less effort, soaked for some time until it was soft and then cooked by boiling the whole grains in a solution of ashes. This practice not only increased the availability of vitamin B_3, but also added many minerals that came from the plants which had been burnt. The resulting dish became known among the Southern settlers as hominy, and it is still occasionally encountered in the South.

The outer edge of the triangular corn grain tends to be stony hard and very difficult to grind, while the inner, pointed part of the grain which is closer to the cob is softer and more floury. The settlers with their stone mills soon learned, perhaps from the Indians, how to separate the soft floury meal which came from the inside of the kernel from the hard, larger pieces of the flint-like remainder. This harder part required longer cooking, and, because of its grainy hard texture, came to be called "grits." The finer meal, which was softer, was that which was used to make cornbread, muffins, and so forth, giving a more fragrant and delicate flavor and texture.* To this day in the North and Midwest, "corn meal" is often made by using both parts of the kernel and usually produces a corn bread which is unpleasantly gritty unless it has been soaked for some time in advance. A lack of traditional

---

* A similar process is traditional in India when wheat is processed at home. The harder and more flinty outer portion of the grain remains in large pieces (delia) and is used for making dishes similar to what would be called in the West "cracked wheat." The softer inner portion which is found in firmer particles, called suji, is used for sweet and more delicate dishes.

understanding of corn preparation may be one reason that corn has remained essentially a field crop, even in the Midwest where it is grown in huge quantities. It may be significant, however, that the corn grown in the Southeast is much richer in niacin (vitamin B_3). This is the nutrient in corn which is most likely to limit its nutritional value.[54]

Because a great deal of energy could be produced on a small amount of land by growing corn, its culture spread rapidly from the New World to Europe, Africa and even Asia. In these areas, unfortunately, its use was not well understood, and it too often became the sole item of diet. Deficiency diseases, especially resulting from lack of protein and, perhaps more importantly, niacin (vitamin B_3) followed. In Italy, for example, where poor farmers in some areas came to rely exclusively on home-made *polenta*, a sort of mush made from maize flour, a chronic disease called pellagra began to appear. The same situation resulted in South Africa among the Bantu and in those areas of India where corn came to constitute the entire diet.[55] Though, as we shall see later, the discovery of niacin and of its role in pellagra eventually eradicated the disease for most of the wealthier countries of the world, there are still areas of Africa and Asia where only small amounts of corn stand between the populace and starvation. Here pellagra, along with other deficiency diseases, is still seen.

It has been suggested that those who eat a predominantly corn diet should include a generous serving of green leafy vegetables each day.[56] The use of dried beans, as demonstrated by typical Mexican cuisine, are an important adjunct to corn diets, boosting the protein as well as the vitamins and minerals. It is interesting to note that none of the indigenous Americans, nor the Europeans who ate their diet, were ever found to develop pellagra. From all evidence, however, none of the Indians ever attempted to live exclusively on corn, but were able to maintain an impressive state of health when the corn was combined with vegetables and beans. When used intelligently, corn remains

a useful grain, and its importance in the world today is demonstrated by the fact that corn production runs only slightly behind
wheat and rice in the amounts grown per year.

Oats

Next to wheat, rice and corn, more oats are grown in the
world than any other grain. Although they have been found
growing wild all over the world, there is no name for oats in the
ancient language of Sanskrit, and apparently the plant was long
regarded as a weed. Oats were known to the Romans and Greeks,
but there is no evidence that they were cultivated by them. They
were used, however, by the ancient peoples north of the Roman
empire in what is now Switzerland, France and Germany. The
Scots, who made oatmeal a sort of national dish, did not really
begin to use them until the 17th and 18th centuries. A large
proportion of the oats that are grown today are used for cattle,
and it is difficult to say on the basis of the amount grown how
commonly oats are used as a food for man. Why oats were
neglected and have been relegated largely to the role of animal
feed is difficult to understand* since they are higher in protein
than any other grain and they are very easy to cook.[57]

A unique characteristic of the whole oat grain, or "groat"
as it is usually called, is its softness. Unlike wheat, rice or corn, it
can easily be mashed between the fingernails. Because it is not
so hard, the time required to prepare an oat cereal is considerably
less than that needed for other grains. This is true even if one
cooks the whole groat. During the cleaning and hulling, oats
are ordinarily exposed to a temperature of around 200 degrees
F. This causes a slightly roasted flavor which is considered
desirable. The richness of the flavor can be further accentuated
by roasting them briefly either dry or with a bit of fat before

---

* The strong feelings against oats as a food may have been based on an awareness
of their pharmacological properties (see Chapter 13).

adding the water to make cereal. When prepared whole this way, cooking time will be 45 minutes to an hour, but there are techniques for processing oats which make them even easier to cook. The most time honored method is to smash them flat with a roller, a task accomplished relatively easily because of their softness. When the whole groats are prepared in this way, they are usually marketed as "old-fashioned rolled oats."

Instead of rolling them, the oats can also be cut with a steel blade into 3 or 4 small pieces which also cook more rapidly than the whole grain. Modern quick-cooking oats, however, combine the two processes and are essentially steel-cut pieces which are, after steam heating, rolled into small flakes.[58] This is what is traditionally sold as oatmeal and what is most commonly prepared as breakfast cereal. Instant oatmeal, by contrast, is pre-cooked in water and then dried out again so that boiling water need only be stirred in to produce the finished dish. While analysis shows little change in nutrient content as a result of these pre-cooking processes, it is likely that oats stored after this are more prone to undergo degenerative processes than those which have been stored as whole, untoasted, live groats. Nevertheless, oatmeal is often the only whole grain food one can obtain if he is forced to eat in the average restaurant, and for this reason, it has endeared itself to many.

Rye

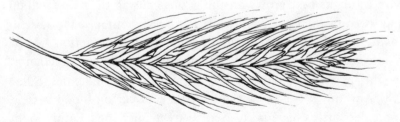

While the volume of rye produced does not compare with that of many other grains, most of it is used for human consumption, since rye has never been a popular feed crop. This doesn't mean that all the world's rye goes to make bread—a significant portion of it is used in the preparation of whiskey and rye whiskey is familiar in America. A similar alcoholic drink called *kvass* is taken in Russia where black bread made primarily of rye flour is also traditional. Rye is especially resistant to cold and for this reason has been grown widely not only in Russia, but throughout the middle European countries and Scandinavia as well. The basic bread of medieval England was probably also made primarily of rye, but it was the immigrants from Germany, Eastern Europe and Scandinavia that brought rye bread to America. A favorite German rye bread was the heavy, nearly black pumpernickel. Today, however, commercial breads sold under that name may be made mostly of wheat and colored dark with dyes.

Rye has a stronger and heartier flavor than wheat, and some prefer it for this reason. It is lower than wheat in gluten content, and is thus well suited to making pastries in which the development of gluten will produce toughness. On the other hand, it is more difficult to work into a loaf that will rise nicely. It is traditionally said that while "wheat makes fat, rye builds muscles," and even today the use of rye bread is an article of faith for many dieters.

One disadvantage of rye is that it tends to become afflicted with a fungus that grows on the grains causing them to swell up and become black. This fungus growth contains a powerful toxin called ergot which produces violent constriction of the blood vessels, hemorrhages, burning pains and violent cramps. In the past, poisoning from ergot produced epidemics called "St. Anthony's fire." Because of their effect on blood vessels, ergot derivatives have been used to treat migraine. Eating foods made from good quality whole rye, however, is unlikely to either cure headaches or to be poisonous.

Buckwheat, Barley and Millet

Technically, buckwheat is not a grain. The plant is not tall and slender like the grass family to which grains belong. Instead, it is branched and low-growing with heart-shaped leaves and fragrant flowers which the bees adore. The little triangular groats are actually the fruits of the plant, but for all practical purposes, they are eaten like grains. Buckwheat grows well in poor soil and thrives in cool, moist climates. It seems especially suited to be a food in those areas since it has a warming and drying effect on the body. For this reason, perhaps, it is favored as a wintertime dish. In the middle European countries, it is traditionally cooked whole or cracked and prepared like rice. There, it is called *kasha* and is considered especially delicious when served with yogurt. Buckwheat groats can be purchased in two forms: raw and roasted. The raw groats are lighter colored while the roasted ones are dark and have a richer taste and aroma.

Most of the world's barley is used as cattle feed or as a source of beer and whiskey, but it is actually a very valuable food grain. Like buckwheat, it comes from colder climes and is especially useful in the wintertime when its warming effects can be appreciated. Its use as a food goes back about 8,000 years at which time it was grown in Egypt. It was a chief bread grain for many middle Eastern and classical European peoples such as the Greeks, Romans and Hebrews. Even today, barley bread is frequently used from Tibet through China, and in Japan it is an important part of many traditional dishes. Sprouted barley has a high content of maltose, a sugar which is the primary ingredient of malt. Malt syrups have been used for making beer and milkshakes and even for sweetening cookies.

When barley is milled to remove the outer bran-like covering, the process is called pearling. Pearled barley is lighter in color and easier to cook, but it is devoid of many of the minerals and much of the protein. Barley is highly regarded as having important medicinal properties, and barley water (the broth produced by boiling the grain in water and straining it) has been traditionally used in both East and West for a variety of complaints from upset stomach and nervousness to teething problems in children.

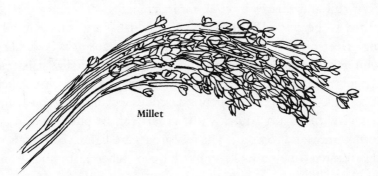

Millet

Millet is better known in the West as an ingredient in bird food than as a grain for human consumption. In many parts of the world, however, including much of Africa and large areas of India and China, millet is the staple grain. Actually, there are many different species of millet, and they are quite different from each other. The three most important in the world today, however, are sorghum, finger millet and bullrush. Sorghum *(Sorghum vulgare)* is grown in South and West Africa and China. It is also important in Central and Northern India where it is known as *juar*. Some varieties of sorghum are not grown for their grain, but for their stalks which are crushed like sugar cane to obtain the syrup which is traditionally used in Southern and Midwestern America. Finger millet *(Eleusine coracana)* is shaped so that each ear consists of five spikes which rise from a central point like fingers from the palm of a hand. It is grown on a large scale in Sri Lanka and in South India where it is the principle grain and is known as *ragi.*

The third major type, bull-rush millet, *(Pennisetum typhoi-deum)* includes a white-seeded variety called pearl millet which is the familiar yellow millet sold in American health food stores. The ear, shaped like a cattail, is born on a stalk much like corn. It is extremely drought resistant and is often grown in the drier areas of India where a dark variety is known as *bajara*. This is valued for its warming and drying qualities and is a favorite food during the rainy season.

OTHER STARCHY FOODS

In addition to the grains which we have discussed, there are other foods that are significant sources of starch in the diet. The first and perhaps most commonly used is the potato. The white potato is a native of Peru. It was discovered there by the earliest European explorers and brought back to Europe where it rapidly became a staple. Since that time, its use has spread across the world, and it is now one of the most common sources of starch in the diet of almost every country. The potato contains not only large quantities of starch, but a small amount of protein as well, and just beneath its skin are a number of vitamins and minerals. A medium whole potato will contain about 22 grams of carbohydrate (about 100 calories). It also contains, however, two grams of protein, 0.7 milligrams of iron, 9 milligrams of calcium, 1.7 milligrams of niacin and 36 milligrams of vitamin C. This means that if an active person were to eat his full 2000 calories a day in nothing but baked potatoes, he would get 40 grams of protein, 14 milligrams of iron, 180 milligrams of calcium, 34 milligrams of niacin and 720 milligrams of vitamin C. Though this cannot be called an ideal diet, it not only contains a significant amount of protein but adequate amounts of some of the vitamins and minerals as well. This is rather surprising since the potato is considered by most people to be a food that is totally starch. In fact, the potato provides a food so nearly complete that after it was brought from the New World, the

Irish were able to subsist on it until the mid-1800's. When the potato arrived in Ireland, it had quickly become popular since the overcrowded Irish could supply their food needs without difficulty on a small plot of land. However, it became so exclusively the diet of the Irish that when the potato blight came, many persons starved, the whole economy was disrupted, and mass migrations resulted. The Irish brought with them to America, however, their acquired taste for the white potato, and for this reason in many sections of the country it is still known as an "Irish potato." According to traditional lore in Asia, however, where the use of the potato has also become common, it tends to create problems with gas in the digestive system. Throughout the world, people use tubers such as the *yucca* and *yame* of Central America and the *shakar kandi* of India which are similar to the potato.

Bananas are another starchy food, and though they are generally considered a fruit rather than a vegetable, unripe bananas are often prepared as a vegetable dish in India. As the banana ripens, much of the starch is converted to sugar and the sweet flavor develops. Before this process occurs, however, the banana is predominantly starch, and for this reason it can be cooked much in the same way as starchy tubers like the potato. In many of the tropical countries, special varieties of the banana (called plantain) are grown solely for their use in cooking. These banana-like fruits are tougher, more fibrous, more starchy and lend themselves better to cooking. In parts of Latin America and South India they are practically a staple.

Beans, peas and other leguminous seed-like vegetables are highly prized for their protein. However, most of them also contain significant quantities of starch. Lentils, for example, contain over twice as much starch by weight as protein. Kidney beans contain almost three times as much, and this is also true of most other beans and peas. Soybeans, by contrast, actually contain more protein than carbohydrate, though they are unique in this respect. However, soybeans also contain about half as much fat per weight as protein or carbohydrate, whereas lentils, for example, contain practically none.

HOW MANY CALORIES?

A calorie is a measure of heat produced when some substance is burned or oxidized. For most people, carbohydrate is the major material which is burned to produce heat and supply the energy needed for the body's functioning. One gram of carbohydrate, when oxidized, will produce about four calories. A gram of fat (which is designed for compact storage) will produce about nine calories. When burned for energy, a gram of protein will also produce four calories (if one is so unwise as to use it for this purpose). A piece of bread provides about 50 to 60 calories, a banana about 85.

Although many popular books have been written in response to the question of how many calories we need in a day, the answer is really quite simple. We need as many calories as we use, or, if we are overweight, we need a few less than we will use. The remainder will be supplied by the use of fat stores. One who consistently eats more calories than he uses may convert these to a storage form (fat) and gain weight. However, the fact that weight is not being gained does not necessarily mean that the proper number of calories are being eaten. Some people do not readily digest or assimilate all of the food that they eat. Unfortunately this does not mean that the undigested food will simply pass harmlessly through the body. In fact, it may provide a good deal of trouble since the large intestine is designed to handle the remainder of digested food, not to serve as a repository for food which has not been digested. Thus it is that a very lean person may overeat and remain thin but feel drowsy, lethargic and uncomfortable.

Counting calories is often a waste of time. One can most accurately judge his caloric needs from the signals his body provides. As long as the calorie-rich carbohydrate is accompanied by the other nutrients which normally are combined with it in nature (protein, fat, vitamins, minerals, etc.) then the taste buds and the sense of hunger become a reliable index of how much should be eaten. It is primarily when empty calories, that is, carbohydrates which have been separated from the other components of food, are taken alone that the problem of excess caloric intake arises. However, it is not only carbohydrates which supply calories, and they are not the only ingredient in foodstuffs which can be empty and non-nutritional. In fact, as we are about to see, in the modern American diet, fats are probably the worst offenders in this respect.

Fats and Oils: Stored Energy

5

Fats and oils, like starches, are made up of carbon chains, but they are simpler and more compact. Rather than being based on complex sugar molecules attached to one another in a series, the fat chain is a simple linear arrangement of carbon atoms. When compared to carbohydrates, which have water added to the carbon skeleton, fats have only hydrogen added to it. Therefore, rather than being a hydrated carbon ("carbohydrate") fats are a hydrogenated carbon, i.e., hydrogen is added. Technically, then, fats and oils are "hydrocarbons" and are structurally related to petroleum.

Each carbon atom has the capacity to attach to four other atoms. In addition to being linked to the adjacent carbon atoms on either side of it in the chain, each carbon may also be attached to two hydrogen atoms. When all the potential hydrogen atom spaces are filled, then the fat chain is "saturated." This does not necessarily happen, however, and when positions are left vacant (see diagram), the fat or oil is said to be "unsaturated." The melting point of a fat is due in part to how saturated it is. The greater the number of open positions, the more likely the fat is to be liquid at room temperature. Highly saturated fats, like

Model of an Unsaturated Fatty Acid

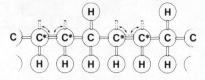

This representation of an unsaturated fatty acid schematically demonstrates how unsaturated carbon atoms* might react with other organic compounds.

animal fat (lard) for example, will be solid at room temperature, while relatively unsaturated and "polyunsaturated" vegetable fats will be liquid. Most animals tend to store their energy in saturated chains, which we usually refer to as fats, while plants tend to store their energy in unsaturated form, which we call oil.

The length of the carbon chains that make up fats may vary widely. In butter, they range from four carbons long all the way up to eighteen, while the carbon chains in beef fat range from fourteen carbons to eighteen in length. Chains which are longer tend to be more solid at room temperature while those which are shorter (see diagram) tend to be more liquid. Butter gets soft when left out of the refrigerator, while beef tallow is hard enough that candles are made from it. Yet both are largely saturated. Therefore, there are two different variables which affect the melting point of a fat: one, the number of unsaturated positions it holds, and two, the length of the carbon chains that make it up.

In their storage form, most of the fat chains are attached in sets of three to a neutral compound called glycerol. The result is a large molecule with three limbs that is called a "triglyceride" or neutral fat. During digestion, these neutral fats are broken down, the chains being severed from the glycerol to float free as "free fatty acids." These fatty acids pass across the intestinal membrane and are absorbed into the blood. Here they are reassembled around another molecule of glycerol to form, once more, neutral fats or "triglycerides." A high level of triglycerides is found in some people who form fatty deposits along the walls of their arteries, and blood tests for triglycerides have taken their place alongside those for cholesterol in recent years.

A Typical Fat Molecule

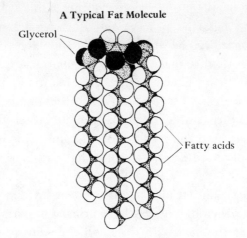

Glycerol

Fatty acids

CHOLESTEROL AND YOUR ARTERIES

Some fat-like substances in the body are different from the simple carbon chains that make up most oils and animal fat. The best known of these is cholesterol. Not a triglyceride, it is a waxy, fat-like compound which serves a multitude of purposes in the body. It is a complex molecule with the same ring structure as many hormones, and it is the base from which estrogen, cortisone and testosterone are made.[1] It is also a component of nerve tissue. One end of the molecule can form a "salt" which is soluble in water, while the other end combines readily with fat. For this reason, cholesterol salts (or "bile salts" as they are called, since they are the major part of bile)* promote the mixture of fats in the small intestine with water so they can be broken down and absorbed through the intestinal wall.

Cholesterol is most likely to cause trouble, however, along

---

* Hence the name *cholesterol: chol* meaning bile and *sterol* meaning hormone-like.

the walls of blood vessels, and it is because of this that it has become famous. As the cholesterol accumulates, a sort of hardening or plaque develops in the vessel wall. If nothing happens to halt the process and it continues unchecked, the deposits can become thick enough and large enough to seriously narrow the space inside the blood vessel. The blood supply to the area where that vessel leads is reduced, and if muscular exertion, which increases the demand for oxygen, continues, then not enough oxygen and fuel will be supplied to the tissue, and the result is often pain. This is what happens when people with arteriosclerotic deposits in the blood vessels leading to the legs try to walk more than a short distance. There is severe leg pain. It also happens when the deposits are located in those smaller blood vessels (coronary arteries) which supply the walls of the heart. In this case, the pain is in the chest, and if the arteries are narrow enough, portions of the heart muscle may actually die because of lack of blood. When damaged or destroyed in this way, the heart wall, or *myocardium* is said in medical terms to be *infarcted*, and the result is called a *myocardial infarction* or a "coronary." When the arteries that become blocked off lead to the brain, the damage that results there affects the ability to walk, speak, write or even understand. This is called a cerebral vascular accident, or, in common terms, a "stroke."

In the 1900's, arteriosclerosis has become more prevalent, especially in Europe and the United States, and heart attacks and strokes have come to be the major cause of death. For decades, conventional medicine felt powerless to deal with this condition, but when it was discovered that severe arteriosclerosis is often accompanied by high blood levels of cholesterol and that cholesterol makes up the bulk of the arterial plaques, it was natural to assume that cholesterol caused arteriosclerosis and that a diet low in it would help prevent this disease. Therefore, eating foods high in cholesterol such as dairy products, eggs and animal fats was discouraged. A great campaign was launched, and the idea that avoiding these foods would help prevent arteriosclerosis became widely accepted by the public. A diet high in animal fat seemed to raise blood cholesterol levels in some people and was thought to increase the formation of plaques. If animal fats were bad, then maybe vegetable fats were good.[2] At least they contained no cholesterol. Lard in the kitchen and butter on the table gave way to vegetable shortening and margarine.

THE MARGARINE STORY

The history of margarine's rise to fame as a product for promoting health is fascinating.[3]   In 1869, when butter was in short supply in France, a prize was offered to whomever could come up with an attractive substitute. M. Hippolyte Mege took first place by mixing lard and the drippings from meat packing, the most inexpensive fats then available, flavoring them with a yogurt-like milk preparation and coloring them so that their taste and appearance bore at least some remote resemblance to good French butter. Of course, nobody was fooled, but the price was right and margarine became an increasingly market-able item. During World War II when food was rationed and butter fat was difficult to obtain, margarine got another boost and became widely known to most Americans. The lard-like white blocks of margarine were sold along with a small packet of yellow dye which was used to make it look like butter. The weekly ritual of stirring a bowl of margarine and food coloring became a familiar routine in many households.

By this time, more inexpensive methods for extracting vegetable oils had been developed, and they were even less costly than the fats obtained from the meat industry. It was also at this point that the process of bubbling hydrogen through vege-table oil developed. This filled the empty spaces on the fat chain with hydrogen atoms, saturating it enough so that its melting point came closer to that of butter. An added benefit of this process is that by leaving fewer unoccupied slots, the fat keeps its flavor longer.   It is the attachment of oxygen atoms to these empty spaces that causes vegetable oils to go rancid. As a result, the proportion of vegetable fat in margarine began to rise, and today most American margarine is almost entirely vegetable in origin.   In other countries such as England, though, it still contains significant quantities of lard, whale blubber and other animal fats.

Margarine is often advertised as being "made from poly-unsaturated oils," but manufacturers neglect to mention that the oil is changed into margarine by saturating it with hydrogen (hydrogenating it).   Though in all fairness, some margarines do contain small amounts of liquid poly-unsaturated oil added to a hydrogenated base, the bulk of the fat must, of necessity, be saturated or the margarine would be liquid like any other poly-unsaturated oil, even in the refrigerator.

Once a vegetable oil has been hydrogenized, however, a "new" fat has been created. Since such artificially hydrogenated vegetable fats are a recent addition to the diet of man, and since the human body has had no experience with them, it seems reasonable to wonder if it has the capacity to deal comfortably with this essentially synthetic food.   In fact, a recent elaborate statistical analysis of the incidence of heart disease and the consumption of hydrogenated fats in England has shown a dramatic and detailed correlation between the two.   Where margarine and solid vegetable shortenings were used in significant quantities, the rate of heart attack was always higher than where they weren't.[4]   Though similar analyses have not been carefully done in America, it is interesting to note that in the Southeastern states, the region where margarine consumption is highest in relation to population and to butter consumption,[5] there is an area where the incidence of heart attacks is so high it has been termed "an enigma."[6]   It seems increasingly likely that eating margarine, instead of preventing heart attacks, actually accelerates the process which causes them.

Population and Table Spread Sales in Food Stores, 1969

POPULATION   MARGARINE PURCHASES   BUTTER PURCHASES

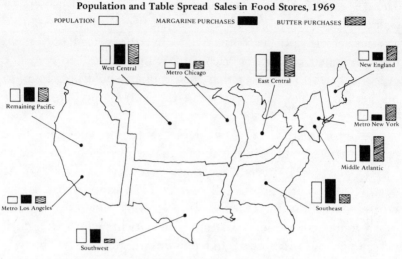

Rjepma, S.F. The Story of Margarine. Public Affairs Press, Washington, D.C., 1970.

POLYUNSATURATES, PRO AND CON

Liquid vegetable oils have not been hydrogenated. They remain unsaturated, and since in most cases there are a number of unfilled positions on the carbon chain, most vegetable oils are said to be "polyunsaturated" (*poly* meaning "many"). While some experiments using margarine have shown it to raise blood fat levels,[7] it was research using polyunsaturates which first showed an ability to lower cholesterol levels and decrease the number of heart attacks.[8] But the evidence was far from clear, and further research has thrown doubt on the long term value of using vegetable oils for this purpose.[9] In some of the experiments, this effect was temporary, and on further follow-up, it was not seen at all.[10] Nevertheless, Americans had been convinced, largely through commercial advertising and the news media, that they should use unsaturated vegetable oils even though no good statistical proof exists that they prevent one from developing a heart attack. In fact, the phrase "polyunsaturated fatty acids" has become "virtually synonymous with heart protection in both popular and orthodox medical thinking."[11]

Though the FDA has stated that it is illegal for advertisers to claim that polyunsaturated oils can be beneficial in preventing arteriosclerosis and heart disease,[12] advertisers need only mention that their product is "rich in polyunsaturates" to convince every reader or TV viewer that the product would be a boon to his health.   The idea persists and the shift to polyunsaturates continues.

Unfortunately, a closer look at the people who have changed to vegetable oils has shown that while deaths from heart attacks decreased, overall mortality rates did not fall.[13]   As deaths from heart disease fell, deaths from cancer began to increase. Recently, there has been a growing number of reports of an increased incidence of cancer in patients who take a high percentage of unsaturated and polyunsaturated oils. This was noted by physicians whose patients showed an unusual frequency of malignant melonama, a rapidly fatal form of skin cancer. Inquiry into their dietary habits showed that in each case there had recently been an enthusiastic switch to vegetable fats and oils instead of butter.[14] Other research supports this impression.[15] Of course, oils are present in most grains, vegetables and even fruits. But as long as they are still an integral part of the whole food they are apparently healthful, assuming that the diet is reasonably balanced. Once the oil is removed from the plant material, however, it seems to become susceptible to a whole host of destructive influences.

DAMAGED FATS AND OILS

When unsaturated, the carbon chains of fats and oils may have their spaces filled with oxygen instead of hydrogen atoms, a process that takes place very rapidly when the oil is heated. The "rancidity" that develops gives the oil an objectionable taste and odor. Moreover, the oxygen atoms which are attached to the rancid oil are not tightly held and have been found to be very reactive. The compounds that hold them are called "free radicals," and the reactive oxygen will readily jump over to other molecules such as vitamins, oxidizing or burning them and changing their structure enough so that they are no longer biologically functional.[16, 17]

In addition, overheating changes fats causing, for example, what is called polymerization. This means that the fat chains link together so that the structure of the fat molecule is altered. This forms new compounds which are probably less useable, handled by the body differently, and which may be, in some cases, harmful.[18, 19] Several experiments have shown that rabbits given a diet containing average amounts of cholesterol but high levels of polyunsaturated vegetable oils that had been

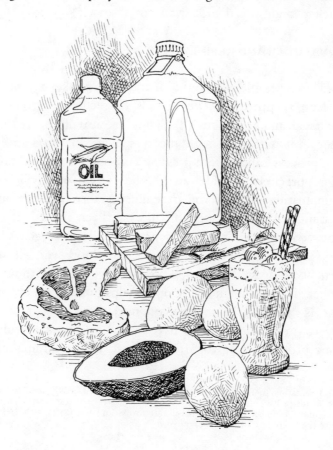

heated to between 375° and 400° F had an increased incidence of arteriosclerosis.[20]   In the case of corn oil, this effect was not seen when it was given without heating it.[21]   The temperature at which most deep frying is done happens to be approximately 375° to 400° F, and if results with experimental animals holds true for man, the popularity of foods fried in vegetable oils may be one factor contributing to arteriosclerosis in America.   Other oils, like olive oil[22] * have caused just as many plaques in the arteries when unheated. In monkeys, who are more like man than the experimental animals used in other studies, peanut oil, given just as it is purchased from the supermarket, caused much more arteriosclerosis than butter, producing "widespread and advanced" disease.[24]

OILS—NATURAL AND REFINED

The vegetable oils found in the supermarket are prepared by a lengthy process.   The kernels or seeds are ground to a coarse meal and then pressed.   They are usually heated before pressing, but with such substances as olives, peanuts and coconuts, a process called "cold-pressing" is possible. If cold-pressed, or more precisely, "cold-drawn," the "virgin oil" will contain few impurities and will be of edible quality without further processing.   Although such oil has not been heated, it is still unsaturated and retains a tendency to collect oxygen and become rancid, producing free radicals.   Moreover, most oils labeled "cold-pressed" are not, in fact, produced without heat. If no heat is used, much of the oil remains in the meal or "cake," and it is therefore a more economical and almost universal policy to press the meal as it is heated.   Even with this hot-pressing process, three to fifteen percent of the oil may remain

---

* It is fascinating to find that garlic, which is almost universally used to spike the copious quantities of olive oil present in most Mediterranean dishes, has been shown to lower blood cholesterol and decrease clot formation, both of which are thought to reduce the likelihood of heart attacks.[23]

in the meal, so in large scale operations, chemical solvents are most often used to extract it. The oil thus extracted, however, contains more impurities and is more highly colored than oils produced without heat and consequently requires further processing and bleaching to produce the light, odorless, clean-tasting oil usually sold in supermarkets.[25]

Clearly the elaborate technology which makes such an economical extraction of vegetable oil possible is strictly a modern development. For this reason, though it is not so unnatural or "synthetic" as margarine, it has been suggested that polyunsaturated oil is a relatively recent addition to the diet[26] and that the human body has not evolved the capacity for dealing with quantities of it.[27]   There may be some truth in this, though the use of certain vegetable oils, such as olive oil, date back to antiquity. Even such famous examples of good health as the Hunzas of the Himalayas have traditionally used oil made from apricot pits in their food. What is not generally recognized, however, is that the Hunzas are careful to prepare only as much oil as they can use in a day or two. After this time, if any is left, they will discard it and prepare fresh. In the middle European countries where flaxseed oil has been used extensively as a cooking fat, housewives are insistent on having their oil fresh and customarily buy it from street vendors who have just pressed it. Refrigerating the oil, putting it in a dark bottle, and keeping it tightly capped slows the process of oxidation, but oils can go rancid inside the body as well as outside.[28] Picking up oxygen present in the tissues, they can form the free radicals that cause damage to cellular components.

The kind of oil may be important, too. Not all oils are the same. As we noted above, heating may make corn oil more dangerous, though olive oil seems to be just as risky when raw. In ancient India, where the effects of various hand-pressed oils were systematically studied, they were classified, on the basis of long experience, according to their effects. Linseed oil was noted for its warming effect, which is in keeping with its use in the cold countries of Eastern Europe. Sesame oil was said to be the least perishable, while safflower oil, which, interestingly enough, is touted in the West today as "highest in polyunsaturates," was said to be excessively irritating and capable of provoking or aggravating a wide variety of disorders.[29]

There is some evidence that large quantities of vegetable oils speed up the aging process in the skin (probably because of the presence of free radicals) causing a dramatic increase in wrinkling about the face. Damaged chromosomes have also been attributed to unsaturated oils and there have been reports of numerous other negative effects from a high intake of them.[30] At least a substantial part of the problems arising from such oils is probably due to the highly reactive oxygen that they carry. Compounds which prevent these little oxygen radicals from doing their damage are called "anti-oxidants." One such anti-oxidant is vitamin C, but vitamin E works more powerfully. Recent research on vitamin E suggests that the need for an anti-oxidant inside the cells is especially high in people who have consumed large amounts of polyunsaturated oils.[31, 32, 33, 34] Vitamin E will help somewhat in such cases though it may not be able to prevent all oxidative damage completely.

EGGS, LECITHIN AND CHOLESTEROL

The story of eggs reminds one of what happened with margarine and polyunsaturated fats. Early on, it was discovered that egg yolks were high in cholesterol. This led, as we have seen, to a general attitude that omitting eggs from the diet would protect one from heart attacks. Later, however, when the subject was studied more carefully, it was discovered that the matter was more complex than had been thought. Egg yolks not only contain cholesterol in significant quantities, they also contain lecithin. Lecithin is an unusual fat-like compound which has the special property of being able to dissolve cholesterol and other fats.   One end of the lecithin molecule is oil-like and combines readily with fats, while the other end tends to have an affinity for water.   Thus it can take hold of fat molecules and pull them into solution.   Lecithin is a natural component of many beans and peas, and the lecithin sold in health food stores which is popular with dieters as well as those who are concerned about heart disease is extracted from soybeans.   It has long been known that beans and peas lower serum cholesterol. This is probably due to a number of factors, including the presence of plant sterols, which are similar enough to cholesterol to crowd it out at the intestinal wall where absorption occurs. The cholesterol-lowering effect of dried peas and beans may also be due in part to the action of the lecithin they contain.   In some experiments, substantial doses of lecithin by mouth have been shown to lower blood cholesterol[35] and based on this principle, it has been used by some physicians to treat arteriosclerosis.

While recent research suggests that dried beans and peas not only lower cholesterol but actually help to prevent heart disease,* it is not at all clear that this is a general principle.   One cannot assume lowering blood cholesterol always prevents heart attacks.   Though some researchers have found a correlation between blood cholesterol and heart disease, others have found none at all.   The plaques that form inside the arteries contain cholesterol, but they contain other substances too, such as triglycerides, connective tissue and sometimes calcium and fibrin— the sticky protein that helps blood clot.   In fact, fibrin usually forms the initial "streaks" in the arterial wall before cholesterol appears.

When it comes to the relationship between diet and heart disease the picture is even more confusing. While we know a few specifics with relative certainty, e.g., beans and peas tend to lower both cholesterol and the incidence of heart attacks, as do the

* See Chapter 6, Protein.

complex carbohydrate and fiber of most whole grains, vegetables* and some foods like onions,[36] other dietary changes that lower cholesterol do not necessarily prevent heart disease. While one study shows a decrease in coronary heart disease on a cholesterol-lowering diet,[37] another suggests that this can't be true.[38] Nevertheless, laboratories continue to measure cholesterol levels, patients are warned that an elevation means increased risk of a heart attack, and to leave off butter, milk, eggs and fats. In the medical journals, however, the issue is far from settled, and the controversy rages on.[39, 40]

Answers may be just around the corner, however. Since cholesterol does not move through the blood in a free form, but "rides piggyback" on various proteins, it is possible for the kind of protein/cholesterol complex that predominates in the blood to vary from person to person. When the cholesterol is broken down into separate fractions according to the kind of protein with which it is combined, very close correlations with heart disease emerge. It has recently been found that some of the lighter complexes are associated with plaque formation, while the heaviest ones seem to actually protect against it. This may explain why it was that for so many years a relationship between blood cholesterol and heart disease was found and sometimes not. The fraction of the cholesterol that protected one from the problem and the fraction that caused it were being lumped together.

If this is borne out by future research, it should soon become easier to find out which foods specifically contribute to and which prevent arteriosclerosis. In the meantime, one can rest easy if he remembers that the bulk of research indicates a diet free of meat,† low in total fats and oils and high in whole grains, dried beans and peas, onions, fresh vegetables and fruits will diminish his risk of heart disease, and as we shall see, tend to create a better state of general health as well.

---

* See Chapter 4, Carbohydrate.

† See Chapter 6, Protein.

FATS AND OILS IN A BALANCED DIET

Detrimental effects from fats may be more likely when one's nutrition is also deficient in other ways. In experiments with rats on ordinary laboratory rations, huge amounts of animal fat (for example, 60%) will promote the deposit of cholesterol in the arteries. If the rats are fed a highly superior diet, however, with high quality protein and an unusually rich supply of vitamins and minerals, no deposits in the arteries result, even though the animals become quite obese, weighing three or four times their usual weight. When instead of animal fats, vegetable fats are used in the same large quantities, the rats do no better and no worse. It would appear that large amounts of fat or of other single dietary factors which have been shown under certain circumstances to promote arteriosclerosis have little or no effect if the diet is very good in other respects.[41]

A study in India, for example, showed that Punjabis in the north of India consumed 19 times more fat than south Indians, yet their rate of heart disease is seven times less. Moreover, the Punjabis in the North eat predominantly milk fats (butter and ghee) whereas the south Indians use mainly unsaturated vegetable oils. It is also true that the Punjabis take more sugar in their diet than do the south Indians.[42] It would be foolish to conclude, however, on the basis of this data that high levels of sugar and fat cannot cause heart disease. The Punjabis are renowned for their strength and vigor, and their diets contain not only sugar and large amounts of fat, but generous portions of fresh vegetables, fruits, milk, whole grains and beans and peas. Decades ago, nutritional experiments with rats demonstrated that feeding the typical Punjabi diet to a group of rats over a long period of time produced a sort of super-race of rodents that were unusually resistant to diseases of all sorts.[43] Unfortunately, most research has not looked carefully at the total diet when investigating the effects of specific nutrients on arteriosclerosis.

WHAT ABOUT BUTTER?

Though the fat of butter and milk is saturated almost as much as other animal fats, (butter is a semi-solid at room temperature) it differs from them in other ways, such as the length of the carbon chains. It therefore cannot be assumed that butterfat will have the same effects on the arterial lining as other animal fat. In fact, there is some data suggesting that butterfat, unlike other animal fats, actually has a protective effect on the heart.[44] When the watery part is removed so that only the clear fat is used, the result is an excellent cooking fat, superior to whole butter which scorches and turns black if heated above a certain point. In the East, however, many other virtues are ascribed to such clarified butter, and it is said that it has the capacity to take on and to magnify the properties of that with which it is combined. For this reason, it is said not only to make foods more nutritious, but is also an important ingredient in the preparation of many natural medicines.

Although butterfat may have certain properties that promote good health, it is not always available. In many areas of the world, dairying is uncommon, and in other cases, dairy cows, instead of being grazed or fed straw and other plant materials that cannot be used by man, are routinely fed grains and other human foods, so that milk products are too expensive to be within reach of the common man. In any case, a great deal of fat in the diet is probably not necessary, so that the inability to use butter does not mean that one must supplement his diet with vegetable oils or other fat. In most parts of the world, dietary fat could be cut considerably with benefit. This is especially true in the West where fat makes up an average of nearly 45% of the caloric intake.[45] Though the fat, if of good quality, may not necessarily have injurious effects in and of itself, it remains essentially an empty food like refined sugar, containing calories, or fuel, but none of the other nutrients which the body needs.

Preparing Cooking Oil
(Ghee)

Butter is not pure fat; it is also comprised of water and of milk solids which are soluble in water. When the water is evaporated by boiling, these solids precipitate, and the oil or ghee remains. This is the basis of the ghee making process.

To make ghee, place one pound of unsalted butter in a saucepan until it boils; then lower the heat. When the white foam of milk solids which will accumulate on the top begins to collapse and thicken, start skimming it off. Do not disturb the bottom of the pan, as some of these solids will also sink and can be left in the pot until after the ghee is poured off. As the butter continues to boil, watch the oily portion to see when it becomes clear, and watch the sediment on the bottom to see when it becomes a golden brown. Be careful that this does not scorch and ruin the ghee.

When all the water is evaporated, the sound of the cooking will change from one of boiling to one of frying, and the bubbling will stop. When only the clear, hissing oil and the golden sediment remain, the ghee is ready. At this point, the temperature will begin to rise quickly, so remove the pan from the heat, and let it sit for a moment. During this time, the hot fat will turn the sediment a little darker.

Pour the ghee off into an earthenware, glass or metal container for use near the stove. Scrape out the sediments and refrigerate them with the skimmings for use on toast or vegetables.

See *Himalayan Mountain Cookery* by Mrs. R. Ballentine, Sr., p. 134.

While small amounts of sugar and fat in a diet otherwise rich in protein, vitamins and minerals is not likely to cause trouble, in the West, where sugar consumption amounts to 120 pounds a year per person, so that refined sugar supplies 20-25% of the calories, the percentage of fat in the diet may be very important. If 45% of the calories are supplied by fat and 25% by refined sugar, as is the case for the average American, then 70% of the diet is empty calories. This is even more risky when many of the fruits, vegetables, grains and so forth which make up the other 30% but must supply virtually all the nutrients, are, as we mentioned earlier, low in many vitamins, minerals and proteins due to soil conditions, storage or processing.

It is interesting to compare the Western diet, containing 45% of its calories in fat with that of most people of China and Japan where fat comprises only 10% of the calories. Besides this radical difference in diet, there is also a radical difference in the incidence of arteriosclerosis: in the Orient, it is quite infrequent, whereas in the U.S., it ranks as one of the most common of fatal disorders. And this is not genetic. The Japanese in America who adopt the diet of their new homeland suffer the same incidence of arteriosclerosis as other Americans. Those who stick with their native diet do not.

Moreover evidence is mounting that large quantities of fat in the diet may be one of the major causes of cancer.[46] This is true not only for vegetable oils, where the mechanism can be explained as we have seen, but also with the saturated fat of meats,[47] especially beef,[48] where the cause is not understood. An association between high fat intake and malignancy is well-documented in the case of cancer of the colon[49] but may also be true of breast cancer as well.[50]

When one eats a diet comprised of 70% empty calories, the other foods he eats must be extraordinarily rich in essential nutrients to make up for his "nutrient debts." That they are not explains how we can have nutritional deficiencies in a land of plenty and probably also accounts for both the popularity and success of vitamin and mineral supplements. It may throw some light on the problem of obesity, as well. If one on such a diet eats enough to supply himself with needed nutrients, he will have to push the excess useless calories aside in order to use the valuable part of the food. Unused calories are, of course, put aside in the form of fat, and if the diet were consistently of this sort, then the fat would tend to accumulate.

HOW MUCH FAT?

For such reasons, one might wonder how far he can safely reduce his fat intake. Nutritionists feel that minimal requirements for fat are probably extremely low. Some years back, a study was made of the dietary habits of the Hos, an aboriginal tribe in Bihar, India; 200 out of 250 families were found to use no fat of any kind in their cooking. Moreover, they drank no milk and ate no meat. Their total daily intake of fat was around 3 grams per person per day, the equivalent of less than a teaspoon of oil. This provided only about 2% of the calories in the diet. Though for various reasons their health was not ideal, it was equal to that of neighboring tribes who ate average quantities of fat, and they presented no signs or symptoms which could be attributed to fat deficiency.[51] For one who eats no meat, about two tablespoons of added fat in the diet will supply about 10% of his caloric intake (assuming he eats 2500 calories a day). If used skillfully, this will usually permit the food to be prepared in a palatable way while reducing drastically the empty calories in the diet.

The situation is much more difficult for those who eat meat, since even lean cuts of the better quality meats (with fat trimmed off) may contain up to 30% fat. This is due to the fact that animal muscle often contains a great deal of fat running through the muscle tissue itself, especially when animals have been lot-fed, in preparation for slaughter. The "marbling" effect in the more expensive cuts of beef, for example, which is considered to improve its flavor and tenderness is due to large quantities of fatty tissue which can be seen interspersed through the muscle fibers. Reducing fat intake below the 30% level often proves difficult for one who eats meat since in order to accomplish this, he must prepare all his other food with little or no cooking fat or butter, and he must eliminate most pastries, desserts and milk products. Possible signs of an excess in concentrated fats and oils in the diet include an unpleasantly oily face and scalp and acne-like pimples on the face or other parts of the body.

Despite the inconvenience, reducing fat intake may be worth it. Evidence is accumulating that arteriosclerosis is not a

permanent condition.   It has been, in some cases, reversed.
Whether this happens or not depends largely on the diet.[52]
Since a majority of adults in the West are already suffering
from some degree of arteriosclerosis, the fact that it can be
decreased or eliminated should come as welcome news.

Reversal can be accomplished by adopting an extremely
careful diet. It should be low in sugars, high in vegetables and
fruits that are rich in vitamins and minerals, and unusually low
in fat. Saturated fat especially should be eliminated or reduced
to extremely low levels. The oils in vegetable foods are preferable, but *only* in their natural form, taken as whole seeds, beans,
grains and vegetables. Cooking and salad oils, margarine and
vegetable shortening must be omitted. When one is on an arterio-
sclerosis-reversal regimen, very small amounts of butterfat may
be occasionally used, but total fat, from all sources should
remain at levels no higher than 10-15% of caloric intake. This
means virtually eliminating meat since even lean cuts invariably
contain too much fat.

Such a strict regimen is only necessary for those already
suffering from some appreciable degree of arteriosclerosis, and
is not necessary for merely maintaining good health. Even
reducing fat levels to 20-30% of caloric intake is a big change
for many people, however, and requires a drastic reduction
in animal foods. For most persons, this brings up the question,
"How can I get enough protein?" The answer lies, as we shall
see, in increasing one's intake of dried beans and peas and whole
grains which not only have their own preventive effects against
arteriosclerosis but also, when taken properly, are a rich source
of protein.

Protein: Building Blocks

Protein is a structural material. It is the protein molecule which provides the rigid structures which enable plants and animals to raise themselves above the surface of the earth. Structures that stretch upward are always built essentially around a protein framework. Protein is the latticework around which calcium and phosphorous are deposited to form bones. Hair and nails are also made of protein. Connective tissues get their strength from collagen, a protein substance that creates the fibers that form tendons and which makes up the sheets that cover the muscles, holding them in place. The long strands of muscle fiber are collections of long protein molecules which can respond to chemical changes by altering their shape or contracting. Blood clots form when, under the proper conditions, red blood cells become entangled in the long strands of fibrin, a protein substance in blood. Even inside the individual cells of "soft" tissues such as the liver or spleen, it is an inner framework of protein that gives them their shape and is the basis of their organization.

Protein molecules are the giants of the biochemical world. If we compare the size of different molecules, we find that while water has a molecular weight of 18, and a molecule of cane sugar has a weight of 342, protein molecules vary from 6,000 to 100,000 or even up to 1,000,000. Some of these molecules are so heavy that they can be made to sink to the bottom of a test tube by centrifuging it, and they are so large that they cannot pass through the membrane which encloses the cell. These larger molecules are the basis of more advanced forms of life. Whereas the molecules of mineral compounds are simple and small, the process of evolution has been, to a great extent, based on the elaboration of more complex protein molecules. Though it is the stuff of life, the body does not have stores of protein like it does of carbohydrate or fat. One researcher studying protein deficiencies concluded that the biochemistry of the body, growth and the continuation of life itself go hand in hand with protein "hoarding."[1] Perhaps this underlies man's hankering after high protein foods, a notion so deeply rooted in our language that we speak of the "meat" of a matter as its essence.

AMINO ACIDS

Each protein molecule is a long chain whose links are the smaller nitrogen-containing units which we call amino acids.

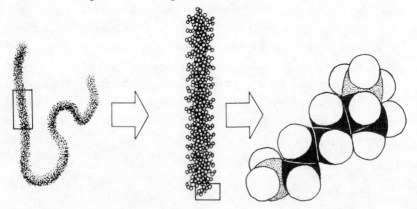

The figure on the left represents the shape of a protein chain. In the center the helical configuration of the amino acids can be seen, while the figure on the right shows the spatial arrangement of the individual atoms in the protein chain.

Each amino acid has a separate composition, but they all contain at least one atom of nitrogen as well as hydrogen, oxygen, carbon and sometimes sulphur. Nitrogen makes up 80% of the atmosphere, and certain microbes in the soil, called "nitrogen fixing bacteria," are able to take the nitrogen in the air and convert it into a form which can be used by plants. Therefore, all amino acids and all proteins depend for their existence on the nitrogen from the air.

A nitrogen-containing compound is called an amine, a word which is derived from the same root as ammonia (NH_3). When proteins break down, the nitrogen atom in the amino acids combine with hydrogen to form ammonia. This is what gives decomposing proteins their characteristic strong odor. People who eat excessive protein, as well as those with severe kidney damage who cannot rid themselves of the breakdown products of protein, may develop a strong ammonia-like body odor. A few of the amino acids, such as those found in eggs, contain sulphur as well as nitrogen. When they break down and the sulphur combines with hydrogen to form hydrogen sulfide, there results the characteristic "rotten egg" odor. Aside from sulfur and nitrogen, amino acids contain only hydrogen, oxygen and carbon, so it is these two elements, sulfur and nitrogen which set proteins apart from carbohydrates.

Most of the approximately 20 amino acid molecules can be converted into others, or manufactured by the body if there is a shortage of one type. However, there are eight which the body cannot synthesize in this way, and it is therefore essential that they be taken into the diet already formed. For this reason, they are called the "essential amino acids."

Any amino acids which are not needed for the construction of new protein molecules can be burned as fuel. This is not a "clean burning" fuel, however, since the nitrogen atom itself cannot be oxidized by the body. Proteins are like bricks. Although one might use them to make a fireplace, he certainly wouldn't attempt to use them as fuel for the fire; they require

too much heat and leave too much residue. The nitrogen fragment of the amino acid molecule and the remains of other
protein substances makeup urea and uric acid. When the kidneys
are unable to excrete all of the uric acid through the urine, it
may accumulate in the tissues and joints and crystallize, producing protein toxicity and giving rise to the symptoms of gout.
In merry old England, gout was the disease of the affluent, and
both Dr. Johnson and Henry VIII, who took wine and meat in
quantity, suffered from it.*

Although meat, cheese, milk and eggs are usually considered "the protein foods," there are many other important
sources of protein. Beans and peas, of course, also contain a
high percentage, and this is especially true of soybeans which
are one of the most concentrated sources known. Nuts are also
rich in protein, and they probably comprised the only high protein item in the diet of primitive food-gathering tribes. Seeds
such as those of the pumpkin and sunflower also contain large
quantities of protein, although the essential amino acids do not
occur here in what is thought to be the ideal proportions. Even
grains contain some protein, and as we shall see, contrary to
common belief, most vegetables and even fruits contain a small
but significant amount.

FLESH FOODS: MEAT, FISH AND FOWL

When protein is mentioned in the highly industrialized
countries of the West, most people automatically think of
meat, fish and fowl. Because they usually contain all of the
essential amino acids in approximately ideal proportion, they are
called "complete" or "high quality" proteins. Furthermore,
because they have no carbohydrate, they are also thought of as

---

* It is traditionally said in the East that much meat may also aggravate the tendency
toward other kinds of arthritis—a concept borne out by clinical experience but not as
yet researched.

"pure" protein, (though in fact they contain variable, and often large, amounts of fat). Because meat has assembled in it the constituents of animal tissue, it is often regarded as the ideal balanced nourishment for similar tissues in the human. Certainly the average American believes that in order to get a healthy balanced diet, he should have a substantial piece of meat daily— or, if not, then fish or fowl.

CAN ONE GET ADEQUATE PROTEIN WITHOUT MEAT?

In reviewing typical menus from around the world that were based primarily on grains, vegetables and legumes with only one-tenth of the protein coming from meat, milk and eggs, nutritionists found that a diet sufficient to supply 2,500 calories would supply 50% more protein than needed by 98% of the population.[2] One of the world's foremost authorities on protein requirements has stated that for adults it is difficult to obtain a mixed vegetable diet which will produce an appreciable loss of body protein without resorting to high levels of sugar, jams, jellies and other essentially protein-free foods.[3] Moreover, dieticians accustomed to computing meatless menus find it difficult not to exceed the protein allowances when caloric needs are met.[4]

Other nutrients are also apparently available in adequate amounts from non-meat foods. A comparison of 200 subjects, some on a regular diet, some on a meat-free diet, showed no evidence of deficiency, and the intake of all nutrients was equal to or greater than the Recommended Dietary Allowances set by the National Research Council as long as some milk was included in the diet.[5] By now all the most respectable and conservative medical and nutrition journals have proclaimed that a good vegetarian diet is wholesome and healthful,[6, 7] and otherwise conservative nutritionists have even begun to speak up about the possible dangers of eating large quantities of meat.[8] A number of studies have shown decreased cholesterol among vegetarians[9, 10] and recent work suggests this represents a reduction in that part of the cholesterol that is most likely to cause arteriosclerosis.[11]

MEAT AND HEALTH

It has been suggested that the positive effects of a meat-free diet on blood cholesterol and the possible benefits for arteriosclerosis are due to a decreased intake of fat in the diet. Though meat is thought of as a protein food, most cuts contain nearly as much fat as protein. A slice of lean ham, in percentage of total calories, will be 25% protein but 75% fat, whereas a choice grade of lean, cooked, trimmed sirloin will contain 65% protein and 35% fat; untrimmed it is 24% protein and 76% fat. A slice of whole grain bread will contain 14% protein, only 9% fat and 77% complex carbohydrate, a plate of cooked beans will contain about 36% protein, less than 6% fat and 58% complex carbohydrate. In other words, even when the fatty parts are carefully removed from meat, using it as a source of protein in the diet still brings a nearly equal amount of fat. Bean and grain proteins bring little fat but 3 or 4 times as much complex carbohydrate.

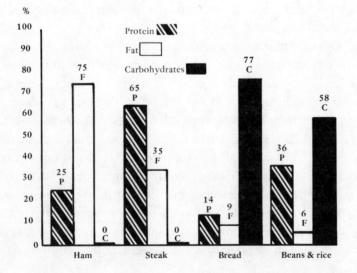

Moreover, the protein itself may have different affects. Vegetable protein has been found in experiments with animals to protect in some way against arteriosclerosis when compared with the protein of animal foods.[12]   Research on groups in America who for religious reasons eat little or no meat has turned up further interesting correlations between the amount of meat consumed and the incidence of several diseases.   Seventh Day Adventists in some cases are pure vegetarians, while in other cases they eat small or even average amounts of meat.   On the whole, however, their lifestyle and racial and ethnic background is essentially the same.   Those who take no meat, however, have much less cancer and heart disease than those who eat the same amount of meat as the average American.[13]   It is also well documented that a vegetarian diet is associated with lower blood pressure.[14, 15]   In addition, it has been found that vegetarians have less osteoperosis than those who eat meat.[16]

There is much evidence that the consumption of meat in the diet increases the probability of cancer of the large intestine.[17, 18]   It was known decades ago that vegetarians have more fiber in the diet[19] since they rely on high fiber vegetable protein instead of meat, and this has recently been correlated with a decrease in such diseases as diverticulosis,[20] and arteriosclerosis.[21] It also seems true that vegetable fiber tends to absorb a variety of environmental pollutants and carry them out of the body.[22] While eating bran could boost the fiber content of a meat-eater's diet, this is probably not an ideal solution.*

Yet a meat diet is not necessarily unhealthy.   When Weston Price traveled around the world, many of the groups he studied were very healthy despite eating diets partially or even totally made up of flesh foods.   The ancient scriptures of India do not prohibit meat, but prescribe carefully which meats are most appropriate for which people.   It is likely that many of the problems stemming from meat consumption today are due in part to

---

* See Chapter 4, Carbohydrate and Chapter 11, Elimination.

the quality of meat eaten.

TROUBLE IN THE MEAT MARKET

Even if one is comfortable with the idea of eating flesh foods, he will find that those available today are generally not wholesome. In the meat departments of many large supermarkets, sanitation is questionable, and much of the meat is contaminated or partly spoiled.[23, 24] During the deteriorization of the cells after death, bacterial growth begins. Meat's tendency to deteriorate causes significant hygienic problems during its packing and marketing which, unfortunately, have not been solved, even in the technologically advanced countries.[25] A great many samples of meat have been found to be infected with *Clostridium perfringens*. Toxins produced by this and other similar bacteria often found in meat are not destroyed by cooking—even though the bacteria are killed.[26] Such toxins can cause serious gastro-intestinal illness. When frankfurters from all over the United States were studied, over 40% had more than enough bacteria growing in them to consider them "spoiled" by accepted standards.[27]

Fresh, uncooked, flesh foods are sometimes considered to be more naturally handled by the body than cooked meat and may be useful in certain extreme situations. Raw beef juice (not to be confused with blood) has long been a home remedy for sick children, and some physicians prescribe it in cases where the patient is unable to assimilate other foods.[28] However, contamination with bacteria can be a problem here and there is also some possibility of parasites, though in beef this is thought to be rare. Trichinosis, transmitted by poorly cooked pork is a more frequent and serious problem, but beef can be contaminated by cutters or grinders when they have also been used for pork.[29]

In America, where large amounts of chemical pesticides, herbicides and other poisons are used in the growing of animal feeds, there is also the danger of accumulation of these toxic materials in the animal tissue.[30]   On a diet of such grains and grasses, combined with polluted water and air, the animal will tend to accumulate such chemicals in his body so that the concentration of poisons in the animal will be many times greater than that in the plants which he ate. The concentration has been found to be particularly high in fat and in organs like the liver which are concerned with filtering out toxic materials.

Exactly how much pesticide residue is found in animal tissue will depend on the animal's food supply. If he eats plants, the amount will be less; if he eats other animals, it will be greater. This is because each animal eats a large quantity of food over a period of time—but the pesticides remain in the body. The animal is in a sense "filtering out" and retaining such chemicals. If he eats plants, his levels will not be extremely high; if he eats other animals the situation is different. Salmon which eat other fish which eat plankton have been known to develop damage to the nervous system from DDT when other aquatic life was unharmed. Some fields have been found to contain as much as 100 pounds of DDT per acre though some animals, like earthworms are fairly resistant and may accumulate an appreciable amount and still survive. Birds, however, which regularly eat such worms will concentrate much larger and more toxic amounts.[31]

Obviously, animal foods have much higher concentrations of pesticides than plant foods and contribute a much larger share of such environmental toxins to the diet of man. Meat, fish and poultry contain 2½ times more DDT and similar pesticides than do dairy products. They contain *13* times as much as the average content of grains and vegetables. As early as 1962 it was found that the levels of DDT in the bodies of those who ate meat was more than double that of those who didn't.[32] Though the use of DDT has been stopped, it and its breakdown products are still present in the environment and probably will be for some time. Moreover, it has been replaced by other often even more toxic substances and the total use of pesticides has accelerated.[33]

Eliminating meat, fish and fowl from the diet goes far toward reducing the intake of pesticides, but the increase in fruits, vegetables and grains that results may have an even more important effect. It has been shown that fiber-rich whole foods help to pull a variety of toxic chemicals out of the body.[34] More fruits and vegetables, grains and beans will also mean more vitamins and minerals as well and the overall improvement in nutrition helps one deal better with any remaining pesticide intake.[35]

Modern methods of raising animals for food further detracts from their quality. In order to raise them more quickly, shorten the time they must be fed, and hasten marketing so as to maximize profits, animals are fed hormone preparations which cause them to gain weight and grow quickly. One of these, diethylstilbesterol, has recently come to the public's attention. It is an estrogen-like hormone commonly fed to steers which causes the animal to gain fatty tissue. This hormone, also known as "the morning after pill," when it is given to women as a method of birth control, has been incriminated in the development of breast cancer, fibroid tumors and excessive menstrual bleeding, as well as impotence in men.[36] The association between the development of vaginal cancer in the daughters of women using stilbesterol has been firmly established. Hogs raised in this fashion and prevented from exercising so they will fatten quickly create problems for the farmer since they sometimes die of heart attacks on the loading platform. In order to keep such animals from falling ill on this unnatural regimen,[37] antibiotics are added to their feed. In 1970 approximately 1,300 tons of antibiotics were fed to animals in the U.S. Though the exact effects of the residues of such antibiotics in the meat supply are not known, a Federal task force concluded in 1972 that there is "an imminent hazard" to human health posed by the low level feed use of antibiotics in food-producing animals.[38] Animals raised in this fashion are obviously far from healthy and some develop malignant growths.[39] While these tumors are removed in the slaughter house before the meat is marketed, it seems clear that such animals cannot provide a high quality food for man.

MEAT AND CONSCIOUSNESS

But what about "organically grown" meats? If they are free of pesticides, antibiotics, etc., are they a healthful food? The answer is a qualified "maybe," since there remains the question of how flesh eating effects consciousness. Many persons note that when they eliminate meat from their diets, a tendency to get headaches disappears. They also note an increase in mental clarity. Yet we know that many groups of peoples, such as certain American Indian tribes, were hunters and flesh eaters who lived close to nature, maintaining a state of health and alertness that far surpassed what most of us enjoy today.* How can this paradox be explained? Although this question may never be fully answered, we might speculate.

It seems that man's ancestors developed in warmer climates where they subsisted largely on fruits, nuts and leafy and root vegetables which could easily be gathered. When changing climatic conditions or migrations compelled them to take up hunting as a means for survival, we might guess that they adapted with some difficulty. How could an essentially peaceful food-gatherer learn the cunning and aggression necessary for stalking and killing his prey? Those individuals whose biochemistry was such that the breakdown products of flesh food stimulated a tendency toward aggressiveness and hunting would have a definite edge on their fellow men and tend to survive and propagate. Such a characteristic would eventually be widespread in those who had survived, having become a definite part of their heredity. Each individual, especially, perhaps, the males who did the hunting, would demonstrate this tendency: when they ate meat

---

* Though violence was not unknown among the American Indians, [40] no one has ever made a careful study on the relationship between the quantities and types of meat eaten by various tribes and the tendency to warfare and destructive aggression.

or flesh, the by-products of its digestion would stimulate in them the hunting instincts and aggressiveness necessary to continue to survive under such circumstances.

Carrying this speculation further, we would find that such groups of early humans would have had a definite advantage over those who had not acquired this biochemical mechanism. They would have been able to survive as hunters or, when conditions so dictated, revert to a life of food gathering (or, later, agriculture). Furthermore, their aggressive capabilities could have easily been turned toward the conquest of more peaceable groups, and it is easy to see how their numbers might have increased and they might have come to predominate in those areas inhabited by early man.

But what would happen to such a man when he, living in an agricultural setting, ate meat and flesh but did not participate in hunting or stalking or killing it? If we follow the logical implications, it would be clear that he would suffer from a stimulation of aggressive feelings and hunting instincts that would have no comfortable outlet in a settled, peaceful community. A civilization of people suffering from this difficulty might be more likely to turn toward senseless warfare with their neighbors, violence on their streets, or experience incessant feelings of anger and hostility. One anthropologist has suggested that warfare in prehistoric Europe became "an everlasting proclivity" only after livestock breeding became common in rural communities.[41] What had been a dual capacity for gathering or hunting with great adaptive potential could have become a major danger to survival.

Although this theory cannot be definitely proven, it is interesting to note in this connection that for millenia in India meat as an article of diet has been traditionally prescribed for the rajputs, the caste made up of warriors and rulers. By contrast, the brahmins, who were to dedicate themselves to study and spiritual advancement and were not to engage in battle, were forbidden the use of meat. This lends a bit more support to the hypothesis that man has a dual biological potential and that he can be geared to more aggressive behavior by eating meat. Perhaps over thousands of years of cultural evolution, the people of India discovered how to harness such potential productively.

In carnivores, the constituents of the meat which are not useful remain as wastes which must be eliminated. This requires a period during which the carnivore is rather sluggish and dull. This state of lethargy is called "tamasic" in traditional Indian thinking and is contrasted with the active aggressive state involved in hunting called "rajasic." The classical Indian culture, which is predominantly vegetarian, puts a high value on the maintenance of a state of calm equilibrium ("sattvic") which avoids either of these extremes.* The lion is viewed as a classical example of the vacillation of this from one extreme to another. Ferocious and aggressive during hunting, after the kill and after feeding, the lion lapses into a long period of dormancy during which the meat is digested. It was perhaps the understanding of the effects of flesh eating on consciousness that lead so many of the ancient teachers to advise against it. Pythagorus, who was a spiritual teacher as well as a mathematician in the Classical Greek period, taught the advantages of vegetarianism, as did Buddha and others.

Closely tied to the effects that meat-eating might have on consciousness are the psychological and moral aspects of eating meat. Some people object to meat-eating on the basis that it is not humane. Another moral consideration is that it is wasteful and not economically sound. Ten to fifteen times more protein can be provided from a plot of land through growing food crops than through raising beef cattle.[42] If one thinks of providing optimal nutrition for the whole of mankind, the economics of land use becomes important. For such reasons it is important to explore the nature of other foods rich in protein since they are not only more economic, but may have quite different

* See Chapter 19, Food Sadhana.

effects on both the body and the mind.

MILK

Since it serves as the link between generations, milk is an especially unique food. Mothers nursing their young provide a typical continuity, such as in the salvation of anything young and delicate. It is the sheltering of young tissues by repetition and familiarity. Milk is, of course, the natural diet of the human infant—human milk, that is. Mother's milk is the food most suited to infants' needs. During the evolution of man, the survival of the race was dependent on milk. It nurtured the offspring to grow up to be healthy, to reproduce, and to pass on the ability to yield such milk. In this fashion, mammals, including humans, evolved a system of feeding their young which permitted a close relationship between the mother and infant and which created a long period of relatively helpless dependency. Through this arrangement, the foundations could be laid for the unfolding of intelligence and human consciousness.

Milk has the unique quality of containing the best that the mother can offer, even at the expense of her own health. In the case of calcium, for example, the infant is assured an adequate supply since the mother's milk will contain sufficient amounts of the mineral even if she is herself malnourished. Her bones and teeth will be demineralized before she will give her infant calcium-deficient milk. In many cultures, milk is, in fact, a symbol of the willingness to give, to sacrifice, and to put the welfare of another above that of oneself. Such expressions as "the milk of human kindness" are to be found in many languages. For this reason, in some areas of India where dairying has been traditionally important, the cow is given a special place of reverence and respect. This characteristic of milk is of practical importance as well, since in a situation where the food supply may be poor quality because of the depletion of the soil or poor agricultural practices, the one item produced on the farm which is most likely to retain its high nutritional value is milk.

Since the grains and other food fed to the cow could be used directly as human food, dairying is often said to be an inefficient and expensive means of supplying protein in the diet, but as in many other dairying cultures, this is not the case in India.   There, cows are fed primarily on leaves, grass and the waste from vegetables, plants and grains, so that the milk is being produced primarily from fiber (cellulose), something which the human can't digest anyway.*   In India, the family cow is almost an integral part of the household. If milk from contented cows is nutritionally superior, then there may be more wisdom than meets the eye in the care and patience that is given dairy animals in India.   Visitors are always astounded to find the pampered cows wandering nonchalantly and unafraid even through the busiest of big city traffic.

Among the many complex protein substances found in milk are small amounts of anti-bodies which may confer some resistance to infection.   One farmer noticed that after grazing his milk goats in a field with poison ivy and then drinking the milk, he no longer broke out in a rash when he came in contact with the plant.[42]   While it is not possible to draw conclusions from one such case, there are probably many properties carried by milk which have not yet been identified. This is especially true in the case of nursing, where the infant takes the milk raw, fresh and as it comes from the breast. It has been said that young animal sucklings do better when breast fed directly than when given the same milk previously withdrawn and allowed to stand.

There is ample evidence that infants who are breast-fed for some time after birth fare much better than those who are given bottle feedings from the beginning.   As early as the 1930's, an extensive study done in Chicago showed that less than one in 1,000 infants who were breast fed died of respiratory infection while over 50 per 1,000 who were artificially fed died from this

---

* See Chapter 4, Carbohydrate and Chapter 11, Elimination.

cause.[44] A 1977 study supports this conclusion.[45] Similarly, it is thought by some experienced physicians that the mother's milk can also transmit tendencies toward certain health problems that she herself has, especially if nursing is continued beyond the earlier stages of infancy. For this reason, in many cases, weaning is recommended after three to six months. If the mother's diet is poor, or if she is emotionally unsettled and frequently upset, nursing is probably best avoided altogether. After an initial three to six months of nursing, cow's milk which has been boiled can be substituted and continued for another several months until the child can begin to add some solid food to the diet.

LACTOSE INTOLERANCE

Fortunately, almost all infants are able to handle milk comfortably, but if they can't, they will have difficulty feeding and will often be diagnosed as having "a milk allergy." Though it sometimes involves a true allergy,* this is sometimes due to a deficiency of lactase, the enzyme involved in the digestion of lactose, which is the sugar that supplies carbohydrate in milk. To be absorbed by the baby, this milk sugar, a disaccharide, must be split by the enzyme lactase into two smaller sugars, glactose and glucose. When this enzyme is missing, the unabsorbed lactose remains in the intestinal tract, feeding certain bacteria which then begin to grow and multiply there. The result can be abdominal pain, diarrhea, gas and so forth. Infants deficient in lactase will often thrive if given a milk preparation in which lactose is absent, such as soy milk or fermented milk products like yogurt.

Research has shown that in certain areas such as Northern Europe, India and some parts of Africa where dairying and a diet containing milk have been traditional for hundreds and even thousands of years, adults will usually retain the capacity for handling milk since it is used as a part of their diet after infancy.

---

* See Chapter 18, Megavitamins and Food Allergies.

In many ethnic groups, however, where milk drinking is not traditional, the enzyme lactase disappears at about the time of weaning. In this case, adults who drink milk find that it strongly disagrees with them. Since most white Americans are descended from Northern European stock where dairying has been practiced for many centuries, only 6 to 15% of them will show symptoms of milk (lactose) intolerance. In a few areas of Africa the people also traditionally take milk as adults, and among the dairying tribes of Uganda, for example, only 20% or less of the adults have difficulty digesting lactose. For the pastoral tribes, however, where milk is not used after infancy, lactose intolerance is seen in about 80% of the people. Since most Black Americans have a mixed ancestry, and are not ordinarily descended from one particular tribe, the picture here is less clear. It is difficult for a Black American to predict whether or not he is intolerant to lactose, but about 70% have this problem.[46]

Up until ten years ago, lactose intolerance was not well recognized, and it was the practice to encourage and even require milk consumption among all racial groups. This led to rather embarrassing situations, both in the ghettos of America and in foreign aid programs abroad, where children were being made sick by the milk supplied them through government assistance.

On the other hand, some careful studies have shown as low as 29% lactose intolerant Blacks. But it was noted that some of those who do absorb lactose well still manifest the same symptoms as those lacking in the enzyme. In other words, some people who get upset stomachs are absorbing lactose. What's even more surprising, some people who did *not* absorb lactose had no symptoms or discomfort of any kind![47] As we shall see later, the bacteria in the intestinal tract that do the fermenting of the lactose and cause the gas, may vary tremendously from person to person.

Moreover, milk is an extremely complex food and one may react adversely to other constituents of it besides lactose.[48] In any case, such problems suggest that unaltered milk may not be an "ideal" food for all adults; that, at least in some ways, they do "outgrow" their ability to handle it. Experiments have shown, however, that both humans and laboratory animals can develop a tolerance to lactose if it is taken consistently in gradually increasing amounts. Part of this may be due to changes in the intestinal bacteria which metabolize the sugar, but there can also be an actual increase in the activity of the enzyme lactase itself.[49] This ability to develop the capacity to handle milk even in those who are "genetically intolerant" may be important. In a cold climate where fresh produce is not to be had during much of the year, wholesome milk products may be preferable to many of the other foods which might be available.

PASTEURIZED, HOMOGENIZED AND RAW

The need to preserve milk so that it can be supplied to the large urban areas in America has led to almost all dairy products being pasteurized. This is also intended to destroy those bacteria in milk which might cause disease. The pasteurization process, however, heats milk to only 145° F (62° C) for thirty minutes or to 161° F (72° C) for fifteen seconds. As a result, some bacteria remain,[50] and the very important question of viral growth in the milk is still a subject for study. Not only does pasteurization fail to destroy all the microorganisms that are present, but it apparently alters the milk in such a way as to render it difficult to digest. This may be due to a partial alteration or denaturation of the protein in it.

In large protein molecules, the amino acid chain is coiled or bent into limbs; these in turn fold upon each other in intricate but very important ways. The folding and coiling is maintained by relatively weak bonds between the amino acids. These bonds must be strong enough to hold the molecule's shape, but not so strong as to make it rigid, for the huge protein molecules often depend for their function on the ability to change their shape. These delicate limbs which shift are very fragile, and heat can alter them. Then the shape of the molecule is changed and its ability to function is impaired. This is called "denaturing" the protein, i.e., its basic nature is disrupted. If too many of the weak bonds are broken, the complex molecule collapses into a broken tangle which may present great difficulties for the digestive enzymes, which are hard put to "get a handle on it" so as to break it down. In this case, further heating may, under some circumstances, complete the denaturation to the point of breaking it into shorter chains, or even down to single amino acid links, in which case digestion is actually facilitated. Something of this sort may happen with milk.

Experiments have shown that when milk is partially heated (pasteurized), it tends to coagulate into a tight mass when exposed to stomach acid.[51] Many diary farmers know from experience with their children that pasteurized milk constipates them whereas raw milk does not. If pasteurizing milk tangles the large and complex coils of the protein molecule, making them difficult to digest, boiling it breaks it down more completely. Fifty years ago it was observed that children who were given milk that had been quickly brought to the boiling point and cooled were healthier and gained more weight than those taking pasteurized milk.[52] In any case, boiling the milk is a much more effective means of sterilizing it. In India where there are thousands of years of experience with milk in the diet, it is never taken without boiling it first, despite the fact that the cows are often cared for personally. Moreover, in Switzerland, another country with a long history of dairying, at the famous Bircher-Benner Clinic where raw food is stressed, boiled milk is nevertheless given to patients, even though fresh raw milk is available.

Some states have provision for certifying dairy herds to produce raw milk for human consumption, and such "certified raw milk" is available in many areas. The health of the herd should be carefully considered, however, since many dairy animals are raised on feeds grown on poor soil and are kept "healthy" through the use of chemical additives. To drink the milk of such an animal is unwise. Boiling raw milk will sterilize it without necessarily destroying its nutritional advantages. Certainly fresh raw milk which has been brought to a boil has a more appealing taste than ordinary pastuerized, homogenized milk.

YOGURT AND CHEESE

In cultures where milk is traditionally used, there is a common method of preparation which not only makes the milk easier to digest, but also preserves it and prevents the growth of undesirable bacteria. This is the practice of making various sour milk preparations. It probably originated with the need to find some way to preserve the milk beyond the first few hours after milking, although it also serves other purposes. The most common method of souring milk is to simply set it aside and allow it to ferment. The texture and taste of the resulting preparation will depend on the particular strain of bacteria which happens to be present in the milk or in the air or in the bowl where the milk is left. In the Balkan states, especially Bulgaria, the local bacteria produce a soured milk which is of fine texture and quite delicious. This is called "yogurt," and even in America the best yogurt is prepared by allowing milk to sour after a small amount—a "culture"—of this Bulgarian product is added. The milk is usually boiled before the culture is added. Besides other possible advantages, this destroys any undesirable "wild" bacteria which might interfere with the growth of the culture or be disease causing, as well as inactivating certain enzymes which would tend to kill the bacteria that are to be added. During the souring process, lactose is broken down to lactic acid, so soured products are more easily tolerated by those who do not tolerate milk sugar well. The rapid growth of the implanted bacteria will crowd out and destroy most disease causing microbes that might find their way into the milk. Moreover, the growth of the new bacteria in milk during the process of souring may supply a strain of bacteria which is beneficial to the intestinal tract.

Years ago in many sections of rural America, it was the custom to take naturally soured raw milk, called "clabber," and, after it had reached a firm consistency, to hang it in a cheese cloth overnight to allow the whey to drip out. This produced a fresh, raw "cottage cheese." In India a similar fresh cottage cheese is made by simply adding lemon juice to boiling milk to curdle it and then hanging this in a cheese cloth to drip. The result, "paneer," is quite delicious and in many ways superior to commercial cottage cheese.* In aged cheeses, such as cheddar, provolone and mozzarella, the aging and the subsequent "improvement in flavor" is a result of the growth of certain bacteria in the milk solids.[53]

IS MILK "MUCUS-FORMING"?

Many persons avoid milk and milk products in their diet because they say they are "mucus-forming," and it is true that some people can notice an increased amount of mucus in the throat, nasal passages and bronchi when they use greater quantities of milk. Milk is a body builder. Its basic nature is to promote the growth of flesh. It is designed to be the most efficient food possible for the rapidly growing animal. In Ayurvedic terms, milk is said to promote *kaph*. This is the solid, substantial aspect of the human being, and when it is deficient, one is likely to be unstable psychologically, and thin and underdeveloped physically. During periods of growth, when recovering from an illness, or when one needs to gain weight, milk can be a

---

* Some commercial cottage cheeses are made with rennet, an enzyme taken from the intestines of calves, where it acts to digest its mother's milk, and for this reason may be avoided by strict vegetarians. However, generally it is the "large curd" cottage cheese which is curdled with this agent, while the "small curd" is not. Moreover, very recently a "vegetable rennet," produced by bacterial cultures, has come into use. Since it is less expensive, it seems to be rapidly replacing animal rennet in making aged cheeses as well as cottage cheese. The exception is Swiss cheese, as it is apparently difficult to get the characteristic "holes" without using animal rennet.

very valuable addition to the diet. If the body does not need to increase in *kaph*, however, or if it is for some reason unable to properly assimilate it, then it is thrown off as waste. Besides, animal milk is not perfectly designed for human metabolism, and some waste is certain to result. Unusable *kaph* is what is known in the West as mucus, and our English word, "cough" takes its origin from the Sanskrit term.

In the East Indies, milk is made less mucus-forming by adding water, boiling it, taking it hot, and sometimes by adding ginger, pepper or other pungent spices. These promote the digestion and assimilation of the milk. Goat's milk also seems to be more easily handled by the body and many people find it to be "less mucus-forming." If the goats are properly handled, goat's milk is also quite delicious and will not have any objectionable odor or taste. Gandhi lived for some time almost exclusively on it, and it is said that when he came from India to London he brought a goat along with him, kept it on the roof and subsisted on its milk.

NON-DAIRY MILKS

While the use of milk is limited and/or unknown in most parts of the world, there is a long tradition of the use of vegetable "milks" among various peoples. The Chinese and Japanese have for millenia used a milk made from soybeans. The beans are soaked until they swell and then ground, pounded or otherwise liquified. This mixture is strained and the pulp discarded. The resulting liquid is a thick, heavy milk, which, though different from animal milk, is quite tasty. It must, however, be brought to a boil before it can be used. Otherwise it tastes "green" and bean-like and contains an enzyme which prevents digestion.[54] In the Far East, this milk is curdled and hung in a cheese cloth to form a solid curd called "soy cheese" or "tofu." This is the major source of protein in the diet of many Chinese and Japanese, and because of its high quality, it is often called "the meat

Tofu

Many people shy away from tofu (soy bean curd) because it is unfamiliar and tastes rather bland when eaten plain. Properly used, however, it is quite delicious, and so versatile that it can be added to almost any recipe, providing a rich protein and mineral bonus. It is low in fat and high in protein. Made fresh in one's own home* it has a delicate flavor, though the tofu from health food or grocery stores is usually adequate. It should be kept as fresh as possible by storing under water which is changed periodically. In Japan, where it is a staple food, it is made daily and purchased every morning from neighborhood vendors. Here are some ways to use tofu:*

Dressings: Blend tofu, lemon juice, salt and seasonings.

Dips: Blend tofu, toasted sunflower seeds and lemon juice to taste. This can also be poured over cooked vegetables.

Mash tofu with salt, pepper and lemon juice to the desired consistency so that it will resemble cottage or cream cheese; excellent for use in salads or in toasted sandwiches with tomatoes, alfalfa sprouts and roasted sunflower seeds.

Fried: Slice tofu and place it in a skillet of hot ghee in which spices have been browned. This also makes an excellent sandwich.

Tofu "burgers" can be made by mashing tofu with chopped celery, onion, green pepper, ground seeds, eggs and bread crumbs and frying in patties until golden brown.

Scrambled: Fry some chopped onions in an iron skillet with ghee and a little browned tumeric, cumin and ground coriander. Crumble in 1/3 to 1/2 cup of tofu per person, stir until mixed, and serve with toast.

Cubes of fresh, soft tofu in a clear broth with a little chopped scallions or chives or a dash of lemon juice have a delicate flavor.

Tofu makes an excellent replacement for cheese or meat in such dishes as lasagna, pizza, chow mein, enchilladas, toastadas or tacos.

Place cubes of tofu on the steaming rack over vegetables a few minutes before cooking is finished or atop breakfast cereal like millet just before it's done to give the meal "staying power."

Tofu gives extra body to casseroles or bean loaves or stir-fried vegetables.

Blend tofu with honey, chopped nuts, raisins and spices such as nutmeg, cinnamon or cardamon for a topping or with fresh fruit to make a "parfait." Tofu can also be used to make frosting, ice cream, cheese cake, puddings, jelled dishes and even cookies.

* A simple recipe for homemade tofu is in *Himalayan Mountain Cookery* by Mrs. R. M. Ballentine, Sr. and detailed uses are in *The Book of Tofu*, Shurtleff, W., and Aoyagi, A., Autumn Press, Ind. Kanagawa-Ken, Japan, 1975.

without a bone."* This process can easily be carried out in the Western kitchen, and tofu is a delightful ingredient in vegetable dishes, pizza or as the basis of cheesecake.

The American Indians in the Southeast collected hickory nuts, and, by means of some process now lost, managed to crush them and prepare a "hickory milk" which was, according to those explorers who sampled it, quite appetizing. In the Middle East, a milk is made from sesame seeds. One of the most delicious of these milk-like preparations is almond milk. This can be prepared by simply liquifying one cup of raw almonds, one quart of water, and one tablespoon of honey and oil in a blender. The milk is best strained and is suitable for many of the uses to which other milk is put. A similar milk can be made from cashews and many other nuts or coconut. Such a milk made from the coconut is important in South Indian cooking where it is added to various curried vegetables to give them a rich flavor.

LEGUMES

Since medieval times, dried beans and peas were known in Europe as "poor man's meat," and even today in America, a bare kitchen and a can of beans is the cartoonist's way of portraying hard times. However, this attitude toward beans is hardly universal. The soybean holds a position of honor in traditional Chinese culture, and beans are consumed by the highest castes in India. Research there has shown that the relationship between income and the consumption of beans and peas is the opposite of that which the affluent Westerner would expect: the higher the income in India the greater the quantity of legumes consumed. The story is told of an ancient Indian raja who was imprisoned by his adversaries. Kept in royal custody, he was asked with great solicitude what he would prefer to eat. His

---

* For detailed information on the nutritional value of soybeans and the traditional Chinese ways of processing them, see Chen, Phillip S., *Soybeans for Health, Longevity, and Economy*, Provoker Press, 1970.

answer was simply, "Green gram" (mung beans). Even today in India, a preparation of dahl made from whole mung beans is considered both a culinary delight and a nutritional treasure, indeed a dish "fit for a king."

Except for parts of Western Europe and America, dried beans and peas have been one of the most highly valued and crucial ingredients in traditional diets since antiquity. Remains of lentils have been found in Egyptian tombs dating back as early as 4,000 years ago, and wall paintings from 1,200 BC in Egypt depict the preparation of lentil dishes. In Mexico, archaeologists have turned up evidence of the use of beans as early as 7,000 BC. In fact, legumes are responsible for a major part of the protein in the diets of most people in the world even today. There is not a peasant cuisine in the world that does not contain its favored bean dish. In Mexico, kidney beans of various descriptions are the favored legume. In China and Japan, soybeans are most often used while Cubans prefer black beans. American favorites include Boston baked beans, New Orleans red beans, Texan pinto beans and Southern black-eyed peas.

While beans and peas usually contain around 20-25% protein, it is often said that this protein is not ideal for human consumption since it does not have a balanced amino acid content. For a protein to be best utilized, it should contain the proper proportion of the eight amino acids which the body is unable to manufacture. While the proteins in such foods as egg white, for example, or milk (casein) are ideal, containing all the eight essential amino acids in the proper balance, the protein of plant foods such as legumes do not, and this led to their being regarded as "unable to support life."

THE HISTORY OF ATTITUDES TOWARD PROTEIN

By the late 1800's, research scientists had succeeded in separating pure protein from whole foods such as cereals, beans, peas, nuts, leaves, meat and milk. Chemical analysis showed that

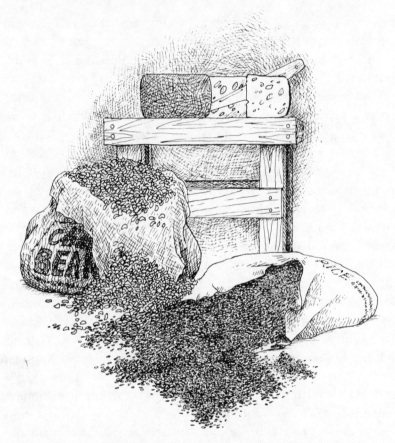

these proteins differed vastly from one another as far as percentages of nitrogen, sulfur, carbon, hydrogen and oxygen that they contained. In fact, there were so many proteins of so many varying and intricate compositions that the picture became very confusing. Around the turn of the century, however, it became understood that the proteins were essentially chains of amino acids. The types of amino acids that were present had something to do with the usefulness of the protein in the diet. Thereafter a great deal of research was done to identify the amino acids that made up the various protein, and experiments based on these discoveries followed. When a balanced diet was fed to experimental animals and only the protein was changed, it could be clearly demonstrated that some proteins were better able to support life than others. Milk protein (casein) and egg white (albumin), for example, supplied all the nutritional requirements of the laboratory animals.

On the other hand, the proteins of corn and wheat were not adequate. Animals did not thrive eating them as their only source of protein in the diet despite the fact that the rest of the diet was excellent. These proteins were "incomplete," lacking in some of the essential amino acids. When the missing amino acids were added to the diet, along with the wheat or corn protein, then the animals did quite well. By 1935 it was clearly established that there were eight essential amino acids and that these must be present in the protein fraction of the diet in certain proportions in order for the protein to be well utilized. Meat, milk and eggs had the eight strategic amino acids in the right proportions to qualify them as "complete proteins." Plant foods did not. They were regarded as "incomplete" and unable to sustain life alone.

This idea became so literal and so ingrained in the academic world that many nutritionists were convinced that one who ate no milk, meat or eggs could not live and would soon perish from lack of adequate protein. Even as recently as thirty years ago anthropologists were of the opinion that if, indeed, the "rice-eaters" of the Orient were able to live without the meat protein required by a European, then they must be somehow genetically different. The point that escaped the academicians, but which is very obvious to one who has dined on the peasant foods of almost any country, is that one rarely eats one food such as a grain, a bean or a simple vegetable alone. These foods are usually taken in combinations so that the amino acids absent in one are supplied by those present in another. This is possible because the deficiencies of the eight essential amino acids are different for beans, for grains and for vegetables. Grains can therefore be combined with legumes, for example, to form proteins which are "complete." Their amino acids are said to be "complementary" since what each lacks, the other supplies.[55] This simple fact has only gradually become recognized by nutritional researchers, and it has been only very recently, almost forty years after the discovery of the importance of "complete protein," that it has been integrated into the theory of nutritional science as taught in modern universities.

BEANS AND GRAINS

Legumes are deficient primarily in methionine. This is their "limiting amino acid." Grains, on the other hand, usually contain ample amounts of methionine but are generally limited instead by their rather deficient content of lysine, another of the essential amino acids. Interestingly enough, lysine turns out to be abundant in legumes, so grains and legumes mesh perfectly as nutritional complements. Combining grains and legumes provides a more ideal balance of the essential amino acids, making the protein more usable so that more of it can be assimilated by the body. Thus it is no accident that the peoples of many cultures have separately, and apparently independently, evolved traditional diets based on a combination of grains and legumes. In Turkey, where some of the earliest remains of wheat have been found, (dating back to about 5,500 BC) traces of peas and lentils were found alongside them. We will seldom find a group of people anywhere in the world who eat bean or pea dishes alone as the sole article of diet. On the contrary, it is considered somehow natural to take such dishes with bread, tortillas, rice or some other grain preparation.

When combined in the right proportions, the protein of the grain and the legume becomes more useful gram for gram than either of these proteins alone. Research with experimental animals has shown, for example, that a diet containing 18% wheat protein would produce an average weight gain of only about 40 grams by the time the animal was five weeks old. A diet of 18% protein supplied by lentils did only slightly better.

If, however, the animals were given a diet containing, still only 18% protein, but this time a protein 1/3 of which was furnished by lentils and 2/3 by wheat, the weight gain by five weeks was nearly 130 grams, three times the amount which was gained on either the wheat-based or the lentil-based diet.[56]   For this

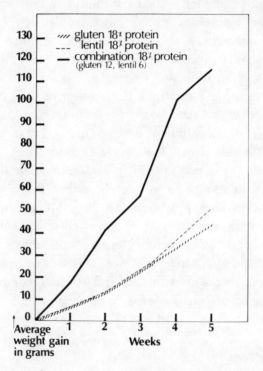

Differences in Growth Rate with Different Protein Sources[56]

complementary effect to occur, however, the grain and legume must be taken together.[57]

For any grain/legume combination, there is a certain proportion that is optimal. Experiments have shown, for example, that rice and black beans, the favorite dish of Cubans, Costa Ricans and many other Latin Americans, provides the most complete and ideal protein when one takes four times as much rice as beans (80% rice and 20% black beans). However, with corn bread and crowder peas, a traditional dish in the South-eastern United States, the most ideal proportion is half and half.[58]   Generally, the best results are obtained when there is more grain than legumes, and the most commonly successful ratio is about 2 to 1.[59]

The experimental evidence on this point corresponds quite well to what is observed among most peoples of the world. It seems to be instinctively understood in the traditional cooking of the more developed cultures that legumes should be used in small amounts. In India and China, for example, the amount of rice that is served is larger than the amount of dahl or soy bean preparation that is taken with it. In India, the dahl or bean preparation is usually diluted, (soupy) and served in a very small container as a side dish. In Chinese cuisine, when tofu or soy cheese is added to vegetables, it is also used in small amounts. For most populations, an average intake of 30-75 grams (dry weight) of dried beans or peas per day is common. This is roughly equal to about a cup of a cooked dish made primarily of beans (more or less depending on how much water is used in the cooking.) More often than not, this will be taken in two separate meals throughout the day and will be accompanied each time by at least twice that quantity of bread, rice or some other grain dish.

BEANS AND HEALTH

Legumes not only supply a convenient complement to the bread or rice that is the staff of life for most people of the world, but they also bring other benefits as well. When compared with meat, they have significant health promoting properties. As mentioned earlier, a number of experiments have shown that dried beans and peas lower blood fats and decrease hardening of the arteries. This is of obvious significance since coronary heart disease is perhaps the major health problem in the West. In one experiment done with human subjects, it was found that sucrose, bread and potato diets caused identical serum cholesterol levels while a diet containing legumes lowered the level by 9% [60] Similar results were noticed in India when comparing the dahl (dried beans and peas) popular among the Indians with other items of diet.[61]

In another study done on persons who died from a variety of causes, the degree of formation of arteriosclerotic plaques in the coronary arteries which supply the walls of the heart were measured. Then detailed dietary histories were compiled by interviewing survivors of the deceased. While less fat and more fiber in the diet seemed to be associated with less plaque formation, there was one factor that seemed much more important. That was the amount of beans eaten. In all races and all socio-economic groups, a high consumption of vegetable protein in the diet was found in those who had the cleanest coronary arteries.[62]

Though inexpensive and healthful, many people shy away from legumes because they find them difficult to digest. They cause intestinal gas and flatulence in those who have little experience with them. The digestive tract must become adapted to such a food before it can be handled comfortably, and those who are not used to eating beans and peas should start by taking only a small amount.

DE-GASSING BEANS

The gas that comes from eating beans is caused primarily by two unusual starches, stachyose and raffinose.[63] They are rather short chains of sugar molecules, but they are joined by a special linkage that cannot be broken by any of the enzymes usually found in the intestine. For this reason they cannot be absorbed, but remain behind in the digestive tract where they are metabolized by certain bacteria that are more common in those who eat meat. Especially in one who is not accustomed to a vegetarian diet, these bacteria break down the short starches into carbon dioxide and hydrogen, the two main components of gastrointestinal gas.[64]

These starchy villains (stachyose and raffinose), responsible for so many unsavory misdeeds, can fortunately be removed from the beans. Soaking overnight helps a little since enzymes in the bean break down the starches into sugars. But this probably eliminates less than a tenth of the problematic starches. Boiling for 20 minutes will remove a third of them, and 85% can be removed if soybeans, for example, are boiled 5 minutes, soaked for a half hour in tap water, rubbed until the hulls float free, then cooked for an hour.[65] Such elaborate processing is not usually necessary, but may be worth while for those who are just learning to take beans in the diet. Actually, soybeans, which are especially prone to cause gas, are, in the Far East where they form a primary part of the diet, traditionally processed extensively to make popular preparations like tofu.

Another important cause of difficulty with the digestion of legumes is the failure to cook them properly. Very thorough cooking is necessary, preferably after the beans or peas have soaked overnight. Seasonings such as herbs, spices, salt, fat and so forth which are used in the traditional preparation of bean dishes are not added simply for flavor. As we shall see later, they play an important role in promoting their digestion.*

The variety of bean or pea is also important in determining whether it will cause indigestion and gas. Kidney beans, soy beans and broad beans are more difficult for most people to digest and cooking them is a special challenge. In their immature form, legumes such as the tiny green limas or "butter beans" favored in the southeast U.S. are much more easily digested than the large, heavy dried limas. This is probably because they have not yet fully developed their starch content and are more like a green vegetable. Moreover, they do not require cooking as long, and because of their lower percentage of starch they contain more of other nutrients per calorie.

* See Chapter 15, Ayurvedic Nutrition, and Chapter 16, Cooking.

Most of the gas-producing starches can be eliminated by sprouting. This also increases the protein content, decreases the starch content, and shortens the cooking time of legumes. (See insert on sprouting, Chapter 7.) During the process of sprouting, some of the stored starch in the legume is used up in forming the tiny leaves and rootlets and in manufacturing vitamin C. Even an overnight soaking initiates this process, "bringing the beans to life" and it is thought by some nutritionists that this is an important way of improving their digestibility.[66]

Before sprouting, soy beans contain large quantities of trypsin inhibitors, one of the substances which can interfere with digestion. These substances interfere with the action of trypsin, a protein digesting enzyme found in the intestinal tract. Raw beans, on the other hand, which contain such substances, may be almost impossible to digest and can even be found whole in the stool if they were not chewed properly. It is understandable that this anti-trypsin factor would have survival value for the plant, since its seeds would then be eaten and transported by animals to other areas where, if protected from digestive juices, they could be deposited and grow. In any case, the enzyme can be inactivated by heat as can other substances found in raw beans that have untoward effects. Kidney beans and black beans usually contain large amounts of another undesirable compound which can cause severe vomiting and diarrhea unless it is destroyed by very thorough cooking.* The smaller and more delicate mung beans (Phaseolus aureus), for example, contain few trypsin inhibitors and are therefore easier to digest and require less cooking.[67]

Since legumes are inexpensive and high in protein and since protein is the nutrient most commonly deficient in today's overpopulated world, they have recently been hailed as the answer to the world's food shortage. We may guess that as urbanization and overpopulation increase, the need for a source

* See Chapter 13, Beyond Nutrients.

of protein and starch, such as legumes, which are easy to grow, which will give high yield on a small amount of land, and which will store well, will likewise increase.

OTHER SOURCES OF PROTEIN

Meat, eggs, milk, cheese and legumes (especially when combined with grains) are the foods usually considered to be "high in protein." When one feels a need for something "solid," it is towards these foods that he will most often gravitate. They are the basis of "main courses" and dishes that are valued for their meaty, hearty appeal. Yet there are other foods which also contain some protein. Though many of them like nuts and seeds, are not used in large quantities, collectively they may contribute significantly to protein intake. The same is true of dietary staples, like grains and vegetables whose moderate amounts of "hidden protein" add, over the long haul, surprising quantities of this basic structural material to the diet.

NUTS: PROTEIN FALLING FROM HEAVEN

Paleontologists tell us that our ancestors were eating nuts even before they became human. Therefore we might expect that, when fresh, well chewed, and taken in the proper proportion with other foods, nuts would be one of the most superb foods for man. Not only do they contain a large amount of high quality protein, but also beneficial fats, some of which are necessary ("essential fatty acids"). In fact, some nuts are extremely oily. Pecans, for example may contain up to 76% fat. For this reason a pound of nuts can contain as many calories as 12 pounds of potatoes; clearly not a food for dieters! Their concentrated, fatty composition, as well as their distribution in nature hint that they should be taken in limited quantities. This is true not only for the weight-conscious since large quantities of nuts can be very difficult to digest. In the East, it is said that two or three nuts at a time is enough, and in traditional dishes they are used frequently but sparingly.

If nuts are not fresh, they are best avoided altogether. When they have been shelled and allowed to stand for a long time, the fats in some nuts undergo oxidation and become rancid. This not only gives them a strong, disagreeable taste but can make them harmful.* Though often this rancid flavor is covered up by oiling, roasting and salting the nuts, they are still best avoided.

SEEDS: PUMPKIN, SUNFLOWER, SESAME, ETC.

Of course nuts, grains and legumes are also seeds, but they are not usually referred to as such, and they are already a familiar part of the average diet. Here, we are referring to those foods which are more called seeds, such as pumpkin, sunflower and sesame, as well as others which are almost unknown in American culture, but which are excellent foods, such as flax seed, squash seed and even cucumber seed. Most seeds contain only two or three times as much fat as protein, whereas nuts contain three to seven times as much. Nonetheless, seeds are more commonly used as a source of cooking oil since they are less expensive.

Sunflower seeds were grown by the American Indians and the plant was introduced into Europe in the mid 1500's. The use of the seeds spread to Asia where they were enthusiastically adopted by many peoples from the Middle East to India and northward to Russia. The czars, it is said, fed their soldiers two pounds of sunflower seeds a day as a staple, and even today the caricature of a Russian peasant depicts him munching on a handful of sunflower seeds. Seeds can be used in many ways in the diet but sunflower and pumpkin seeds are especially good with green salads.

The major difficulty with the use of seeds in the diet is that they are sometimes difficult to get fresh after they have

* See Chapter 5, Fats and Oils.

been shelled and are usually too tedious to shell at the time they are eaten. This is less of a problem when they are raw and properly packaged. The roasted sunflower seeds, however, which are sold in health food and grocery stores are often remarkably rancid. Their flavor is noticeably inferior to freshly roasted sunflower seeds, which are delicious. Though it is often more convenient to eat sunflower seeds raw, a light roasting is worthwhile since the heat makes them more usable and therefore increases their nutritive value.[68]

Sesame seeds are a staple protein among many peoples, especially in Africa and the Middle East. One method of preparation is to shell them and grind them into a paste which is called "tahini" in Arabic. There is also another form of sesame paste made from whole roasted sesame seeds and sold in this country under the name of "sesame butter." One advantage of sesame seeds is that they can be used in their husk and therefore keep well. This is not true of sunflower, pumpkin, or squash seeds. Sesame seeds are difficult to chew, however, and if used whole are often found in the stool unchanged. Even when ground, sesame seeds are difficult to digest and are said in the East to be a very complex food with strong effects on the body.

Flax seeds are important in the diets of some European countries and are used in the preparation of a delicious German bread called "leinenbrot." One can easily make this bread by simply kneading a handful of flax seed into whole wheat bread dough before it is shaped into a loaf. In India, cucumber seeds are a delicacy and are mixed with roasted legumes to form a dish called *dahl bizi* which is served with tea. The amino acid deficiencies of most seeds and nuts are similar to those of grains, so they are complemented nicely by legumes.

GRAINS: MORE THAN STARCH

Contrary to the common notion, grains are more than simply starch. Besides containing vitamins and minerals, they also contain a significant amount of protein, though not so much as other "seeds" like nuts or sunflower seeds. An average grade of Canadian wheat contains about 14% protein.[69] If we accept the usual estimate that a person on an average 2,500 calorie diet needs about 60 g of protein a day, we can see that one would get nearly half again this much (87 g a day) by eating only Canadian wheat! On English wheat he'd have more trouble, getting only about 44 g of protein, since it usually contains only half as much protein as its Canadian counterpart.[70]

This protein is, however, not "complete." That is, it does not contain all the essential amino acids in what is thought to be the proper proportions. Even with the inefficient utilization resulting from this improper balance of amino acids, 87 g of protein would probably meet most people's requirements.[71] This is no doubt why some peoples of the world seem to maintain surprisingly good health in a diet that is almost completely wheat. This is also probably why exhaustion of the soil, such as that which has occured in England and the Eastern U.S., decreasing the protein content of grains,[72] can wreak such havoc on the health of a population that is already taking a borderline diet.

If even a small percentage of the wheat is replaced with a legume (such as dried beans and peas), useful protein is greatly increased since their essential amino acids complement each other so well. This accounts for the success of those breads to which the flour of legumes is added. Clive McCay, a highly respected contemporary nutritionist, developed a wheat loaf which contained a small amount of soy flour ("Cornell Bread"). In experiments, it has supported the growth and health of experimental animals much better than commercial bread.[73] The idea is not new, however. The Medieval European's dark barley, rye and wheat bread often had pea flour added. Even today many people of North India continue the traditional practice of adding a small amount of gram flour (the flour of a garbanzo-like pea) to wheat flour before kneading it into the dough from which they roll their unleavened *chapattis.*

HOW MUCH PROTEIN IS ENOUGH?

Americans are often said by observers from abroad to be obsessed with protein. Although only 7% of the world's population, North Americans consume 30% of the world's animal foods.[74] Protein supplements, protein tablets, protein powders and high-protein foods like meat, cheese and eggs are the pre-occupation of most nutrition-conscious people in this country. While protein deficiency is a very real problem in certain impoverished areas, the preoccupation of affluent Americans seems hard to understand.

As a result of reading popular books on nutrition, many people have the idea that with protein, there's no limit—"the more the better." In fact, one well known writer suggests that many people, especially those whose health has not been good, should take 150 grams of protein a day for some time.[75] This is about as much protein as is found in a dozen eggs or nearly two pounds of roast beef. In addition, the author of another popular book on diet, himself a physician, advises readers that he often starts his day with an egg, a chop or a chicken leg, has a broiled steak, pork or lamb chops at noon and for dinner recommends "a really large piece of meat, a pound or a pound and a half.[76]

In contrast, one reputable nutritionist states that convincing studies have shown that an ounce a day of pure protein of good quality is minimally sufficient for the average adult woman "and that men require only a bit more."[77] This was, in fact, proved in experiments at MIT where 100 young men were given experimental diets which allowed regulation of protein intake. Generally an amount less than 30 g (one ounce) was sufficient.[78] In such countries as Peru, populations have been studied who live to an advanced age while maintaining their health and working daily in the field. Their diet, consisting largely of vegetable protein, contains only 30 grams of protein a day. Other researchers have found that even amounts as low as 3.9 or 6.8 g a day were enough to prevent net protein loss from the body.[79]   This is less than a hundredth of the protein contained in the doctor's menu mentioned above!

With such varying ideas of what is needed, planning the protein in one's diet can be confusing. International groups of experts have tended to settle, however, on about 0.8 g per kg— which amounts to about 48 g of protein for the average man.[80] One reason recommendations may be so far above or below this middle of the road estimate is due to the way they are calculated. Most official recommendations attempt to cover the needs of the majority of people. Actually there is a great variation in individual needs. Most RDA's are as high as they are because they are set to the needs of those whose requirements are considerably above the average.[81]

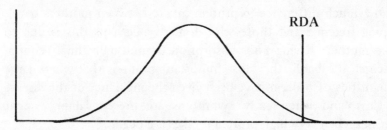

The Recommended Dietary Allowance is set high enough to account for the needs of 98% of healthy people.

If one sets the "recommended allowance" high enough to provide what is needed by the one person in 20 or 100 whose needs are unusually high, then the RDA runs higher than we've mentioned above. Thus recent official figures from the National Research Council are 70 g for an adult man and 60 for a woman. The average person, however, will find 50 grams quite adequate. Certainly there are times when more protein is required, however. When children are about a year old, they are building protein tissues and require nearly twice as much protein per unit of body weight as an adult. Infants require as much as three times the adult's.

PROTEIN REQUIREMENTS DURING PREGNANCY

Probably the most dramatic increase in protein requirements is during pregnancy. During the last three months, a huge
amount of protein tissue is being constructed in the rapidly
growing body of the developing baby. This requires a great
increase in protein intake. If the mother absorbs protein poorly
or for other reasons her requirements are particularly high, she
may run short and serious problems begin. There is a steadily
accumulating body of evidence that this leads to decreased
protein levels in the mother's blood, which robs it of its ability
to draw fluids from the tissues.[82] Accumulation of water in the
space around the cells produces the swelling that heralds toxemia
or eclampsia, a serious disease that is responsible for much infant
and maternal mortality. Some studies have, however, failed to
show much difference in protein intake between mothers developing toxemia and those who don't.[83] Perhaps this is due to
the mothers having poor absorption or unusually high requirements. Probably the most important point is that where large
quantities of protein have been given the incidence of the disease
is less, and when early symptoms are present, improvement
ensues when very high protein intakes are begun.

PROTEIN-CALORIE RATIO

For the average person, one simple way to ensure adequate
protein intake is to calculate the grams of protein needed for the
amount of calories that one burns. The number of calories in
most foods is information that is easily available and common
knowledge among the weight conscious. Protein is most
commonly measured in grams. Though energy requirements
vary, recommended intakes of calories run from 1,900 to 2,700.
Estimates of protein requirements run from 46 g to 70 g. We
should guess, then, that one who took 1,900 calories would need
46 grams of protein and one who takes 2,700 calories needs 70.

Since it is generally true that those who use less calories need less protein,[84] this means that the ratio is about 50 grams of protein for one who consumes 2,000 calories—a nearly average energy intake for those who don't make their living by physical labor.* The ratio then is one g protein for every forty calories. As long as one gets a gram of protein every time he eats 40 calories, he's on solid ground. By the time he has eaten 2,000 calories, he has taken his full complement of 50 g of protein.

Beans, peas, grains, vegetables and fruits contain a variety of nutrients. Besides protein, most whole natural foods contain complex carbohydrate (starch) which serves as fuel. This, as we have seen, is a more ideal source of fuel than fat, so that for maintaining a good protein/calorie ratio, vegetable foods are preferable to meats (which are protein/fat).

HOW TO MAINTAIN THE PROTEIN/CALORIE RATIO

Whole foods, beans, peas, grains, vegetables and fruits all contain a complex of nutrients. Mixed with their carbohydrate are vitamins, minerals, fats and, as we have seen, protein. But how much protein does a vegetable, for example, bring to the diet?

Looking at the chart on the next page, we see that a cup of cooked broccoli contains 40 calories, but it contains over four grams of protein. Therefore, from this point of view, broccoli is a rather "high protein" food. It contains more than one gram of protein for every ten calories. If one ate enough broccoli in a day to supply his 2,000 calories, he would have taken in over 200 grams of protein, much more than necessary

---

* Some estimates are of 5% of calories as protein which would be about 25 g of protein for a 2,000 calorie diet. Others are 15% which would be 75—a middle of the road position would be 10% of calories as protein—or 50 g for 2,000 calories. Such a ratio is probably reasonable until one reduces caloric intake to 25-50% of what he's actually using. At this point efficiency of protein utilization drops and larger percentages must be supplied.[85] Therefore, those on stringent weight loss diets need, as one may expect, more protein per calorie.

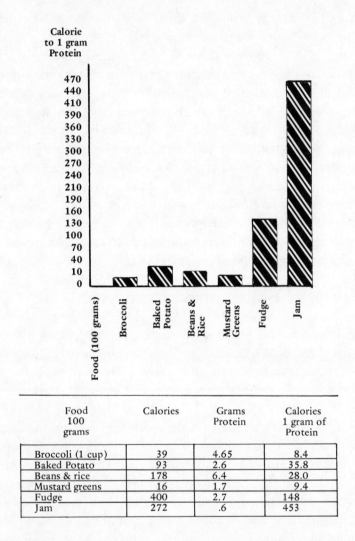

Food 100 grams	Calories	Grams Protein	Calories 1 gram of Protein
Broccoli (1 cup)	39	4.65	8.4
Baked Potato	93	2.6	35.8
Beans & rice	178	6.4	28.0
Mustard greens	16	1.7	9.4
Fudge	400	2.7	148
Jam	272	.6	453

by anyone's standards!

One baked potato contains 93 calories, but it also contains 2.6 grams of protein. Looking at the right column of the chart, we see that the ratio of calories to grams of protein is about 36 to 1. Potatoes then contain a barely adequate amount of protein. A plate of beans and rice (1 cup rice and ½ cup beans) will supply about 178 calories and 6.4 grams protein. That is 28 calories for each gram of protein—a very favorable ratio and one reason that combination is one of the world's most common sources of both energy and protein. Leafy greens by contrast are, like broccoli, surprisingly high in protein. A cup of cooked mustard greens contains 16 calories but 1.7 grams of protein, again a 10 to 1 ratio. A brief glance at the foods listed indicates that most of them actually have more than enough protein to maintain this ratio. It is perhaps for this reason that dieticians find it difficult to plan a diet of wholesome non-meat foods without going over protein allowances. Though constitutions vary and requirements are different from person to person, as long as food is not over-cooked or damaged, one can clearly get enough protein by eating whole, natural "non-protein" foods. The protein in fruits and vegetables is often ignored, not being considered enough to bother with. When most people calculate the protein in their diets they only count milk, meat, eggs, fish, etc. As one can see, however, when all the "hidden" sources of protein in the diet are added up, the sum is impressive.

The only catch here is that as soon as there is a departure from a diet of whole, natural food and, for example, a piece of fudge or two is taken or a bit of jam with bread, one is in trouble. A piece of fudge has 150 calories for every gram of protein. A tablespoon of jam will give one essentially no protein for its 50 calories. As soon as one eats such sweets, he has destroyed the balance. An immediate nutrient "debt" is incurred. In this case it is a "protein debt."* Several hundred calories have been taken with absolutely no protein. If this is done too often in a day, one will never be able to restore the balance and pay off the "nutrient debt" by eating those whole fruits, vegetables, grains and beans which are richest in protein. He must instead resort

---

*   And in the case of sugar or refined flour, a vitamin and mineral debt, as we shall see later.

to concentrated protein foods like cheese, eggs or meat in an effort to get the amount of protein needed.

It has become increasingly accepted in the West that a vegetarian diet can be very nutritious as long as one avoids "calories only" foods such as sugars, refined starches, fats and oils and alcohol. If these are taken in large amounts, one will find it necessary to resort to meat as a concentrated source of protein and other nutrients despite its disadvantages and liabilities. It supplies the protein, but ordinarily at the expense of considerable fat, which comes along with it. And the content of other nutrients such as minerals or vitamins in meat is variable. B_{12} supplements or yeast containing B_{12} may be necessary if one omits all traces of milk and eggs.* Small amounts of milk products may be advisable, but it's best to rely for the bulk of one's protein on one or two good servings a day of high protein vegetable foods, especially combinations of grains and legumes.

THE PROTEIN SPARING DIET

Protein is a structural tissue, and even in healthy adults there is no protein storage such as exists for fats and carbohydrates. Getting the right amount of protein regularly is therefore very important. When this fails, many problems will follow as is sometimes the case when people go on very restricted diets to lose weight. If they eliminate too much protein, they must begin to break down vital tissues to supply what is missing. The supply of fuel, of course, is still adequate, since fat stores remain to be used. But the body also requires carbohydrate, e.g., to keep the blood sugar up. Certain organs, like the brain, demand carbohydrate rather than fat. Since carbohydrate cannot be made from fat, it will be made from protein unless carbohydrate is eaten. For this reason dietary protein should always be accompanied by carbohydrate in the same meal, if

---

* See Chapter 7, Vitamins.

it is to be used most effectively. This is called the "protein sparing action" of a carbohydrate. When this is neglected, as during starvation or when fasting is done improperly, e.g., taking only water,* then tissues must be broken down, both to provide the carbohydrate needed as well as to provide protein.† Of course, at such times other nutrients are needed, too, such as vitamins and minerals. Concern with protein requirements, or eagerness to reduce dietary fat and carbohydrate sometimes leads one to go on extreme diets that ignore his needs for the "micronutrients" which, as we shall see, play a strategic and fascinating role in human nutrition.

* See Chapter 12, Fasting.
† See Chapter 17, Interaction between Diet and Mind.

Vitamins

7

Carbohydrate, fat and protein: these are the bulk of man's diet. Excluding fiber, together they make up 98% of the dry weight of what we eat, but what comprises the other 2%? In order to answer this question, man's way of life had to become artificial enough to create a situation where all the necessary nutrients would not be present. Such unplanned experiments as this occurred in the Middle Ages when walled cities were under siege and encircled by hostile forces. The lack of fresh provisions and the inability to obtain a balanced diet could then produce dramatic pictures of deterioration and death.

Around this time, in the early 1500's, the full development of the mast and sail began to make long ocean voyages possible, and deficiency diseases became widespread, vivid and well known. For the first time, a group of men was separated for a protracted period of time from contact with the earth, plants and a fresh supply of food. It was an accidental but bold experiment in dietary deprivation done up on a grand scale. A non-perishable diet had to be developed, and the standard ration in the British Royal Navy was designed to supply 4,000 calories a day. It consisted of a pound of "hardbread" biscuits, about a pound of salt meat or dried fish, several ounces of butter, cheese or dried peas and a gallon of beer. This provided ample quantities of fat, carbohydrate and protein, all the food elements thought necessary to maintain good health. Yet during the twenty years of Queen Elizabeth's reign, it was estimated that the lives of 10,000 men on Her Majesty's ships were claimed by a dread disease called scurvy.

One of the clearest descriptions of this illness was written by James Lind, who was a naval surgeon during the reign of Queen Elizabeth. The "seafaring men who fell sick of the scurvy had rotten gums, loose teeth, hard and swoolen cheeks, painful jaws and breath of a filthy savor." Their legs were cold, hard, swollen and so feeble that "they were scarce able to carry their bodies."[1] They were full of aches and pains and their skin was splotched with large purplish bruises. Many writers of that era mention treating these complaints by administering a green leafy plant called "scurvy grass." Lind also used ale in which watercress had been cooked, as well as fresh currants, raisins and grape juice. These treatments were found to cure the symptoms of scurvy. The effects of fresh vegetables on the horrors of scurvy showed the nautical experimenters that a lack of contact with fresh plants could not be extended indefinitely.

The following passage from *Two Years Before the Mast* describes the reaction to a large supply of fresh onions and potatoes by a crew which had been a long time at sea and deprived of all but the hard biscuit and salt meat. The onions and potatoes were a Godsend.

> We ate them raw, and a glorious treat they were. We were perfectly ravenous after them, but their chief use was for the men with scurvy. One of them was hardly able to open his mouth, and so the cook took the potatoes raw, pounded them, and gave him the juice to drink. After drinking it, a shuddering and an acute pain ran through all parts of his body, but he persevered, and, so rapid was his recovery that after ten days he was at the masthead furling a royal.

Advances in technology were simultaneously making similar grim experiments possible on the other side of the world. Japan, another small island country, had also developed a mighty naval force, and Japanese ships were likewise venturing far and wide. The Japanese had, like the British, inadvertently launched another large-scale experiment in basic nutrition. The results were tragic. In many cases, two-thirds of the crew was found to be afflicted with a wasting and fatal disease called beri-beri. A change in diet was found to prevent this problem and the Japanese discovered, as had the British, that something else besides fat, carbohydrate and protein was needed in the diet.

In 1906, Sr. Frederick Galen Hopkins published an article which proposed that besides these basic elements, small quantities of some unknown "accessory nutrients" must also be required for the maintenance of good health. Six years later, in 1912, one of these, the substance that could prevent beri-beri, was isolated from rice polish by a Polish chemist. Since it was vital for the preservation of life and was an amine (amino acid-like substance) it was called "vitamine."

Scientists were finding it easy to reproduce such dietary deficiencies using pigeons in the laboratory. A contorted and convulsing bird may be near to death, "but if one takes a glass tube, puts into it the pulp of some sprouting pulse or grain, pries open the pigeon's beak, and blows the pulp down its throat, the miracle happens. In a very short time the pigeon is its usual self, on its perch, and preening its ruffled feathers."[2] The tiny amount of the "vitamine" present in a little bit of sprouted grain could reverse the otherwise fatal disease. Small wonder that these new and miraculous compounds would capture the public's imagination. When so little of a substance can dramatically rescue one from the jaws of death, its power is apparent.

In view of our earlier discussions, the existence of these substances should not be surprising. If it is true that the animal cell and the plant cell evolved together, it seems reasonable to expect that the animal cell would not develop the biochemical equipment necessary to synthesize what is already present in his plant food. The plant cell, then, contains something essential which man can't manufacture. In the years that followed, other such substances were to come to light as man's inquiring mind gradually identified one by one the multiplicity of nutrients that together make up a healthful diet.

VITAMIN A (RETINOL)

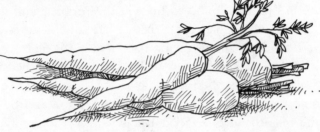

By 1912, Hopkins had shown that young rats died when given a diet of only protein, starch, sugar, fat and inorganic salts, but thrived when less than half a teaspoon of milk a day was added to their food. In this milk, he concluded, was some "accessory food factor" which was responsible for life. Laboratory scientists around the world began to search for this mysterious food factor. Within a year, two groups of American researchers had extracted a fat-soluble substance from butter, egg yolks and fish livers which promoted growth in rats. If it was taken out of the diet, the animals' eyes became diseased.

Two years later another team of scientists separated the water solution from rice bran which though it contained no fat, carbohydrate, or protein, reversed beri-beri. To distinguish the two food factors, the substance that had been extracted from butter and fish liver was called "fat-soluble A" while the second was called "water-soluble B." Five years later the term "vitamin A" was attached to the first and when it was finally identified, it was named "retinol" because of its importance to vision and the role that it plays in the retina.

NIGHT BLINDNESS

Vision occurs when light from the outside passes through the lens and strikes a light-sensitive cell located in the retina. Inside this cell is a special molecule called a photopigment made by the combination of a protein and retinol. Light breaks this down, initiating a nerve impulse that registers in the brain. One of the photopigments, "visual purple" or "rhodopsin," is found only in the rod-shaped cells. At night when we have trouble making out distinct objects, we sometimes find ourselves looking a bit to one side, focusing the light away from the center of the eye where receptors for bright light are located and toward the outside where the rods are.

In the center of the retina is where the light is normally focused during the day for color and detail. The eye can be thought of as similar to the headlights of an automobile, with two separate systems—one for bright light and one for dim. The system for dim light is the more primitive, and its receptor cells, the rods, register small quantities of light. To our prehistoric ancestors as well as to ourselves, this has had great survival potential. First, it permits vision at night, and second, it will be the most sensitive to visual stimuli from the periphery, where one is most vulnerable.

The cone receptors or color system, located at the center of the retina and used in bright daylight, is a more modern evolutionary achievement. When the lights are dimmed and the color receptors don't work, we fall back on our more primitive black and white system. It's functioning depends on the ability to quickly replace the pigment in the rods, rhodopsin, which in turn depends on vitamin A (retinol). Rhodopsin, bleached out and used up during its reaction to light, begins to dwindle if the vitamin A needed to make it is missing in the diet. At this point, a flash of light, like the headlights of a passing car, blinds us and we do not very quickly regain our vision. This difficulty is called "night-blindness," and has been described since ancient times.

An Egyptian medical papyrus of 1,500 BC mentions night-blindness and recommends the liver of black cocks or roast ox-liver as a remedy, as did Hippocrates. Fish liver oil is used today as one source of vitamin A. Most animals store vitamin A in the liver and some polar animals store such huge quantities that eating liver from them can be extremely toxic. Whereas ox liver may contain up to 45,000 International Units (IU)* of vitamin A per 100 grams, cod-liver oil contains up to 400,000 IU and polar bear liver may contain as much as 1,800, 000 IU. Arctic explorers who ignored the advice of the Eskimos and ate polar bear liver came down with abdominal pain, nausea, vomiting and a severe headache. A day or two later there was a generalized peeling of all the skin and a full recovery. One such serving (8 oz) of polar bear liver would be equal to 480 vitamin A capsules of the usual 10,000 IU size.

Since it is in the liver where vitamin A is stored, healthy individuals have been shown to store large quantities of vitamin A (retinol) there, a sufficient amount to meet requirements for months or even years without taking in any through the diet.[3] When dietary intake is consistently low for a long period of time, however, liver stores can be exhausted. In autopsy measurements done in America, it was found that as many as twenty to thirty percent of people had low stores of vitamin A.[4]

This widespread depletion of liver stores of vitamin A in the United States is probably explained by an inadequate dietary intake. A survey of people in ten states carried out by the

---

* One IU equals 0.3 mcg of retinol. The quantity of a vitamin is sometimes stated in units, and sometimes in metric weight, (e.g., milligrams). Because of the way vitamins were discovered, the activity of foods containing them was often measured before the exact identity of the active compound was known. A certain quantity of the food that produced the vitamin effect was designated as a "unit," and other foods were standardized against this. Often such units were named after the different investigators who originated them, but gradually international units were adopted. The chemical nature of the vitamins is now known, however, and scientists generally prefer to measure them in milligrams or micrograms. But in some cases, like vitamins A and E, it is convenient to stay with the familiar IU for non-technical purposes.

Department of Health, Education and Welfare in 1968-1970 showed substandard intakes of vitamin A in pregnant women, in people over sixty years of age, and in a large percentage of teenagers and infants.[5]   Such a pervasive dietary deficiency of vitamin A is of great interest because vitamin A has recently been shown to have something to do with resistance to infection and perhaps even to the development of cancer.

VITAMIN A AND INFECTION

When one group of mice were treated with four consecutive daily injections of 3,000 IU of vitamin A and then injected with different strains of virulent bacteria and fungi, 90% of the vitamin A treated mice survived while only about 35% of those unprotected lived. When the same bacteria were grown on a culture plate, adding vitamin A had no effect on their growth. It was clear then that vitamin A must induce some resistance on the part of the host to infection.[6]   In fact, a correlation between vitamin A deficiency and an increased frequency of respiratory infections or gastrointestinal infections in humans has recently been found.[7]

Even as early as the 1930's, it was known that vitamin A deficiency had something to do with susceptibility to infection. In 1934, Sir Edward Mellanby described in his book *Nutrition and Disease* an experiment in which rats were fed a diet deficient in vitamin A. Almost all had "areas of infection." The most frequent site of the infection was the urinary organs, after which came the ears, nose and last the stomach and intestines and lungs. "If a source of vitamin A such as butter, cod-liver oil or egg yolk formed a part of the diet," infections were never seen in the rats. Adding such foods to the deficient diets, unless the animals were too severely ill generally resulted in rapid improvement and ultimate cure."[8]

It is interesting to note that all of these infections occurred in the protective covering of the body, not the outer skin of which we're accustomed to think, but rather the "inner skin," the lining or mucous membranes that serve as a barrier between oneself and what he comes in contact with inside, such as the air he has inhaled or the food he has swallowed. These mucous membranes line the respiratory passages, the gastrointestinal tract, the urinary passages and even, of course, the eyes, ears and nose, protecting against invasion and infection. A major site of vitamin A's action seems to be such protective barriers, both internal and external. Externally, vitamin A is related to the health of the skin whose primary function is that of protection. It even seems to have a special function in those sense organs whose purpose is to serve as a sensory interface with the outside world: the eyes and the ears. These are also, in a sense, protections or barriers.

Social Barriers

Of all the protective barriers of the body, the face is probably the most strategic interchange between man and his social environment. Teenagers, particularly during their years of awkward readjustment, are prone to develop acne of the face. This condition may in part be due to the endocrinologic changes of adolescence, but it is unlikely that these are the only important factors since it often occurs even in adults who are having problems adjusting to social relationships.

All the coverings and linings of the body are made up of a tough, resilient sheath of several layers of cells called "epithelium." The skin—the outer coating of the body—is made up of a dry epithelium, one whose surface is covered with layers of thin, flattened cells that become relatively dry and seal off the moist inner layers. This outer layer can sometimes scale or flake, but it normally remains relatively stable and gives the skin its smooth, dry texture. When the skin becomes unhealthy with, for example, the build-up of squamous cells that plug the pores, then there is an accumulation of oils and the resulting infection of these clogged pores is called "acne." Both unhealthy epithelium and an increased susceptibility to infection can be related to vitamin A deficiency, and, not surprisingly, vitamin A has been found to improve acne.

Teenagers, as we have seen, are a group whose diet is often deficient in vitamin A, but acne may not be due to a simple dietary deficiency of it. Zinc is necessary for the stored vitamin A in the liver to be released into the blood,[9] and in the treatment of acne, zinc has been even more effective than vitamin A.[10]

VITAMIN A AND CANCER

Inside the body, the linings of the gastrointestinal tract, lungs, etc., are made up of cells different from the flat, scale-like "squamous" cells covering the skin. Instead of being flattened and layered, cells of the inner linings are deep and lined up in vertical rows like columns. Many of them are specialized to secrete mucus, which helps them maintain a moist surface. When vitamin A is deficient, the inner, moist, columnar, mucus-secreting epithelium may lose its ability to maintain itself, and areas shift or degenerate into thin layered cells, much as are found on the surface of the outer skin. In medical terms this is called "squamous metaphasia," meaning that the cells become flattened when they should not be.

This becomes important when we discover that the cervix or entrance to the uterus is lined with glandular epithelium. When these cells shift and begin to become more flattened and squamous in nature, then they are detected as unusual on the "Pap smear," and the patient is told that she has "atypical cells" or is in danger of developing cancer. In fact, the common form of cancer of the cervix, one of the most frequent malignant diseases in women, is simply an overdevelopment of invasive squamous cells.

It has recently been shown that squamous cell cancer could easily be produced in vitamin A deficient experimental animals, whereas giving vitamin A protected them to some extent against this.[11]   These findings are interesting in view of the low intake of vitamin A in the United States and the frequent depletion of its stores.   An association between low intake of vitamin A and lung cancer, the most common cancer occurring in men, has also been reported.[12]   Lung cancer usually arises in the epithelial linings of the respiratory tract by a process of "squamous metaplasia" similar to that which results in cancer of the cervix in women.

This does not mean that everyone should dash out and buy a big bottle of vitamin A capsules. Success with experimental animals does not prove conclusively that more vitamin A will prevent cervical and lung cancer in humans. Besides, "to increase everyone's intake of vitamin A irrespective of their requirement for the vitamin might do more harm than good."[13] Rather, it is important for each person to try to understand how much vitamin A is appropriate to his or her diet. Unfortunately, this matter is not so easy to settle as one might think.

NOT ENOUGH OR TOO MUCH?

Over forty years ago, a large company in America offered a reward to any investigator who could determine the vitamin A requirement of human beings.   Thirteen years later, the judges advised the donors to withdraw the award because no one was able to clearly define the optimal daily requirement. In 1966, one prominent researcher made a fresh attempt and did an experiment on 200 rats. He concluded that, "the variation in rat needs is not a mere 25%, 50% or 100%, but much larger, perhaps forty-fold or more.   Some rats at the lower levels of vitamin A intake gained very little weight, and several died within a few weeks."   Yet others survived and were healthy.   Each group, whether the doses given to it were high or low, had some animals which were healthy and well developed.   "From the standpoint of vigor and appearance, the healthiest animals from the various groups[14] could not be distinguished from each other." In other words, the dose of vitamin A which was life-saving for one rat might be many times more than is needed by another. In fact, it is possible to conjecture from this data that what is a vitamin A requirement for one person might be near toxic for another. This would seem then, to leave one in quite a quandary.

Actually, there is a simple solution: carotene, which is found in vegetables and which the body is able to convert into vitamin A, does not have the tendency to accumulate or to cause toxicity.[15] Carotenes, so named because of their prominence in carrots, are widely distributed in nature and serve as pigments, lending a bright orange, yellow or red color. Not all of the carotene-like pigments can be transformed into vitamin A. Recent research has demonstrated that the body selectively absorbs beta carotene, the most useful of the carotene pigments when green and yellow fruits and vegetables are eaten.[16] This is important for vegetarians since meat-free diets are low in pre-formed vitamin A. Most of it must therefore come from the conversion of beta carotene. Even in Europe and America where most people are meat eaters, it has been estimated that half the vitamin A comes from this source.[17] Surprisingly, green leafy vegetables are even richer in useable carotenes than are carrots.[18] This is because carotene has a particular predilection for cholorphyll. In view of all of this, it is not surprising to find that clinically one of the most successful remedies for facial acne is a daily intake of fresh carrot juice or the juice of a combination of fresh carrots and green leafy vegetables. Though massive doses of carotene may bring a yellow tinge to the skin, this can be distinguished from a true jaundice since the whites of the eyes are unaffected.

Preformed vitamin A is different. Cases of toxicity, resulting from preformed vitamin A, usually taken as capsules of the concentrated supplement, rather than in animal foods, have been described in children and adults in both acute and chronic forms. Acute symptoms usually develop from one large dose, and generally pass off with no permanent effect. Chronic intoxication, however, may be more serious. Most patients who have suffered from chronic vitamin A intoxication have taken at least 50,000 units of vitamin A a day for a long period of time.* The principle symptoms of chronic vitamin A intoxication are bone or joint pain, fatigue and insomnia, loss of hair, dryness and fissuring of the lips and epithelial involvement, loss of appetite and weight and liver enlargement. Usually relief is prompt and nearly complete when vitamin A is stopped.[19] However, if long term vitamin A overdose occurs during child-hood, it may cause premature closure of the epiphyses of the bones, limiting their normal growth.[20] Furthermore, congenital anomalies can be produced in the offspring of rats who are receiving very large doses of vitamin A. In all of these cases, it should be noted, the untoward results were produced by giving preformed vitamin A (retinol), and there is no indication that there is any risk whatever as long as one's source of vitamin A is beta carotene (i.e., vegetable foods).

VITAMIN B COMPLEX

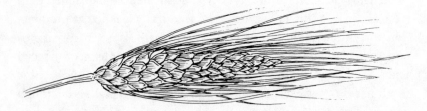

When "fat-soluble A" became "vitamin A," the water soluble extract from rice polishings which had the power to

---

* This amounts to five standard 10,000 IU capsules of vitamin A.

reverse beri-beri began to be called vitamin B. The scurvy-preventing factor in lemon juice, which would not be isolated and identified for another twenty years, was called vitamin C and the factor which could prevent rickets was called vitamin D. A new idea was gaining ground: there were substances, probably simple chemical compounds, present in food, tiny amounts of which were necessary for health. Moreover, when these substances were absent from the diet there occurred definite diseases. No doubt there would emerge for many of the great disease pictures a single compound or "vitamin" which would have the power to reverse and cure.

Though the theory was shaping up, scientists still had not identified the water soluble anti-beri-beri compound present in rice polishings. It had been found, however, that the water soluble "B" could be separated into two parts: one which was easily destroyed by heat and one which was not. The heat resistant factor failed to cure beri-beri but still had the power to reverse certain symptoms of deficiency. It was called vitamin B_2, while the term "B_1" was reserved for the anti-beri-beri compound which was as yet unidentified. Actually, this was only the beginning. As we shall see, the heat-resistant fraction turned out to contain a number of substances, so soon there was a vitamin B_3, B_4, B_5, etc. Up to the present time, twenty-five B vitamins have been identified, though in many cases the terms were later discarded, either because the substances so designated turned out not to be essential or because they were found to be identical with others which had already been recognized and named.

The term "B complex" continues to be useful, however, since to a great extent these substances are found together in nature. Those foods which are rich in one member of the B vitamin complex are very likely to be rich in several of the others. Consequently, pure deficiencies of a single B vitamin are rare in man.[21] Moreover, since the functions of various groups of B vitamins are often closely related, the symptoms of deficiency of the different members of the group overlap to some extent in terms of the enzyme systems which are involved. Since the functions of various groups of B vitamins are often closely related, deficiencies of the B complex are especially likely to result in malfunctions of the nervous system. Anemia is also likely to occur. A sore mouth with cracks at the corner, a burning sensation inside the mouth and a tongue which is swollen, shiny, purple and cracked are all symptoms of vitamin B deficiency. Others are breathlessness, mental problems, defects in memory, insomnia, dizziness, headache, lack of appetite, weakness in the legs, lethargy and burning sensations in the feet.

Probably the richest source of the B complex is the germ and the bran of seeds such as cereals, nuts, beans, peas, etc. Leafy green vegetables and milk are also good sources. Some meats such as pork contain significant quantities of some B vitamins, while other meats, such as beef, are extremely low. Liver of almost any kind, however, tends to contain high quantities of the B vitamins and is one of their richest sources. For those who do not wish to take animal food or who are leary of eating liver because of its tendency to concentrate contaminants from the environment, nutritional yeast, if properly grown, is a rich source of all the B vitamins. Unfortunately, research has shown that taking large quantities of yeast can also create problems. Uric acid levels have been elevated after taking three tablespoonsful of yeast (45 grams) a day.[22] This could lead to such problems as gout, especially in those individuals who already have a tendency toward that. If one wishes to use yeast as a dietary supplement it should usually be limited to one or two tablespoons a day.

Moreover, the exact vitamin and protein content of nutritional yeast will vary according to the strain of the yeast and its freedom from harmful contaminants will depend on the kind of substance on which it is grown. Some yeasts contain adequate amounts of B_{12}, for example, while others contain none at all. It is more important, if one wishes to take yeast as a supplement,

to have a complete analysis of its vitamin content to make sure
that it contains all of the vitamins for which it is being taken.

B_1, THIAMIN

In 1926, pure crystalline thiamin was finally isolated and
proved to be the anti-beri-beri factor in water-soluble B that had
so long eluded researchers. Beri-beri has always been thought to
be primarily a disease of rice eaters and endemic in the Far East.
Actually, it is not widespread among all rice eaters but only
among those who have for one reason or another adopted the
practice of eating polished rice. Even so, as we have seen, this is
not true in India where large portions of the population subsist
on polished rice. Here beri-beri is essentially unknown because
tradition dictates that the rice be boiled before it is milled.
Twentieth century researchers have found that this ancient process drives the B complex from the bran into the center of the
grain. After this, though the bran may be removed during milling,
the B complex, including thiamin, largely remains in the rice.[23]
On the other hand, outbreaks of beri-beri have also been
documented in wheat eaters. This has happened when people
were cut off through a long winter from sources of fresh provisions and their stores consisted mainly of refined wheat flour.
Such was the case, for example, in 1916, when the Third Indian
Division was besieged by the Turks at Kut-el-Amara. During this
siege, the Indians ate whole wheat chappatis and remained well.
The British troops, however, ate white bread made from refined
white flour and beri-beri broke out amongst them.*

Beri-beri in the Emergency Room

Though photos of exhausted Orientals or prisoners of war

---

* In the U.S. today, this would not happen of course, since white flour is "enriched"
with added thiamin.

who have swollen limbs might immediately bring to mind the diagnosis of beri-beri, this disorder is not ordinarily thought of when a patient with high blood pressure and heart failure enters the emergency room in a Western hospital. Such symptoms, however, along with swelling and accumulation of fluid in the limbs, are typical of the wet form of beri-beri. Some patients who responded poorly to the usual treatments for heart failure have improved dramatically as soon as thiamin was adminis- tered in large doses,[24] suggesting that thiamin deficiency may be at the root of some of these cases.

A second variety of beri-beri is called "dry beri-beri." In this case, there is no swelling or accumulation of fluid in the arms and legs. The primary effect seems to be on the nervous system. The nerves to the limbs often degenerate and there results a wasting of the muscles. The thin, wasted, nearly paralyzed arms and legs are another familiar feature of classical prisoner-of-war beri-beri. Before the disease has reached this advanced stage, however, the symptoms are less dramatic. One early sign is a sort of numbness of "pins and needles" sensation found in the legs which may be diagnosed as "peripheral neuropathy." Though it is often attributed to diabetes, alcoholism or advancing age and is generally not considered treatable, thiamin may help.

A third thiamin deficiency disease involves degeneration of the brain (the Wernicke-Korsakoff syndrome). Symptoms include unsteadiness, a staggering gait, and a state of disorienta- tion and apathy. The disease progresses to the point of death unless thiamin is supplied, but to be effective, it must be given early in the disease and in high doses.

Anxiety and Neurosis

The above, of course, are pictures of extreme thiamin deficiency, but research suggests that less dramatic symptoms can result from a continual low intake of thiamin. Some years back, a group of research workers at the Mayo Clinic put eight subjects on 0.15 mg of thiamin per day. (This is equivalent to about one-sixth of the recommended minimum daily requirement). The result resembled what is commonly called "anxiety neurosis," though there was a gradual worsening, ending in an even more severe state.

Later, in a similar experiment, thiamin intake was restricted only as far as 0.45 mgs., about half the minimum daily requirement. Surveys had shown that this level of thiamin intake was frequently found in American diets. The diet given in the experiment was hardly unusual. It was white bread, corn flakes, potatoes, polished rice, sugar, skim milk, beef, cheese, egg white, gelatin, butter, vegetable fat, canned fruit, canned vegetables, coffee and cocoa. Within eight to twelve weeks, most of the patients showed a disinclination to be active and an inability to adjust in a group. There were "unmistakable, easily demonstrated changes in personality which were reflected in attitude, behavior and effectiveness in performing tasks which previously had been performed readily. All subjects became irritable, depressed, quarrelsome, uncooperative and, without knowing why, fearful that some misfortune awaited them." Two of the patients became very disturbed and threatened suicide. "All became inefficient in their work . . . all subjects lost manual dexterity. Their hands and feet frequently felt numb." The authors concluded that physical and mental efficiency as well as a sense of well-being were maintained when one mg of thiamin per day, the RDA* was provided.[25]

It is interesting to note that all the subjects in this study had previously been treated in the Rochester State Hospital for psychiatric illness. Though they had been considered recovered, one cannot help wondering if such persons might not be especially susceptible to the effects of a lower intake of thiamin. In fact, experiments since then have demonstrated clearly that the

* Recommended Daily Allowance. This and other figures are based on RDA as proposed by the Food and Nutrition Board, National Academy of Science, National Research Council.

thiamin requirements of persons vary.[26]

Sources, External and Internal

Nine young men were put on a diet of purified protein, vegetable shortening, sugar and a mineral and vitamin mixture so that their thiamin intake could be gradually decreased. After they had remained on very tiny doses (0.2 mg a day) for months without exhibiting any neuritis, edema, loss of appetite or vomiting, thiamin was cut out altogether. In the course of the next month, only four of the nine youths developed an obvious deficiency disorder. Another was borderline but the remaining four showed no signs of deficiency even when the experiment was continued another seven weeks. This puzzled the researchers. In the first place it seemed surprising that persons could go so long on such a low intake of thiamin. But after such a gradual depletion, to remain perfectly well for seven weeks with no thiamin at all seemed unbelievable. Looking for possible sources of thiamin in these "resistant" individuals, the investigators analyzed their feces. They found that on the average those who remained well had about twenty times as much free thiamin in the stool as the others. Apparently thiamin was being manufactured by the intestinal microbes.[27] We may conclude that considerable variation exists between people as far as their thiamin requirements go, and this difference may be based at least in part on differences in their intestinal microbes which, as we shall see later, are extremely important. Antibiotics can upset the balance of bacteria in the colon, and could in this way play some part in B vitamin deficiencies, perhaps making one more dependent on external sources.

Thiamin, the original heat-susceptible factor in "water soluble B," is of course both susceptible to destruction by cooking and easily dissolved in the cooking water. Therefore, much thiamin is lost by discarding cooking water. Baking powder and soda also destroy thiamin in muffins, breads and cakes.[28] Beef is relatively low in thiamin—a hamburger containing only an unmeasurable trace. Even a glass of milk will contain only a 1/10 of a milligram. Pork, however, is remarkably rich in thiamin, one reason perhaps, why the Chinese are so fond of adding bits of pork to their polished rice dishes. Though the daily minimum requirement of thiamin is thought to be only a milligram a day, it is easy to see how many people could get less than this. Since an excess cannot be stored in the body and since thiamin is crucial to the metabolism of carbohydrate, the ratio of this vitamin to carbohydrate in the diet is important. It makes sense to take carbohydrate foods along with their proper complement of thiamin. Such considerations, along with the widespread deficiency of the vitamin in a diet based on beef, canned fruits and vegetables and refined grains, led in 1941 to the mandatory enrichment of flour by adding thiamin. This has helped offset its lack in refined flour so that the effects of taking an overprocessed diet do not show up as the symptoms of thiamin deficiency. Sugar and sweets, however, are not "enriched" with thiamin, and among those who avoid breads in order to lose weight but go on sugar binges, the weakness, irritability and "neurotic" symptoms of thiamin deficiency are not uncommon.

B$_2$, RIBOFLAVIN

Riboflavin is another vitamin which has been shown to be sometimes synthesized by intestinal organisms, supplying enough of it to meet one's needs.[29] Intestinal synthesis may explain why dietary deficiency of riboflavin, an important constituent of a tissue oxidation co-enzyme, does not produce more dramatic symptoms. Many nutritionists have been puzzled by the infrequent appearance of severe riboflavin deficiencies, especially in view of the fact that nutritional surveys show that riboflavin intakes are often substandard.[30] Sir Stanley Davidson, a British authority on nutrition, notes that there are many people who live for long periods on a very low intake of riboflavin. Though minor signs of deficiency are common in many parts of the world, why these conditions do not progress and lead to a serious illness remains a mystery[31] in view of the importance of riboflavin to cell respiration. Whereas thiamine deficiency produces the classical picture of beri-beri and vitamin C deficiency produces classical scurvy, there is no dramatic, life-threatening disease that emerges when riboflavin is restricted in the diet. It has been shown, however, that riboflavin levels were very low in some children with heart disease,[32] and it is still possible that a lack of it plays a subtle part not yet identified in some other diseases.

Symptoms of riboflavin deficiency are cracking and peeling of the lower lip with splitting at the corners of the mouth. It has also been suggested that vertical wrinkles, radiating up from the upper lip, as well as "disappearance" of the upper lip are related to riboflavin deficiency.[33] Riboflavin is also important in the health of the eyes, and sensitivity to light is one symptom of riboflavin deficiency. When volunteers stay on diets low in riboflavin for some time, they develop a greasy scaling on the chin, forehead and especially in the creases between the nose and cheek [34] as well as little whiteheads accumulating under the skin.

The richest sources of riboflavin are brewers yeast and organ meats, but milk contains significant quantities, as do whole grains, especially wheat and dried beans and peas and seeds such as sunflower seeds. Leafy green vegetables can also provide generous amounts of riboflavin.

B_3, NIACIN

Pellagra is another of the serious, widespread diseases seen where diets are poor. The picture of pellagra is one to rival scurvy and beri-beri in its severity. It is sometimes called "the disease of the 4D's:" dermatitis, diarrhea, dementia and death, since the major symptoms of pellagra are found on the skin, in the bowels and in the mind, and since, if untreated, it is ultimately fatal.

Perhaps the most important symptoms are those involving the nervous system. In mild cases they may be only weakness, tremor, anxiety, depression and irritability. In the more severe and acute cases, however, there is a more dramatic disturbance, with the classical signs of acute psychosis. But physical symptoms can be serious, too. Digestive upset is usual and diarrhea is common. Cracks appear in the corners of the mouth and the tongue looks like raw beef. A disordered stomach with a lowered level of stomach acid is also common and worms may invade the gastro-intestinal tract. There is often a redness of the skin resembling severe sunburn which appears on all parts of the body exposed to sunlight. The skin there becomes rough and thick and dry, hence the Italian name *pelle agra* which means literally, "skin that is rough." This can be seen especially on the backs of the hands, on the face and most strikingly on the neck. The classical "redneck" appearance sometimes seen in poor white rural southerners who have spent long hours in the sun may be related to this disease since deficient diets in that part of the USA were historically associated with a high incidence of pellagra.

By the first decades of the 1900's, pellagra was appearing regularly among such impoverished people, especially where corn (maize) made up the principle part of the diet. By the twenties and thirties, it was so widespread in the Southeastern United States that it seemed to be an epidemic and for this reason it was thought that pellagra might be an infectious disease. The Federal government sent a physician, Dr. Goldberger, to investigate, but he established clearly that the origin of the disease was nutritional, not infectious, and he demonstrated that it could be cured with a boiled extract of yeast. This was an awkward treatment, but it worked. What it was in this extract that did the job, however, remained a mystery. Obviously, it was water-soluble and resistant to heat. But all efforts to separate out the active compound were in vain, so it was simply called the "PP factor" (pellagra-preventing factor). When riboflavin was finally isolated from the heat-resistant B, it was naturally assumed that this was the substance that would cure pellagra, and it was eagerly used to treat the disease. But the researchers were in for a disappointment. Their B_2, purified riboflavin, had no effect on pellagra.

Years went by. Pellagra ran rampant not only in the southeastern United States but also in Italy, South Africa and India. Identification of the pure compound that could reverse the disease and that might be cheaply synthesized eluded researchers. The answer came only with the rediscovery of nicotinic acid, a compound which had been isolated and discarded a full twenty years earlier during the search for the anti-beri-beri factor. It was this nicotinic acid which turned out to be the "PP" or pellagra-preventing factor, providing a long-awaited, simple and inexpensive treatment for a disease which had reached such epidemic proportions. Because it was present in the water-soluble B after B_1 and B_2 were removed, it was soon dubbed "B_3."

But actually, the history of nicotinic acid goes back much further. It was first produced in 1867 by oxidizing nicotine, the principle alkaloid found in the leaves of the tobacco plant, imported from America to France by Count Nicotin whose name it took. Much later, in 1942, the term niacin (which is an abbreviation for *Ni*cotinic *Ac*id vitam*in*) was originated so that there would be no confusion between the nutrient and tobacco.

Niacin is found in large quantities in organ meats, peanuts and in brewer's yeast, Goldberger's standard treatment of pellagra until the discovery of niacin. Niacin is also found in large quantities in whole grains and in significant quantities in dried beans and peas. But the human body is not completely dependent upon outside sources of niacin since it can be manufactured from one of the essential amino acids, tryptophan. In a sense, then, it is not a "vitamin" at all, as, strictly speaking, it is not necessary for it to be present in the diet. What is needed can be made by the body if there is a high intake of the kind of protein that contains ample quantities of this amino acid. Unfortunately, some of the foods which are low in niacin such as corn (maize) are also low in tryptophan.

Niacin and Corn

Surprisingly, however, the amount of niacin found in corn is not particularly low. In fact, whole corn may contain more niacin than other grains such as oats. Nevertheless, as we have seen, pellagra has been almost uniformly a disease of corn eaters, much as beri-beri has been most often a disease of rice eaters. Once more, however, this is a result, not of any intrinsic defect in the grain itself, but rather in the failure to prepare it properly. The niacin in corn is found in a bound form and is not available for absorption unless it is properly prepared. Much as the traditional cultures of the Orient understood the use of rice and used it either unmilled or milled after parboiling, so did the traditional cultures whose diet was based on maize cultivation understand its use.

Maize originated among the American Indians where it was the basis of their agriculture. Upon visiting America, Sir Walter Raleigh wrote:

> I tell thee 'tis a goodlie country, not wanting in victuals. On the banks of those rivers are divers fruits good to eat and game a plenty. Besides, the natives in those parts have a corne, which yields them bread; and this with little labor and in abundance. 'Tis called in the Spanish tongue "mahiz"[35]

Though various tribes of American Indians have consumed huge quantities of maize and in some cases have subsisted primarily on it, pellagra has been unknown among them. This is because the corn was customarily treated in a special way to release the niacin. Most often this was accomplished by soaking the grain in water that had been mixed with ashes. This ash water would soften the coating and make the niacin available for intestinal absorption. Sometimes the grain was pounded into a meal and then ash water was added. The result was not only to liberate niacin but also to add significant quantities of other useful minerals from the ash.[36] This was and still is the custom among some tribes in the southwestern states.

In the Southeastern United States, settlers learned this technique from the Indians, and a nineteenth century recipe for hominy runs—"Take a peck of good corn and add two quarts of hardwood ashes and soak overnight." A similar custom persists today in Mexico where lime water is added to soften corn and make it into a dough which can be patted into tortillas. This practice also makes niacin more available.[37, 38]

In the last 200 years, corn, or maize, has been adopted in the north of India, especially in Punjab, as part of the customary diet. A special chapatti is made from corn meal and served with mustard greens, a dish favored by native Americans as well as the Europeans who settled in the New World. In India it is recognized, however, that corn has a "vatic" tendency, which means that it tends to provoke mental instability if not prepared properly. This is remedied through certain cooking processes. For example, the fresh green ears, "corn on the cob," are boiled and then afterwards roasted in ghee. Perhaps the extreme heat which sears the part of the grain containing the bound niacin helps in some way to release it.

Just as industrialization made milled rice cheap and available in the Orient and paved the way for epidemic beriberi, so did the less expensive and more convenient commercially ground corn meal alter the cooking habits of the southeastern United States. Making hominy in the traditional way by soaking in an alkaline solution and cooking for hours was too time consuming. The pre-ground corn meal was cheap and easy to make into "quick corn bread." Where the economic situation was bad and other foods fell out of the diet, such corn meal often came to make up the bulk of the diet, but it was not able to sustain health.

Niacin as a Medicine

Patients with pellagra, especially those with mental symptoms, responded dramatically to niacin. This led eventually to the attempt to treat other severely disturbed psychiatric patients with niacin even though they did not have the classic signs of pellagra. When low doses approximating the usual daily intake produced no results, doses were pushed much higher—a hundred times more, for example. Then some patients showed definite improvement.* Subsequently, other disorders such as elevated blood cholesterol,[39] cholesterol deposits in the skin,[40] as well as similar deposits in the arteries to the legs that obstruct blood flow [41] have been successfully treated with extremely large or "mega" doses of niacin. Large doses of niacin prolong blood coagulation time, an effect which may be helpful in preventing heart attacks and strokes. [42] It has even been claimed that niacin can help regulate blood sugar level in hypoglycemic patients,[43] and it is the most frequently used nutrient in the "megavitamin" treatment of schizophrenia.†

Meanwhile, the possible dangers of taking high doses of certain vitamins is an extremely important issue and one which is still controversial. Even some of the foremost advocates of vitamin therapy have warned against taking unbalanced doses of vitamins, especially the B complex.[44] As we shall see later, there are definitely some cases where taking excesses of one B vitamin may eliminate more obvious symptoms while the basic disorder becomes progressively worse and even crippling.** There has been a recent report of high doses of vitamin C destroying vitamin B_{12}.[45] In addition, very high doses of B_6

---

* See Part V, Food and Consciousness.
† See Chapter 18, Megavitamins and Food Allergies.
** See Vitamin B_{12}.

can cause liver damage according to some studies, and it is clearly established that niacinimide, one form of vitamin B_3, also causes damage to the liver.[46]

Niacinimide, a compound closely related to nicotinic acid, is sometimes used in preference to niacin since it can play the same role metabolically and it does not cause the flushing produced by high doses of niacin. This rush of blood and heat to the skin can be frightening though, as far as is known, it is not harmful. Despite the fact that it may be more pleasant to take niacinimide, it is not without its drawbacks. Besides the possibility of liver damage, high doses of niacinamide have also caused depression in some persons.[47] Niacin, on the other hand, is generally said to be non-toxic even in the extremely high doses that are sometimes used. Yet when very large doses of niacin are given, liver tests often become abnormal. Though investigators at the Mayo Clinic performed liver biopsies on patients who had been under treatment for a year with high doses of niacin, and found no abnormalities.[48] Disruption of the delicate functioning of the liver would not necessarily be visible on microscopic examination of the tissue until some structural changes had occurred. In any case, pushing niacin doses higher and higher in order to get further improvement may be an error. Deficiencies of other nutrients may in fact be what is preventing progress.

As mentioned earlier, chronic cases of pellagra not uncommonly demonstrate loss of sensitivity in the extremities with odd and unusual sensations. There may also be a lack of balance and difficulty walking. These symptoms are not those of niacin deficiency. Rather they are symptoms of a degeneration of the spinal cord due to a deficiency of vitamin B_{12}. By 1952, nutritionists had recognized that, "While lack of nicotinic acid dominates the picture, pellagra is in truth a disease of multiple deficiencies: nicotinic acid, protein, riboflavin," and perhaps other nutrients.[49] Perhaps it is necessary to give such high doses of niacin to get a response because a lack of other nutrients is preventing one from doing well on more normal amounts of it.

In such a case, the answer is to supply the other needed nutrients rather than to force a response by giving higher doses of niacin.

B₆, PYRIDOXINE

Pyridoxine was first isolated in 1936 as the substance in the "water soluble B" that could cure a skin disease in rats which had been produced by a poor diet. It has been recently discovered that there is some relationship between vitamin B_6 (pyridoxine) and shifts of hormones in the female. Alterations in hormonal balance occur just prior to the menstrual period and this has often been thought to be the origin of the acne that so often flares up at this time. Early in pregnancy the "morning sickness," that classically occurs during the first trimester, may also be the result of pyridoxine deficiency.[50] The severity of the deficiency increases during the course of pregnancy and more serious disorders later on may also be related to this.[51] Recently, the use of pyridoxine supplements has greatly reduced the incidence of pre-eclampsia and toxemia,[52] a severe condition which endangers the life of the mother and leads to a loss of nearly half of the pregnancies. It is now hypothesized that this disorder may be at least in part due to pyridoxine deficiency,* as is the diabetes occurring during pregnancy.[53]

No one knows exactly what impact pyridoxine deficiency during pregnancy has on the developing infant. However, it has been recently shown that pyridoxine is extremely important for the development of the nervous system. Certain disorders of central nervous system functioning like epilepsy have responded to pyridoxine supplementation, especially in those infants who have demonstrated a higher than normal pyridoxine need.[54] Not only pyridoxine, but also most of the other members of the

* See also Chapter 6, Protein.

B Complex are important for the development of the nervous system.

In addition, pyridoxine is intimately tied up with the problem of arteriosclerosis. Research seems to indicate that it plays a crucial role in fat metabolism and that a diet high in animal fats is more likely to cause cholesterol plaques when intakes of B_6 are low. An arteriosclerotic condition has been repeatedly produced in experimental animals by putting them on a pyridoxine-deficient diet. Though it is certainly true that other factors play important roles in the development of arteriosclerosis, it would seem that its prevention would be difficult if not impossible without adequate amounts of vitamin B_6 in the diet.[55]

Though pyridoxine is widely distributed in nature, and most foods contain significant amounts, much of it is lost in processing. About half is lost during the refining of flour, for example. Unlike thiamin, riboflavin and niacin, this is not replaced by "enrichment," so commercial white flours remain deficient. Canned vegetables also contain little pyridoxine so that those who eat a meal containing the white bread and canned vegetables served in most restaurants will likely come out lacking. Also deficient in B_6 were the canned rations consumed by Korean soldiers who, interestingly enough, were found on autopsy to have advanced arteriosclerosis even though many of them were only in their twenties.[56]

Unfortunately, the optimal amounts of pyridoxine are not known, though estimates run around one to three mg a day. Moreover, reliable measurements of the amounts in most foods are not available. Except for organ meats, the amounts contained in most foods are so small, however, that one cannot afford many low-B_6 foods like white flour, sugar or fat without building up a "pyridoxine debt" that would be difficult to pay off. High levels of B_6 are often found in the stool, suggesting that it is manufactured by intestinal bacteria. Though it is not known to what extent this is absorbed, it seems possible that this could contribute to pyridoxine intake. Diet, then, may affect B_6

intake as much by its effect on intestinal microbes as by the amount it supplies directly.

Pyridoxine deficiency probably causes symptoms similar to those of thiamin and niacin deficiencies, and it can produce a sort of depression. Thus depressed persons occasionally improve on high doses of pyridoxine, though this is the exception rather than the rule.[57] Oral contraceptives, again probably because of a disruption in hormonal balance, seem to somehow create a pyridoxine deficiency, and this is often associated with depression. In these cases, response to pyridoxine is especially good.[58] Frankly toxic symptoms can be observed by the time dosages of 600 mg or more are given, but the long term effects of lesser quantities of the substance are not known.

VITAMIN B$_{12}$

Vitamin B$_{12}$ is unique in many ways. First of all, it is the vitamin which is needed by the body in the tiniest amounts. Only a few thousandths of a milligram* per day are necessary to prevent the symptoms of deficiency. Even more important for many people is the fact that vitamin B$_{12}$ is the only vitamin which is not found in strictly vegetarian diets (those without dairy products). It is present in milk, eggs, meat and is manufactured by many bacteria and yeasts. Any food which is strictly of plant origin, not fermented, and free of all bacteria and insects, will be found to contain no vitamin B$_{12}$. In cultures where food is grown organically and processed little or not at all, deficiencies of B$_{12}$ are uncommon, even when there is no meat, milk, eggs or other animal food in the diet. This is thought to be due to the fact that organically grown foods will often contain traces of bacteria from the soil or even tiny bits of insects which are difficult to see or remove completely. These alone may be enough to provide the extremely small doses of

* 3 to 4 micrograms

vitamin B_{12} that are necessary. When foods are grown with the use of pesticides, however, insects and bacteria are likely to have been thoroughly exterminated, and the processing of food to render it suitable for long storage or shelf-life will be even more likely to remove any traces of vitamin B_{12}.

Though our understanding is limited, some authorities feel that the bacteria in the intestines may also produce certain amounts of vitamin B_{12} which may find their way into the body. But in our culture, where the use of antibiotics is common and the population of microbes in the intestine is unstable and variable, this would still not be a dependable source of vitamin B_{12}. Therefore, there are cases of vitamin B_{12} deficiency among those vegetarians of the West who strictly avoid not only meat, fish and fowl, but even all eggs and dairy products.[59] With proper understanding, this situation can be prevented, but where there is ignorance or neglect, the results can be disastrous.

A severe anemia develops in B_{12} deficiency which leaves the skin and mucus membranes pale. The tongue becomes red, raw and sometimes ulcerated, eventually losing its papillae and becoming shiny and smooth. The symptoms are not limited to anemia, paleness and an unhealthy tongue, however, Before treatment was available, the disease would inevitably progress from numbness and tingling in the fingers and toes, to loss of balance, shooting pains and weakness in the arms and legs, and inability to walk without the feet far apart. These symptoms are due to a degeneration of the spinal cord and brain which is steadily progressive and leads inevitably to death. The unrelenting course of the disease made it notorious. It was certainly more than simply a case of anemia. The name that came to be attached to it, "pernicious anemia," reflected the grim neurological degeneration that followed the pallor and low blood count.

This disease was as much feared as cancer until 1926 when two researchers demonstrated that relief could be obtained by taking large quantities of liver in the diet. For this discovery they won the 1934 Nobel prize. But some patients had to eat two pounds of liver a day in order to control the anemia. Clearly there was some difficulty in absorption. Patients with the disease were often found to have too little hydrochloric acid in the stomach, as well as little or none of the special factor that assists in the absorption of vitamin B_{12}. Thus pernicious anemia can occur even in persons whose diet is rich in this vitamin. Why some people are deficient in the stomach acid and other substance needed to absorb B_{12} is not known, but probably hereditary and constitutional factors play a part. Acid secretion is also related to emotional factors and, interestingly, mental symptoms are present in most cases of pernicious anemia. There is often irritability or refusal to cooperate in treatment, paranoid thinking, confusion especially at night and a failing memory. Moreover, it has been demonstrated that psychiatric symptoms may occur long before anemia or neurological problems appear.[60] This fact, as we shall see, makes vitamin B_{12} deficiency even more intriguing.

FOLIC ACID

in 1931, a doctor working in Bombay noted in her pregnant patients a high frequency of an anemia in which the red blood cells looked just like those in pernicious anemia. Yet it did not respond to the liver extract which had so dramatically cured the pernicious anemia patients. It did, however, respond to an extract of yeast which had no effect at all on pernicious anemia. Apparently there were two different anemias only superficially alike, the one anemia of pregnancy responding to yeast and the more dreaded pernicious anemia responding only to liver. The anemia of the pregnant women never seemed to develop the same horrible neurological symptoms of pernicious anemia, but the diseases were otherwise quite similar. In 1945, when a group of American chemists finally succeeded in purifying the substance in yeast that could reverse the anemia of pregnancy, it was natural that this was immediately tried on pernicious anemia.

The results were startling. The dreaded anemia improved dramatically. This new substance extracted from spinach, called "folic acid," was hailed enthusiastically as a new and simpler cure for pernicious anemia. No longer would one have to choke down the pounds and pounds of liver that the pernicious anemia patient had previously been forced to eat. The enthusiasm, however, was short-lived. Whereas the anemia disappeared, the neurological symptoms did not improve. In fact, sometimes they got worse. The doctor from Bombay had been right. There really were two distinct anemias.

While folic acid completely and totally cured the anemia of pregnancy, it only touched the surface of the more serious disease, pernicious anemia. It restored the blood, but did not stop the deeper process—the degeneration of the nervous system. Rather than helping patients with pernicious anemia, treating them with folic acid simply covered up the disease, eliminating the one symptom, anemia, which might serve as the earliest clue that something serious was going on. For this reason, folic acid is only sold in very tiny amounts even today. If large doses were available, it is feared that some people might unknowingly mask the symptoms of pernicious anemia.

Obviously, the biochemic roles of vitamin B_{12} and folic acid overlap to some extent. This overlap involves the synthesis of DNA, the complex protein chain which is the basic substance of chromosomes and which carries the genetic coding that governs the cell's metabolism. When either B_{12} or folic acid is missing or deficient, then the duplication of chromosomes cannot occur at the normal rate and the reproduction of cells is slowed. Pregnancy is a time when cells are multiplying quickly and a great deal of new tissue is being formed. This requires large amounts of folic acid and may be one reason why it is often deficient during pregnancy.

Such a deficiency can have serious consequences. If folic acid is withheld from the diet of experimental animals very early in pregnancy, the fetus simply stops developing and is re-absorbed. If deficiency begins a bit later during the pregnancy, the young are born, but 95% of them have abnormalities. Skeletal deformities, undeveloped organs and malformations of the heart and blood vessels are seen. Some of the offspring are born with extreme deformities of the nervous system such as the brain being outside the skull or the brain cavity being distended with fluid [61] (hydrocephalus). Such experiments strongly suggest that some of the birth defects and mental retardation which occur today are due to poor diets during pregnancy.[62]

In one recent study, 55 out of 250 pregnant women were found to be folic acid deficient.[63] Though all such deficiencies may not be severe enough to create structural defects that are apparent at birth, it is possible that more subtle disorders result that may not cause problems until later in life.

A pigmentation of the face that develops during pregnancy (called melasma) has been attributed to folic acid deficiency.[64] A similar pigmentation occurs sometimes on the faces of patients who are taking birth control pills, and research has often turned up folic acid deficiencies among them.[65] But prolonged folate deficiency, whether it comes from birth control pills, other drugs, or simply a poor diet can result in mental deterioration. In studies involving 75 psychiatric patients, nearly half were found to have low levels of folic acid.[66] This is even more common among elderly psychiatric patients, folic acid deficiency being found in over 80% of them in one hospital.[67] Their most common symptoms are indifference, withdrawal, lack of motivation and depression. The World Health Organization has recommended that the aged, pregnant women and those on birth control pills should have extra folic acid. " The average balanced diet contributes 0.15 to 0.2 mgs. per day of folic acid which . . . is less than half the recommended allowance of 0.5 mgs."[68] Thus many people who eat an "average balanced diet" are suffering a mild deficiency of the vitamin.

When folic acid was originally isolated in spinach, it was

given its name from the Latin *folium*, which means "leaf," and subsequent studies have shown that it is very abundant in bright green foliage and green and leafy vegetables, a food many people seldom eat. Other fresh vegetables and fruits are also excellent sources of folic acid. Unfortunately, canning, overcooking or discarding cooking water can result in serious losses of folic acid. One nutritionist suggests that if everyone were to eat one serving of fresh vegetables or fresh fruit each day, the folate deficiency that results from an inadequate diet would be "wiped off the face of the earth."[69] Dried beans and peas are also a relatively good source, and even whole grain bread can supply fair amounts of folic acid. By contrast, a diet high in fats and refined carbohydrates is likely to lead to folic acid deficiency.

Though folic acid is not toxic, large doses of it may relieve the tiredness, weakness and anemia of B_{12} deficiency, while deeper and more serious problems continue. This raises the possibility that something similar though less dramatic might occur with other B vitamins when large doses of them are given to remove symptoms without a thorough understanding of what's going on. If the problem is simply that of a poorly balanced diet, then one can easily correct this. If a deficiency occurs in the presence of an adequate diet, such as may happen with pernicious anemia in those persons who lack the ability to absorb vitamin B_{12}, then the expertise and understanding of a skilled physician is required. Supplying the vitamin in high doses may be a temporary answer, but it cannot be a completely satisfying solution to the problem. What prevents the system from being able to absorb or utilize the usual amounts of the vitamin should, if possible, be corrected, then one's health can be put on a firmer foundation and huge doses of the vitamin will no longer be needed.

PANTOTHENIC ACID

Pantothenic acid is a recently discovered vitamin of the B group. When absent from the diet of rats, they showed graying of the hair, failure to grow, and most significantly, hemorrhaging and destruction of the adrenal glands. Perhaps the reason that this new substance had not previously been identified is because it is so universally present in all living matter. This characteristic led to its name which means literally, "that which is everywhere."

The wide distribution of pantothenic acid in most natural foods is also probably one reason that a clear-cut deficiency disease resulting from a lack of it has never been well documented in man except under experimental conditions. When it was eliminated from the diet over a period of time, subjects developed vomiting and abominal pain with burning cramps. Later they began to complain of tiredness, difficulty sleeping and tingling sensations in the hands and feet. Many of the symptoms of pantothenic acid deficiency are thought to be related to exhaustion of the adrenal glands, which are apparently highly dependent on this particular vitamin. The adrenals are involved, of course, in the response to stress, whether that stress is physiological, emotional, psychological or all three. Though the symptoms produced by experimental deficiency of this vitamin, such as weakness, cramps and difficulty sleeping, are familiar to many people, the possibility that a lack of such nutrients as pantothenic acid may be involved is usually overlooked.

However, after observing that pantothenic acid in natural food stuffs is so widespread that deficiency of the vitamin is unlikely to occur, one standard text on nutrition adds: "Except when processed foods form a large proportion of the diet."[70] Rather than an "exception," having processed foods form a large proportion of the diet is the rule in America, for example, where 40-45% of the calories are fat and up to 20-25% are white sugar. Moreover, much of the remaining 30-40% of the diet is also likely to be processed, at least to some extent, since it will ordinarily consist of canned or frozen vegetables, breads made from refined flours, and frozen meats. About 50% of the pantothenic acid in wheat is lost in processing and 33% of that in meat during cooking. Frozen meats also lose much of their pantothenic acid in the drip that occurs with thawing. Moreover, the typical American diet includes many highly processed dressings, desserts, snacks and sweets. One recent research study of pantothenic acid in the diet, blood and urine of a group of teenage girls showed that nearly all of them consumed what appeared to be inadequate amounts of pantothenic acid. Though minimum requirements have not been clearly defined, the Food and Nutrition Board suggests that 5 to 10 mg per day are probably necessary. Only one girl in the group studied was shown to have consumed that much.[71]

It has been suggested that a difficulty in responding to stress, which may be related to a deficiency of nutrients like pantothenic acid, is involved in the aging process. Research done in Japan found that pantothenic acid levels in the blood decreased year by year after age 60. Moreover, those who, judging by their outward appearance, seemed older had less pantothenic acid in the blood than others who were actually of the same age, but looked younger.[72] In a laboratory experiment, forty-one mice on a regular diet were compared with 33 that were given .3 mg of extra pantothenic acid per day in their drinking water. Those on the regular diet lived 550 days while those receiving the small dose of extra vitamin lived an average of 653 days. This is like comparing a life span of 75 years in humans with one of 89.[73] Yet simply taking pantothenic acid tablets is probably not the answer. Even so ardent a vitamin enthusiast as Adele Davis has warned that pantothenic acid taken alone over a prolonged period may increase the need for vitamin B_1 and thus cause neuritis.[74]

There are certainly many natural foods rich enough in pantothenic acid that most people need not resort to swallowing quantities of vitamin pills. The best sources are liver and other organ meats, yeast, egg yolks and fresh vegetables. Even eating liver or taking large quantities of such foods as yeast and eggs which are high in pantothenic acid is probably not necessary except in unusual circumstances, as long as the diet is made up principally of whole foods, each containing its proper complement of the vitamin. In fact, we might think of the pantothenic acid distributed so widely through almost all natural foods as a sort of nutritional tag so that the appearance of a deficiency is an indication that the diet has come to contain large quantities of stripped and unnatural foods. Taking pantothenic acid alone would be of little help, of course, since the stripping will usually remove many other nutrients besides it.

Once we come to understand this, it is clear why pantothenic acid deficiency is rarely if ever seen as an isolated phenomenon. When it is deficient, it is likely that other vitamins as well as minerals and protein will also be deficient. Such a mixture of multiple borderline deficiencies may underlie many of the vague complaints and feelings of fatigue that commonly occur but don't fall into any of the classical vitamin-deficiency disease categories like scurvy, beri-beri or rickets.

OTHER B VITAMINS

There are a number of other essential nutrients that were eventually isolated from the original B_2 factor in food, and the chemical structures of most of these have been identified. In some cases the necessity of these substances in the diet is still disputed, and not all authorities agree on whether they should in fact be called "vitamins." Biotin is perhaps the best established of these. Its role was clarified primarily because it is destroyed by a protein in raw egg white. When experimental animals or men are fed large quantities of uncooked egg white (about 30% of the diet), fatigue, depression, nausea, pains and lack of appetite begin to appear after a couple of months. All these symptoms are reversed by injections of biotin.[75]

Inositol and choline are two other B vitamins which are constituents of lecithin, and both have to do with the metabolism of fats, the regulation of blood cholesterol and the nourishment of the fat-like sheaths of nerve fibers. It is said that inositol can prevent thinning of the hair and baldness, but this is apparently true only when it has been deficient in the diet or has been poorly absorbed. It appears to be of little use in cases where hair loss is hereditary.

PABA is an abbreviation for the intimidating name "para-minobenzoic acid." This B vitamin also gained a relatively undeserved reputation on the basis of an appeal to vanity. For some years it has been acclaimed in popular literature as a cure for gray hair. Actually, in one of the research studies most often quoted, PABA was given on an experimental basis in quite large doses as a last-ditch treatment for a variety of grave and terminal illnesses. It was observed incidentally that these doses, in the range of 6,000 to 24,000 mg per day, seemed to cause some darkening of gray hair in five of the twenty patients who were being treated. While no definite daily requirement for PABA has been established, tablets used as supplements for therapeutic purposes, which are much higher than the average daily intake, contain only 30 mg. In other words, 1,000 times this dose produced some degree of darkening of the hair in only 25% of patients.[76] It's safe to say that PABA is hardly a practical or advisable treatment for gray hair. Nutritionists generally agree that when graying of the hair is due to nutritional deficiencies, it is likely to be a variety of nutrients that are needed. PABA has also been used in topical ointments to protect the skin from sunburn, and it seems to be effective and non-toxic when used for this purpose.

Another substance sometimes classified as a B vitamin is orotic acid, called vitamin B_{13}. While it is not acknowledged officially in the United States as a vitamin, it has been synthesized in Europe where it is thought by some to be helpful in the treatment of multiple sclerosis. It occurs naturally in root vegetables and whey.

Although it was originally isolated and identified here, vitamin B_{15} or pangamic acid is another substance little discussed in the United States. Most of the research on the use of this nutrient has been done in Russia where it has been shown to promote oxidation and cell respiration and has been found particularly valuable in patients who have inadequate blood supply to the brain, heart or other areas.[77] Like the controversial vitamin B_{17} (laetrile), pangamic acid (B_{15}) is found in large quantities in apricot pits. It also occurs in whole grains and seeds such as pumpkin seeds and sesame seeds.

VITAMIN C

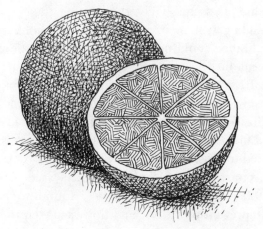

By the time that James Lind finally demonstrated that scurvy could be prevented by citrus juice, it had already become a serious problem. For example, one ship leaving England in 1739 for the Pacific started out with a crew of 961 men. Within a year, 626 were dead, the greater part as a result of scurvy. At the English Naval Hospital where Lind worked, he often saw between 300 and 400 cases a day. Although citrus juice had been advocated as both a prophylaxis and treatment for scurvy as early as 1616, it was Lind who performed a well-controlled experiment, documenting beyond doubt its effectiveness: He gave two oranges and one lemon a day to two sailors afflicted by scurvy while offering ten other, equally ill patients different popular remedies such as cider vinegar and sea water. The results were dramatic and indisputable. The two sailors on the citrus juice recovered sufficiently within a few days to take over the nursing care of the other ten men.

Nevertheless, it was almost fifty years later that the British admiralty finally introduced the mandatory daily intake of lemon juice by the Royal Navy. Within two years of this, scurvy had virtually disappeared from English ships. Perhaps it was this which gave the Queen's Fleet the edge it needed to control the seas. It seems likely that during the Napoleonic wars "the blockading system of warfare which annihilated the naval powers of France could never have been carried on unless scurvy had been subdued." English ships were able to maintain the blockade of the French coast because the sailors were using the juice of a small green lime grown extensively in the British West Indies. This less expensive citrus juice ration had replaced the lemon of Lind's experiments and led to the slang term "limey" being applied to British sailors.

One constituent of the citrus juice, ascorbic acid, identified in 1928 by Szent-Gyorgyi, was found to be extremely powerful in preventing scurvy, and this was taken to be the active ingredient. It was soon called vitamin C. Having fought valiantly to convince the English Navy and the public at large of the value of citrus juice, James Lind would be pleased to see that ascorbic acid is commanding increasing attention from the medical profession today. He would probably be a bit perplexed, however, by the vast difference between the doses currently used and those he suggested. Whereas Lind advocated a teaspoon or two of lemon juice a day, modern physicians are using 500 mg and 1,000 mg doses of ascorbic acid, 25 to 50 times as much as is contained in a whole lemon!

Disorders such as bed sores have responded well to treatment with such high doses (1,000 mg a day) of vitamin C[78] and patients with inflammation of the bowel who developed open draining wounds were found to have very low levels of vitamin

C in the blood.[79]   It was felt that the absence of sufficient vitamin C had impaired the formation of collagen, the fibrous connective tissue that is so important in the repair and healing of wounds.   It is interesting to remember that an inability to heal wounds was one of the ear marks of classical scurvy. Vitamin C, along with related compounds, (often called bioflavonoids or "vitamin P") have also been shown to be effective in a variety of bleeding disorders such as hemorrhage and bleeding gums.[80] Again, of course, spongy, bleeding gums were one of the features of scurvy that most impressed physicians of the sixteen and seventeen hundreds.   But vitamin C is being used in other ways that are apparently unrelated to classical scurvy.

VITAMIN C AND THE COMMON COLD

In 1970, Nobel laureate Dr. Linus Pauling published a book suggesting that high doses of ascorbic acid could prevent colds or that it could at least decrease the severity of symptoms in those who did develop colds.   At first, however, research failed to demonstrate any overall statistically significant benefits from vitamin C.[81,82]   In response to this, advocates of vitamin C for the treatment of the common cold claimed that the researchers hadn't given the vitamin in large enough doses,[83] and that when the doses were adequate, results were better.[84]   It is true that the doses given in some of the early experiments were lower than those popularly used to treat colds.[85]   To make matters more confusing, recent studies using "adequate doses of vitamin C" have produced equivocal results.[86, 87]   Strangely enough, in another study where small doses were given, there was very good protection.[88]   Therefore the subject remains controversial.

It is officially estimated that the minimum daily requirement for vitamin C is about 45 mg. Nowadays, however, vitamin C is usually being sold in tablets no smaller than 100 mg., and the most popular size is 500 mg. Some proponents of the use of megadoses of ascorbic acid speak of its being used as a pharmacologic agent, not a nutrient. What is needed is "medication" not "alimentation," they say.[89]   Many people now self-medicate themselves for colds with one or two of the large vitamin C tablets every two or three hours. This is quite a bit more than the 150-500 mg per day administered in most research studies, and far beyond the 30 to 45 mg a day officially recommended for adequate nutrition. Most people who try the larger doses, however, are soon convinced that vitamin C does have the power to control the symptoms of colds. Success with colds has led to the use of very high doses of vitamin C in the treatment of other complaints, such as flu. Several distinguished scientists, including Drs. Pauling and Szent-Gyorgyi, have publicly advocated the use of large doses of vitamin C to help protect the body not only against colds and flu, but against viral infections in general. When cultures of human cells were bathed in a solution containing vitamin C, they were able to produce larger quantities of a substance ("interferon") which is known to interfere with the ability of viruses to invade cells.[90]

There is also evidence that vitamin C plays a role in the protection against bacterial infections.[91]   It was shown as early as 1943 that proper levels of ascorbic acid maintained the activity of white cells—the "bacteria destroyers" of the bloodstream. More recent studies support this,[92] but indicate that if levels go too high, the effect is reversed, and the white cells become sluggish.[93] Very high doses of vitamin C have been used with apparent success in the treatment of a variety of acute and life-threatening infectious diseases ranging from meningitis to viral pneumonia. Though no controlled studies have been done, a number of case histories showed dramatic improvement within hours when mammoth doses (on the order of 45,000 milligrams of vitamin C per 24 hours) were given intravenously.[94]

A case has been made that vitamin C acts as an intermediary which facilitates electron transfer. In the eye of the chemist, the biochemical reactions of living matter consist essentially of an orderly, step-wise and enzymatically controlled transfer of electrons. When something goes wrong in the cells of the body, this flow is in some way blocked. The details of the breakdown will of course vary according to the particular disease process, infection or injury which is involved. An agent, like ascorbic acid, that floods the cellular fluids promoting the flow of electrons might indeed prove to promote a smoother and more healthy progression of biochemical processes. Those substances which facilitate electron transfer have been called an "oil to the machinery of life."[95]

A number of more specific roles for vitamin C have also been suggested. It is thought, for example, that large doses of ascorbic acid inhibit the action of the histamine that is released in allergic reactions[96] and can therefore be helpful in such problems as hay fever. It is certainly true that smokers have low vitamin C levels and benefit from taking regular doses of it.[97] Huge doses of vitamin C have even been used with some success in treating cancer, but here it is especially important to remember that in such quantities it is being used as a medication, and precautions must be taken accordingly. Though in some of the cancer patients the tumors were destroyed, a number apparently died from the toxins and hemorrhage that resulted when there was such sudden and massive tissue destruction.[98]   One can barely begin to list the numerous diseases where treatment with vitamin C has shown varied but at least partial success.

It has been suggested that while 45 mg or so of vitamin C a day is sufficient to prevent the symptoms of scurvy, it is not adequate to insure optimal functioning of the body. Man, his ape relatives, and, for some unknown reason, the guinea pig are practically the only animals who are not able to synthesize vitamin C for themselves. For the guinea pig and the ape, this is not much of a problem since their diets are high in green leafy foods that contain generous quantities of vitamin C. Gorillas, for example, who make a habit of munching on the leaves of jungle trees, consume about 4,500 mg of vitamin C in an average day. As long as vitamin C was plentiful in the diet, it made sense

to eliminate the biochemical machinery necessary for its production. If the gorilla is going to eat vast quantities of vitamin
C anyway, he hardly needs to cart about the equipment needed
to manufacture it. However, when man departed the jungle,
shifting his diet to grains, beans and less leafy vegetables, the
daily intake of vitamin C gradually dropped. Originally, elimination of the ability to synthesize vitamin C had been in the
interest of efficiency, but it was a different story once the leafy
green foods and their large quantities of vitamin C fell out of
man's diet. Following this line of reasoning, man has been called
a mutant, a species of animal afflicted by a genetic change that
makes his biochemistry defective. On the basis of such thinking,
it has been suggested that humans can only maintain health by
taking extremely large daily doses of vitamin C. One might be
tempted to discount such an idea by saying that it is a recent
concept and that the practice of taking large quantities of ascorbic acid is a modern folly. Surprisingly, however, there are
precedents for this extending far back in history.

Up   until   a   generation   ago,   boneset   (*Eupatorium
perfoliatum*), a plant that grows wild in North America, was a
favorite family remedy among country folk. A bundle of the
dried plants was hung in the attic, and from them a very bitter
tea "would be meted out to the unfortunate victim of a cold or
fever." Those who used it swore by it, and it was felt to bring
the symptoms of a cold or flu to an abrupt halt. Recently an
analysis of the tea reported that the two or three cupsful ordinarily given to an adult may contain from ten to thirty thousand
milligrams of vitamin C.[99] It is intriguing to discover, moreover,
that in India there is a whole series of traditional medicinal
preparations based on a sour, walnut-sized fruit called *amla*,
one of which may contain more vitamin C than a dozen oranges.
A concentrated paste of the partially dehydrated *amla* fruit
is the principle ingredient of many Indian medicines, most
notably a traditional Ayurvedic preparation that is used for
revitalizing and rejuvenating, especially during the winter season

when fresh fruits and vegetables are more scarce.

Judging from the flood of testimonials from the public at large regarding the usefulness of vitamin C, it would seem likely that the claims made for it are at least partially true. In fact, there is a huge volume of often conflicting literature, some of which supports the effectiveness of vitamin C in the treatment of such diverse problems as the prevention of arteriosclerosis,[100] prickley heat,[101] polyps[102] and schizophrenia.[103] There is also evidence that vitamin C exerts some protective effect in those who have been exposed to toxic levels of heavy metals like lead[104] and experimental animals exposed to cadmium.[105,106] In fact, requirements for high doses of vitamin C may actually be created by high doses of toxins in the environment. Moreover, drugs, such as birth control pills,[107] and aspirin[108] have been shown to deplete the tissues of vitamin C. High doses of vitamin C seem to have a protective effect not only against such heavy metals, but also against such toxins as pesticides[109] and such food additives as nitrates whose use have been associated with cancer.[110]

For those who find themselves requiring more vitamin C, however, simply taking high doses may not be the most ideal solution. This is borne out by the side effects that have been observed from high doses of the vitamin. Large doses are said to deactivate B_{12}.* In some animals, large doses of vitamin C have produced demineralization of bones.[111] Similarly, it has been suggested that in man, large doses can interfere with calcium absorption. There is also some evidence that vitamin C is sometimes converted to calcium oxalate in the urine and that for some people this can result in the formation of kidney stones. One young man, for example, who had been taking 1,000 mg a day for many months to prevent colds passed a stone in his urine which, on analysis, proved to be calcium oxalate. His urinary oxalate level at this time was 126.†[112] When he stopped

* See vitamin B_{12}.
† Normal is considered to be less than 40.

taking vitamin C for three weeks, the level dropped to 56. Another such case has been reported where a young man taking higher doses of vitamin C (4,000 mg a day) showed urinary oxalate levels that were even more dramatically elevated (622 mg after 7 days and 478 mg after 4 days on the vitamin C).[113]   It seems very likely that such levels might produce stones, though proponents of vitamin C claim that oxalic acid will only form stones when the urine is alkaline. In any case, this second person was one of a series of subjects studied and the only one to react this way. The researchers felt such a marked tendency to convert vitamin C to oxalic acid is probably rare, but that those who react this way should be identified, and not given high doses of the vitamin.[114]

Besides citrus fruits and green leafy vegetables, there are other foods that are also high in vitamin C. Most fresh fruits are rich in it, especially those that are tart. A cup of fresh strawberries, for example, will contain half again as much vitamin C as an orange. Most muscle meats contain little or none, though organ meats will have variable quantities. Milk contains small amounts. Grains and beans have very little vitamin C until they are sprouted when they become excellent sources of it, and it has been known since the 18th century that bean sprouts would cure scurvy. These can be an especially important source in the winter time when people in some areas have difficulty getting fresh fruit or vegetables. Tomatoes, squash and even potatoes are rather good sources of vitamin C, and cabbage contains enough ascorbic acid so that when fermented in northern Europe to make sauerkraut, it serves to stave off deficiencies through the long winter months. Perhaps the richest vegetable source is the green pepper, one of which will have more vitamin C than an orange. In Mexico, the common folk rely on chili peppers for their vitamin C as well as for other strategic nutrients in a diet that is otherwise only corn and beans.

Growing and Using Sprouts

Sprouts are available year round, inexpensive and high in vitamin C. Yogis living in the caves of the Himalayas have been known to subsist almost entirely on them. Each variety is different. Alfalfa sprouts, for example, are very delicate and best used raw in fresh green salads. Mung sprouts, on the other hand, are more appropriately cooked briefly with a vegetable dish or lightly steamed, as are lentil sprouts. Soy sprouts require even more cooking, and although they are the most difficult to grow successfully they are nutritionally among the best.

Seeds for sprouting should be untreated (commercial seeds sold for planting are often coated with toxic chemicals to prevent their molding.) To germinate, simply sort out any dirty or damaged seeds, place the remainder in a large wide-mouth glass jar, cover the top with mesh or thin cloth, seal with a heavy rubber band or ring lid, and rinse until clean. The amount of dry seeds used to make a batch of sprouts will depend on the variety. Alfalfa seeds, for example, need more room to expand, so about one tablespoon will easily make a quart. After washing, cover the seeds generously with warm water for several hours. After the seeds have become plump, rinse gently in lukewarm water. Let the jar drain in a bowl or pot at a 45° angle, and either cover it loosely or set it in a dark, ventilated place such as a cupboard. Alfalfa sprouts should be rinsed twice a day. Mung beans and lentils will usually do well with only one rinsing while soybeans must be rinsed every three or four hours to prevent their spoiling, especially if the weather is warm and humid.

After three to four days of germination leafy sprouts like alfalfa require exposure to indirect sunlight for several hours to a day, being kept moist and being rotated so that all the areas are given light. This greening process allows the chlorophyl to develop in the leaves and increases vitamin C and flavor. Others, when clean and dry and after hulling (when necessary) can be directly refrigerated in a covered jar. Once a seed has reached its nutritional peak, allowing it to mature further will ruin it. Although sprouts keep well when refrigerated, it is best to use them in three to four days and start a fresh batch every so often. The cloth and jar used for sprouting should be scalded to avoid spoiling later batches. Uses: salads; sautée sprouts with onion, mushrooms and spices for a tasty side dish; add sprouts whole or ground to breads, cereals, soups, casseroles, stuffings, dinner loaves, sandwiches and "vegie burgers."

VITAMIN D

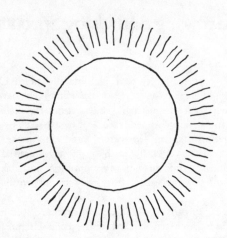

Vitamin D is not ordinarily taken in significant quantities with food. For the most part, one depends on manufacturing his own vitamin D through the action of sunlight on certain oil-like substances in the skin which are related to cholesterol. These are transformed in the presence of sunlight to a molecule whose structure is similar to many of the hormones in the body. It acts in conjunction with the parathyroid hormones to regulate calcium metabolism. The fact that the substance which we call vitamin D is manufactured in the body, that it is structurally related to such substances as cortisone and estrogen, and that it serves to regulate metabolic processes has led some people to suggest that it shouldn't be called a vitamin at all. Perhaps it would be more accurate to call it a hormone. In any case, vitamin D is unique and differs from the other vitamins in a number of ways.

The normal function of vitamin D is to promote the absorption of calcium from the intestinal tract, or if this source is not adequate, then from the bones themselves. It is crucial to maintain blood calcium levels since calcium is, of course, used by the body for other purposes than simply forming bones and teeth. The muscle fibers, for example, will not pull together or contract without calcium ions being present. Calcium also plays a role in the functioning of the nervous system. When vitamin D levels are low, irritability as well as problems with the bones may develop. The deficiency in vitamin D which causes these problems is called rickets.

Since vitamin D is a fat-soluble vitamin, it does not dissolve in water and is not easily excreted in the urine. Consequently, when it is taken in large quantities, it tends to accumulate, and there may be difficulty in getting rid of excesses of it. Large amounts of vitamin D are therefore liable to be toxic. When vitamin D is in excess, so much calcium can be absorbed and removed from the bones that it begins to form deposits that damage the tissues of the heart, blood vessels and lungs. If a large amount is taken suddenly, there will be nausea, vomiting, diarrhea, dizziness and weakness.

When sunlight shining on the skin strikes the cholesterol-like substances from which vitamin D is formed, synthesis will take place whether one needs more vitamin D or not since the process is apparently not enzymatically controlled. It seems that the major way the body regulates the rate of vitamin D synthesis is by shielding from the sun the deeper layers of skin where the reaction takes place. This is accomplished by pigmentation. The black skin of a typical African reflects only 24% of the light which strikes it. The rest is absorbed and will tend to raise body temperature. The skin of a typical European, on the other hand, reflects on the average 64% of the light so that he becomes overheated less rapidly in the hot sun. This is the reverse of what one would expect, and on the basis of these facts, one would think the equatorial areas of the world would have been inhabited by light-skinned people. The paradox is resolved, however, when we take into consideration the danger of vitamin D toxicity.

It is estimated that 100,000 units of vitamin D taken in a short period of time can cause symptoms of toxicity. A fair-skinned adult who exposes most of his body to sunlight during the whole of a tropical day would synthesize up to 800,000 IU of vitamin D,[115] eight times a toxic dose. However, melanin, the pigment which gives the skin of some races a deeper color, lies in the more superficial layers of skin and serves to filter out the ultraviolet rays and thereby slow down the manufacture of vitamin D. When there is no pigment present to prevent these rays from going to the deeper layers of skin where vitamin D is synthesized, then extended exposure to the tropical sun would certainly be enough to produce dramatic symptoms of acute toxicity such as nausea, weakness and dizziness. This no doubt explains why an albino, one who is born with no pigmentation, becomes quite ill if he is exposed to the sun. Many fair-skinned persons will recall having experienced some of these symptoms, which they may have referred to as a "sunstroke," when they were too long in the sun without any previous preparation.

If exposure is increased gradually, most people are able to build up a protective barrier of pigmentation so that they can withstand the sunlight more comfortably and not produce an excess of vitamin D. The results of this adaptive process are called suntan. As the skin darkens, one absorbs more light and consequently more heat, but the light rays will not reach the layers of skin where vitamin D synthesis occurs. One will there-fore be protected from the nausea, dizziness and weakness of vitamin D toxicity and he will be able to stay in the sun more comfortably, despite the rise in body temperature. It would seem that heat is a less important consideration in surviving the tropics than is vitamin D toxicity.

Conversely, fair skin may be a very valuable asset in northern climates where sunlight is less intense, and peoples of the far North who are native to inland areas, such as those of Scandinavia, tend to be quite fair. Research has shown that a patch of white human skin smaller than a postage stamp can synthesize up to 20 units of vitamin D in three hours when exposed to the sun. On the basis of these figures, one can calculate that a dose of vitamin D sufficient to prevent defi-ciency, about 400 units per day, can be synthesized by three hours daily exposure of the nearly transparent pink cheeks of

European infants.[116]

It would seem at first unlikely that the Eskimos, who have a rather dark complexion and cover themselves thoroughly with fur-lined clothes, could manage to survive in a far northern climate, but there is a second route through which the body acquires vitamin D. This is through the diet. The richest dietary source of vitamin D is in the oils of fish, especially that of fish liver. This is the case because fish eat plankton which thrives near the surface of the sea and is constantly exposed to the sunlight. The microscopic plants and animals of plankton contain sterols which, when struck by ultraviolet rays, are automatically changed into vitamin D-like substances. This carries over to fish, and the Eskimos' diet, which contains large quantities of fish, supplies several times the minimum dose of vitamin D. It may be that these people of the Mongolian race were able to survive for generations as they migrated from Asia to North America because their route along the Aleutian Islands and down the coast of Alaska, although it was in the far North, kept them constantly near the sea which amply supplied them with fish rich in vitamin D.

In northern climates then, vitamin D deficiency has often been a problem. It has been said that certain colonies of settlers in Greenland died out because pelvic deformities of the female, which interfered with childbirth, presumably developed from vitamin D deficiency. It is thought that this happened because the settlers were unwilling to eat the fish livers which were part of the diet of the local inhabitants who had thrived there.[117]

American Negroes are other notable examples of dark-skinned people who migrated north and are therefore especially prone to develop vitamin D deficiency. In the ghettos of northern cities, where even the small amounts of sunshine available are obscured by smog and tall buildings, rickets, the result of vitamin D deficiency, is not uncommon. When vitamin D is in short supply, the bones cannot grow properly since not enough calcium is absorbed in the diet to properly calcify them. The bones also become deformed, and the typical child with rickets develops a large bulging forehead and a chest which is collapsed near the mid-portion while the lower ribs flare out. The legs are often bowed, and height and weight may be below normal. Unless such a child is supplied with sufficient amounts of calcium and vitamin D, he will carry these deformities with him into adulthood, whereupon they become irreversible.

The estimated adult daily requirement of vitamin D is approximately that of a growing child, about 400 IUs a day. This can be obtained in one quart of milk which has had vitamin D_2 added. However, the vitamin D_2 which is included in milk to provide this calcium is chemically somewhat different from naturally occurring vitamin D. This synthetic form of vitamin D is made by taking a substance produced by yeast called ergosterol and exposing it to ultraviolet radiation. The ergosterol is converted to ergocalciferol or vitamin D_2, which is then separated, purified and added to the milk.* Many adults are found, on close examination, to show a mild degree of flaring of the lower ribs, which suggests a lack of calcium and/or vitamin D during their formative years. This problem is often prevented by providing adequate milk which has been fortified with vitamin D_2 or, more ideally, plain milk and sunshine. As we have seen, however, milk is sometimes difficult for Negroes to tolerate, and although they require the larger quantities of the vitamin D it contains, it may not be a particularly appropriate source of this for them. If fish does not form a sizeable part of the diet, then vitamin D capsules are probably justified.

A softening in the bones is also often seen in Muslim women in India.[119] Their custom is to veil their faces at adolescence and to wear a dark, tent-like garment which covers them from head to toe. Even thus attired, they rarely go outdoors,

---

* The natural form of vitamin D is vitamin D3 or cholecalciferol. It is the predominant form of vitamin D found in the skin, and it is also the main source of vitamin D in evaporated milk.118

normally remaining in the home. Since their diet is not especially rich in calcium, and fish are not available in the inland areas they inhabit, both calcium and vitamin D are often deficient. Calcium is subsequently pulled out of the bones of these women to keep blood levels up so that the nerves and muscles can function normally. Although their bones may be well-formed in childhood, and they may reach adolescence in good health, they eventually suffer excruciating pain as their bones become soft, fracture readily and are easily crushed by the weight of their bodies.

It has been suggested by some nutritionalists that vitamin D synthesis may also be hindered by the removal of oil from the skin during bathing with soap and water,[120] but this seems unlikely since most of the synthesis occurs beneath the pigmented layers of the skin. Though the small amounts of vitamin D synthesized in surface oils[121] is at best only a minor source in man,[122] it is important for some animals like birds and mammals with heavy coats or plumage since the sunlight cannot penetrate to their skin. For them the preening and licking of feathers and fur is probably less of a cosmetic matter than a nutritional one. Quite likely it is only by swallowing these irradiated oils that such animals are able to get their necessary complement of vitamin D.

VITAMIN E

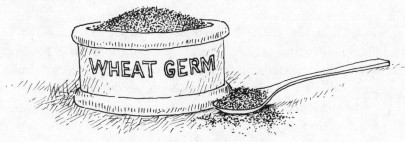

Probably the most controversial vitamin, with the possible exception of vitamin C, is vitamin E. It has not even been universally accepted that vitamin E is a necessary nutrient for man, and yet it is being taken in large doses by millions of Americans for an extraordinary array of human ailments ranging from warts to menopause. However, vitamin E is seldom prescribed by physicians, and the official attitude in academic medical establishments is that it is of doubtful benefit.[123, 124] Medical scientists base their skepticism on the fact that frank vitamin E deficiency diseases have never been observed in adults, although the intake of vitamin E is relatively low in the general population.

Vitamin E was discovered when rats on a diet in which this substance was absent failed to reproduce. The females, when pregnant, miscarried, and the male rats eventually became sterile. In 1936, the pure substance which could prevent this from happening was isolated, and given the name alpha-tocopherol, which means, literally, the substance required to "bring forth normal births." For some time vitamin E was known as "the fertility vitamin," and laboring under the misapprehension that it would increase sexual prowess, middle-aged men made it a popular item in neighborhood drug stores. Over the years, vitamin E has to some extent lost this image, and instead it is now firmly fixed in the mind of the public as a valuable measure for treating heart disease.

AS A MEDICINE FOR HEART DISEASE

Though a great deal has been written, both for the lay public and in the medical literature, about vitamin E for heart disease and related problems, its use remains controversial. Many studies done since the 1940's have shown no difference in the incidence of heart attacks or the severity of chest pain between patients who were given vitamin E and those who were given a blank capsule.[125, 126, 127] A number of clinicians, however, who have been using vitamin E with apparent success for decades have insisted that the doses used in the experiments were not high enough, that they were not continued for a long enough period of time, or that researchers ignored slight but significant degrees of improvement.[128]   It is true that medical researchers have recently realized that clinical studies are sometimes not sensitive enough to detect important positive effects. Another reason for less than spectacular results in clinical trials is that tocopherol may be partially inactivated by the hydrochloric acid in the stomach.[129]   Therefore, if the 400 or more units necessary for a clinical effect is to reach the tissues, then that dose must be given in especially coated tablets that are protected from stomach acid. It is claimed that this would double its effectiveness, but experiments to confirm this haven't yet been done. While many patients claim remarkable improvement and some physicians have been famous for their treatment of heart disease with vitamin E, these results are only anecdotal, clinical and not statistically documented. There are not properly controlled studies done in double-blind fashion which show the benefits of vitamin E in heart disease.

However, in another disease which involves cholesterol deposits in the arteries, results have been more clear cut. Where the obstruction is in the arteries that go to the legs reducing blood flow and producing severe pain when one attempts to walk more than a short distance, there has been a good response to vitamin E therapy.[130, 131] Some research, however, has shown that in experimental animals at least, large amounts of vitamin E can actually induce cholesterol deposits in the linings of the arteries.[132]

Another problem related to heart disease is that of blood clotting. When the coronary artery, which supplies the heart, is only partially obstructed by cholesterol deposits, a tiny blood clot (thrombus) can become lodged in it so that the blood flow to the heart wall is suddenly interrupted. Such a coronary thrombosis, or heart attack, is sometimes treated by giving an anti-coagulant to "thin the blood" so that new clots are less likely to form. Unfortunately, these anti-coagulants, for example, Warfarin, (which is otherwise used as a rat poison) are quite toxic and may overdo the job bringing significant risk of hemorrhage. There is good evidence that vitamin E may reduce the stickiness of the blood, diminishing its tendency to form abnormal clots.[133]   Perhaps vitamin E will be able to replace the more toxic anti-coagulants in the treatment of heart disease. But if it is simply added to anticoagulant drugs it may accentuate their effects triggering serious bleeding,[134] a danger among patients who are being treated with conventional drugs and add vitamin E themselves without their doctor's knowledge.

It should be noted that when alpha-tocopherol is used in this fashion, it is, like vitamin C in megadoses, not actually being used as a vitamin.   Such large doses would certainly not be needed to treat a deficiency, if indeed such a deficiency existed. Rather, vitamin E or alpha-tocopherol is used in these cases as a pharmacologic agent.   This is a matter of medical treatment and not of nutrition.   It is for this reason that the layman is ill-advised to take into his own hands the administration of high doses of alpha-tocopherol or other vitamins.   There can be dangers involved.   For instance, a patient who is taking digitalis may find that the effect of the digitalis is magnified by as much as a factor of two when he takes vitamin E along with it.   This could cause serious problems, including fatal arrythmias.[135] Besides the possibility of interaction with medications, there can be other problems associated with the use of high doses of vitamin E, (for example, iron metabolism can be impaired by vitamin E supplements[136]) despite the fact that it is often said that it is "harmless" and virtually non-toxic.[137]   Nausea and intestinal distress have been reported in some cases where more than 300 IU of the vitamin were taken daily.[138] Others have noted fatigue and weakness minicking symptoms of flu on doses higher than 400 IU a day.[139]   This may be accomplished by abnormalities in the urine,[140] but the whole picture promptly clears up when vitamin E is stopped.

Like vitamins A and D, vitamin E is a fat-soluble vitamin.

It can be found primarily in the oily portion of whole grains, seeds, beans and so forth. In wheat, for example, vitamin E is present mostly in the wheat germ. During modern milling processes, however, the wheat germ is removed, and as a result, white flour retains as little as 14% of the vitamin E found in whole wheat.* It has been said that the increased use of refined flour, along with the decreased use of grains in the diet, has led in the last 100 years to a decrease in vitamin E intake from approximately 100 to 150 IU a day to the present level of about 15 IU. This may account in part for the reason that people with such a wide variety of disorders have reported improvement after taking vitamin E. It seems possible that while a decrease in vitamin E level may not produce any consistent and easily identifiable "deficiency disease," it may lead to a weakness on the cellular level that makes one more susceptible to many problems.†

AS AN ANTI-OXIDANT

It is now believed that vitamin E acts as an anti-oxidant, preventing important molecules and structures in the cell from reacting with oxygen. When the delicate components of living protoplasm are attacked by oxygen, they are often injured (literally "burnt"). Probably the most active form of oxygen is ozone, a rather metallic and unpleasant smelling gas which can sometimes be noticed around electric motors when due to some defect in machinery the oxygen is being converted from O_2 to O_3. Most of the oxygen in the air is found as the more stable O_2 while ozone is produced by the merging of three oxygen atoms

---

* Estimates vary from 55% to 14%. It seems likely that the discrepancy is due to the fact that a great deal of vitamin E can be destroyed in the bleaching process. Thus vitamin E retention in "70% extraction flour" is given as 55% while that for "white flour" is said to be 14%.

† A similar concept is developed for the B vitamins. We do not yet know which cells don't require vitamin E, so the range of symptoms a deficiency of it can produce can not be well postulated.[141]

into one molecule to form O_3. It very easily loses its third oxygen atom, however, reverting to the more stable O_2 state. This single oxygen atom, when released, is very reactive and has a special propensity for damaging the fragile molecules of living tissue. In recent years, industrial processes have produced increasing amounts of ozone, and it has tended to accumulate in polluted areas. Weather bureaus in some parts of the country regularly broadcast an "ozone count" for the day, and many people are able to see a relationship between the ozone count and respiratory problems. This is because the delicate cells lining the lungs come in contact with the air since the nose and throat have no mechanisms for removing ozone. It is thought that many lung diseases such as emphyzema, asthma and so forth, are aggravated by ozone in the air.

In one experiment, two groups of rats were given different doses of vitamin E over a period of 8 weeks. They were then exposed to ozone concentrations in the air similar to what occurs in actual air pollution. The animals' lungs were examined for signs of damage, and it was found that the greatest injury occurred in those who had been given the least vitamin E. There was essentially no damage in those receiving the larger doses.*[142] Oxides of nitrogen are also present in smog and are similarly prone to oxidize tissues, causing cellular damage. It has been suggested that vitamin E may help to protect the cells from this chemical as well.[143] Heavy metals like lead and cadmium, which are often present in polluted air, act as catalysts in the oxidation reactions. Air which is polluted with the frequently occurring combination of ozone, oxides of nitrogen, cadmium and lead, is especially reactive, and puts extra demands on protective antioxidents such as vitamin E.[144]

As we have seen earlier, these damaging oxidating reactions, also called peroxidation, come not only from the air, but can also enter the body through the diet. The principle source of reactive

* A dose which would be equal to twice the RDA.

oxygen atoms in food is vegetable oils which have become rancid. Here again, heavy metals serve as catalysts, and when the oils have been overheated for extended periods and have been in contact with metal frying baskets and so forth, they are especially likely to cause trouble.

Since vitamin E is a fat-soluble vitamin, it finds its way primarily to those cellular structures which are made up of fats and oils. This especially includes the membranes which surround the cell as well as the tiny structures inside the cell itself. If peroxidation occurs, these membranes and intracellular structures bulge like damaged inner tubes, thereby disrupting and interfering with cellular functioning. If vitamin C or other substances such as selenium, which work in the same way, are present in sufficient quantities in the cell and its membranes, the integrity of the cell and the molecules inside each compartment will be protected against the invasion of oxidizing substances. If not, vital molecules are oxidized.

This reaction produces a kind of pigment that accumulates causing discoloration in the tissues. These deposits can be seen in the fatty tissue and the skin of most people who are advanced in age. It has been proposed that if cellular structures could be protected from damage by peroxidation,[145] the aging process could be retarded or perhaps even prevented to some extent. Some years ago, in a well-known medical center, experiments were done to investigate the effects of oxygen on aging. Rats were exposed to air containing much higher concentrations of oxygen. Oxygen is, of course, necessary for life, and proper oxygenation in the tissues promotes good health, so under these conditions, one might expect that the rats would be unusually healthy, but actually quite the contrary was observed. They aged rapidly, their white fur becoming yellowed and scraggly. Apparently too much oxygen caused peroxidative damage of vital structures. When a similar group of rats was exposed to the same high oxygen concentrations, but were simultaneously fed generous quantities of wheat germ oil which is rich in vitamin

E, aging was not accelerated, and they lived their normal life span in good health. Such experiments of course do not prove anything definite about human aging, but the researchers privately drew their own conclusions. The anti-oxidant effects of vitamin E must retard aging. Though vitamin E supplements were not yet available, each of them quietly stocked his refrigerator with a jug of wheat germ oil from which frequent gulps were surreptitiously taken! Even in quest of a fountain of youth, the general public too is now enthusiastically embracing the possibility that vitamin E can slow the process of aging. While aging is probably due to many factors and could never be totally prevented without controlling all of them, it seems possible that vitamin E could have some effect in retarding the process, especially in industrialized areas where environmental conditions (such as smog, pollution and so forth) conspire to aggravate the tendency to peroxidative damage. This is even more true if the diet includes large amounts of unsaturated vegetable oils which tend to bring reactive oxygen radicals into the body.[146] It has been frequently suggested that the necessary intake of vitamin E depends on how much polyunsaturated fat is consumed*[147] In America, where fats comprise an average of over 40% of the caloric intake and where the use of vegetable oils has increased, especially in preparing fried foods, it would be expected that requirements for vitamin E have likewise increased. Unfortunately, this change in dietary fat has come at precisely the time when carbohydrate intake has shifted from whole grains rich in vitamin E to refined flour and sugar, [150] which contain little or none. This increase in need for vitamin E coupled with the decrease in its sources in the diets of most people, may well account for why so many people have found that taking 400 to

---

* While some writers have insisted that polyunsaturated vegetable oils are rich in vitamin E[148] and contain sufficient quantities to make up for the actual demands they create, this does not take into account the rancidity of the oil which increases tremendously the need for anti-oxidants.[149]

600 IU's of vitamin E a day has made them feel better and has relieved a wide variety of ills.

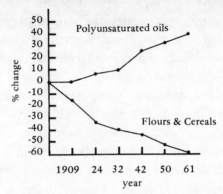

Percent of Change in Consumption of Oils and Grains [156]

If one's fat intake is limited to a couple of tablespoons of saturated fat (butter and ghee) and the polyunsaturates that are taken as natural constituents of whole vegetable foods, then his vitamin E needs should not be high. They should be easily met by the vitamin E contained in a days quota of whole grains, beans, vegetables, etc. It seems likely that vitamin E supplements are only useful or helpful for those who eat foods cooked with large quantities of extracted polyunsaturated oils such as those ordinarily used for frying, for salad oils, and in making many cookies, pastries, cakes, pies and so forth.

OTHER VITAMINS

"Vitamin P" is a term sometimes used to denote the bioflavonoids, a group of compounds related to vitamin C and usually found in nature along with vitamin C. A fair amount of research has been done on vitamin P, especially in the Soviet Union from where reports come of successful treatment of many problems that have to do with fragility and weakness of the blood vessels such as some kinds of bleeding tendencies.[151]

Vitamin K is normally manufactured in the intestinal tract by certain bacteria. It is found in green plants and leafy green vegetables and is an important component of a system that produces blood clotting. Small doses of naturally occurring* vitamin K sometimes reduce the nausea of pregnancy.[152] Interestingly enough, vitamin K has been used to some extent as a food preservative since it prevents fermentation.

Vitamin F was a term once used for "essential fatty acids." The body is unable to synthesize three essential unsaturated fatty acids. They are contained in vegetable oils which are naturally found in whole grains, seeds, nuts and vegetables. Small quantities of these particular fat chains are also found in butterfat, and it would seem unlikely that one could become deficient in them unless his diet was high in refined carbohydrates and meat (the fat and cholesterol of which increases the need for vitamin F)[153] and devoid of all grains, beans and vegetables. Vitamin F supplements have apparently helped some cases of prostate disease.[134]

VITAMINS: SUMMING UP

As we have seen in our discussion of the individual vitamins, they can be taken in various ways. First of all, they can be taken in very small quantities to prevent the occurrence of a "deficiency disease." Small quantities of vitamin C, for example, will prevent the appearance of scurvy, though slightly larger quantities of the vitamin may be necessary for optimal functioning. If health is not good or nutrition is in other ways substandard, it is sometimes possible that even higher doses of the vitamin may help in some way to compensate. Exactly how much of the vitamin is needed for optimal nutrition may vary since each person's requirements are different. Thus it is that extremely high doses of vitamin C have been used to treat people who have certain diseases and who may be suffering from the effects of a diet inadequate in other nutrients besides

---

* Synthetic vitamin K can be toxic.

vitamin C itself. In this case, we are using the substance not really as a vitamin but as a pharmocologic agent, that is, as a medicine.

Unfortunately, taking one nutrient in extremely large quantities may change the requirements of other nutrients in ways that are as yet little understood. Moreover, there is the question of safety since high doses of some vitamins can be toxic. As we have seen, for example, high doses of vitamin C can in some few people, aggravate the tendency to form kidney stones and in other cases even relatively low doses of vitamin D can be extremely toxic. It appears that there is a great deal of individual variation not only in the requirements for certain vitamins, but also in the susceptibility to their toxic effects. Taking such large doses of a compound, even those which occur naturally in foods, takes us far afield from issues of food selection and the common sensical question of how to establish whole-some eating habits and we can begin to sense the fallacy of thinking in terms of "vitamins" as something that can be taken separately from food.

It is really not so clear what it is that makes a substance a "vitamin" in the first place. Generally we say "a vitamin is a necessary compound the body can't synthesize." But by this definition vitamin D turns out to be more of a hormone than a vitamin, since it can be synthesized in the body. Niacin, too, can be synthesized from tryptophan, so its claim to being a vita-min in the classic sense is questionable. Vitamin C has been said not to be a vitamin at all, but to be required because of an inherited defect in man. Thiamin, on the other hand, has been shown to be manufactured in the large intestine of many people so that for some it is unnecessary to take it in the diet and the same is probably true of other B vitamins. Even in the case of the classical deficiency diseases like scurvy and beri-beri, some people came down with the disease while others didn't. What is a "vitamin" anyway? How did we ever get stuck with such a cumbersome notion?

Historically, as we have seen, the concept arose because persons confined under unusual circumstances developed diseases that were related to the unusual and bizarre diets forced upon them by their isolation. The aura of magic and power surrounding the dramatic cure of such diseases by a simple compound set the stage for a growing popular conviction that nutrition could be reduced to a manageable number of similar chemical compounds. Uneven distribution of the substance may well have been a key factor in its coming to be termed "a vitamin." If there are enough foods that don't contain any of it or contain very small quantities of it, then there is the possibility of putting together a diet in which it will be deficient. This is unlikely to happen, of course, where one has access to a great variety of foods, since he will eventually "develop a taste" for some food which contains the needed substance and break the unconsciously self-imposed "vitamin deficient diet." In times of famine or aboard ship, however, a variety of foods may not be available for long periods, and the vitamin deficient diets may be enforced due to these circumstances. When such diets happen to eliminate almost completely one of the more crucial nutrients that are unevenly distributed in this way, then an accidental experiment is performed and a classic deficiency disease is produced.

Diets of today comprised of highly refined and processed foods may be compared in a sense to the early "experiments" that resulted from isolating sailors aboard ship with inadequate food supplies. By contrast, however, modern diets may eliminate across the board a large number of nutrients, some which were so uniformly distributed in natural foods that deficiencies of them had not even been seen before. There results a complex of many borderline "deficiency syndromes." These may well lead to a significant portion of our common health problems today. Untangling which vitamin is deficient to what extent can be an overwhelming job, but actually, the situation need not be so complex. The result of our discussions about individual vitamins should make it clear by now that one can obtain generous quantities of all the known vitamins if his diet is rich in whole fresh vegetables, especially green ones, and whole grains. If these form a significant portion of his diet, 50-75%, then he is assured of sufficient quantities of vitamin A, C, D and E and all the B vitamins except B_{12}. Small amounts of milk or eggs comprising as little as 5% of the diet would take care of this latter problem.

Though this provides for the known vitamins in a quite adequate fashion, how many other substances and less tangible properties of food remain unidentified but nevertheless important for vibrant health remains to be seen. It is unlikely that we have identified all the factors in food which are ideal for optimal functioning. A diet of "new," highly processed and synthetic foods may be virtually devoid of many such as-yet-unidentified nutrients. We might imagine that the result of this would be a sense of craving, of weight gain due to the inability to satisfy such cravings, or of vague symptoms such as nervousness, premature aging and so forth. Such problems would be difficult to relate to nutrition by the classical research approaches based on deficiency diseases and the present concepts of vitamins as "essential nutrients."

As we have seen before, the plant and the animal evolved together, and what the animal cell needs for food is whatever is contained in the plant cell. This includes certain substances which we have identified as "vitamins," "protein," "carbo-hydrate," "fat," etc. But it may well include other substances which we have not identified, or even subtler qualities or energy states of the protoplasmic constituents that our technology is not yet sophisticated enough to pick up. As one well known nutrition-ist has said, "One thing of which my colleagues and I are certain is that nutrition still has its secrets."[155] Some of these, he adds, are minerals about which we are only beginning to learn.

Minerals

8

When plant or animal tissue is burned, the nitrogen, sulfur, hydrogen and carbon that make up the fats, carbohydrates and protein go off as gases, and the minerals alone remain as "ash." The minerals that will be found through such a process to be in the body are primarily sodium, potassium, calcium, phosphorus and magnesium. But there are also a number of other minerals found in very tiny or "trace" amounts such as zinc, iodine, manganese, copper and even arsenic. The list continues to grow as with increasingly sophisticated technology we discover that minerals which we had considered only accidentally present in tissues actually play important metabolic roles. They are often the key ingredients in the large protein molecules we call enzymes, on whose action most of the metabolic processes of the body depend.

Though one atom of a trace element like zinc or manganese may be very small in comparison to the huge, complex enzyme molecule, its role is crucial. Something about it is unique, so that bringing the chains of carbon, nitrogen, oxygen and hydrogen into contact with it allows them to be transformed into new compounds. Such specific and subtle properties recall the alchemist's teachings about the power of the metals. In any event, the inner workings of a cell reveal reactions between the trace elements that would cause even a medieval alchemist to raise his eyebrows in disbelief.

During the one second that the blood is racing through the tiny capillaries of the lung, the single atom of zinc that is set in the center of the enzyme carbonic anhydrase is brought into contact with 600,000 of its target molecules (carbonic acid). The result is that each is broken into one water and one carbon dioxide molecule. Only because of the rapidity of the enzyme's action can the carbon dioxide be freed fast enough from its compounds to leave the blood during that moment in the alveolus when it is separated from the air by only the thinnest of membranes. Our ability to rid ourselves of CO_2 through the exhaled air is then utterly dependent on the presence of these critically located atoms of zinc. Yet the total amount of this mineral in the body is so little that it was, up until a few years ago, considered to be of no significance! Though such trace elements as zinc generally play a very subtle (though crucial) role in the body's functioning, other minerals present in larger amounts, like calcium, may make up the bulk of such tissues as bone.

Minerals are so called because they are found in the earth. It is mineral salts such as calcium carbonate (limestone) that make up rock formations. Where rocks and stones have been broken down into tiny fragments by millions of years of weathering, there exists an accumulation of dust or sand which is the basis of soil. Besides these tiny crystals of mineral salts, the soil is teeming with microbes which begin to "bring the minerals to life," a process that continues when they are passed on to the plant and culminates when they are offered for the nourishment of animal and human tissues.

CALCIUM

Of all the minerals in the body, calcium is the most abundant. The skeleton of the body depends on calcium just as the more rigid, supporting structures in the earth's crust rely to a great extent on calcareous formations like limestone. The deposition of calcium in the bones is a structural process. It is almost as though the bones stretch up against the pull of gravity, raising us from the earth's surface. Without gravity, in fact, the bones begin to lose calcium. During the eight days the astronauts were confined to their space ship, they lost 200 mg of calcium a day, in spite of cleverly designed and vigorous exercise programs. The absence of gravity in space makes it impossible to walk so that the bones begin to lose calcium and continue to do so until the natural forces of gravity, walking, lifting and human activity, which shaped the skeleton, are resumed.

When a bone is fractured and set askew the limb will not necessarily be deformed. As long as the parts unite, the forces of gravity and the forces created by exertion during the use of the limb will gradually cause the bone to reshape, returning toward proper alignment as calcium is deposited along the lines of gravity or the lines of force.

By the same token when gravity is not exerting its effect and one is at rest, then calcification of the skeleton ceases, and calcium tends to be pulled out of the bones to be used for other purposes. Special efforts are made to get bedridden patients on their feet as soon as possible. Old people particularly will become more susceptible to fractures if they remain inactive too long.

Even during the night when one is inactive and lying in bed, calcium can be lost from the body by excretion into the urine if the diet is not rich in it or if the last meal, even though adequate in calcium, was taken many hours before. This is especially true in older people who are prone to eat less of the mineral, absorb it less well, and tend to exercise less.

After the hormonal shifts of menopause, women seem to be more susceptible to the action of the parathyroid hormone, which promotes the removal of calcium from the bones, and they come to lose more of it in the night than they can restore during their waking hours.[1] The result is a gradual demineralizing

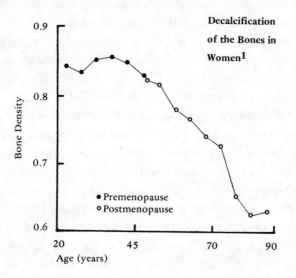

of the bones with increasing age and a growing incidence of fractures. Often there is a collapse of the vertebrae from the weight that they must bear. It has been estimated that such softening of the bones, called osteoporosis, is a major orthopedic disorder in about one out of four women who have passed menopause.

Until recently it was assumed that osteoporosis was a natural part of the aging process and that is could not be prevented, much less reversed. Evidence is accumulating, however, that osteoporosis is more frequent in those with low calcium intakes and that the condition can be improved in some cases, though large amounts of calcium may be necessary to do this. When a group of women between ages seventy-nine and eighty-nine were surveyed, it was found that they were getting only about 450 mg of usable calcium daily from their regular diet—hardly more than half the recommended daily allowance of 800 mg. When they were given a calcium supplement of 750 mg each day, along with 375 units of vitamin D, the bone density *increased* over a three year period. In similar women who were not treated, bone density continued its usual downhill course over that same time period.[2]

Unfortunately, very high intakes of calcium may reduce the absorption of other important minerals, such as manganese,[3] zinc[4] and iron.[5] Properly timed intake of calcium-rich foods (e.g., milk before bed), regular exercise and overall good nutrition stressing fresh, tender vegetables are probably better ways of dealing with osteoporosis than taking huge amounts of calcium supplements. There is also some evidence that osteoporosis is less common and less severe in those who don't eat meat. A recent research study on twenty-five persons who had lived for ten or more years on a meat-free diet showed them to have better mineralized bones than a matched group of men and women who were similar in other respects but took a meat-based diet.[6]

HOW MUCH CALCIUM AND FROM WHERE?

A quarter liter of milk (a little less than 8 ounces) contains about 300 mg of calcium. Most other foods supply much less, though some of the leafy green vegetables are very rich in calcium. A cup of mustard greens (cooked) contains about 310 mg, more than is in an equal amount of milk, and collards 280, a little less than milk. Even broccoli contains nearly 200 mg of calcium in a one cup serving. Probably the richest non-dairy source is "lambs quarters" (*Chenopodium album*), usually regarded as a weed in Europe and America. One cup of its cooked green leaves supplies 400 mg of calcium, more than is required by some people in a day. In North India where this weed is removed from crops to be used as food and is even cultivated, it is the most universally popular leafy green vegetable eaten, and is prepared in a variety of delicious ways.

Sesame seeds are often said to be rich in calcium, and a cup contains 1,000 mg, but since they are rather difficult to digest, one is not likely to eat large quantities at a time. Grains may supply a small but consistent amount of calcium in the diet, though it would be necessary to eat an entire loaf of whole wheat bread to get 450 mg of calcium. Moreover, as we have seen, grains contain a substance in the bran (phytic acid) that may tie up calcium, preventing its absorption. This has led to a number of publications declaring that white bread is more healthful than whole wheat, that brown bread can cause rickets, etc.*

Actually, a number of other factors probably have more important effects on the absorption and utilization of calcium in the body. It has been shown, for example, that lactose enhances the ability to absorb calcium in animals.[7] Of course, in man this depends on the ease with which he is able to handle lactose itself.† The presence of butterfat is apparently also helpful and promotes the absorption of calcium.[8] For this reason it is probably best, especially in children, that nonfat milk be avoided. Two percent butterfat, the so-called "low-fat" milk, is probably preferable for those who should be careful about calcium absorption, but want to avoid a large intake of fat.

The amount of protein that is taken in the diet along with the calcium is another factor which may influence to a great extent one's ability to absorb the mineral. Too little protein will result in reduced calcium absorption.[9] On the other hand, a very high intake of animal protein can also depress calcium retention,[10] which may explain why vegetarians tend to have stronger bones.

These factors suggest that milk would be an ideal source of calcium, since it contains both lactose, butterfat and a moderate amount of protein. It has been said, however, that some people get less usable calcium from drinking milk than from

* See Chapter 4, Carbohydrate.
† See Chapter 6, Protein.

eating leafy vegetables. In days past, it was not unusual for the family doctor, seeing a child with poorly developing teeth but who drank large quantities of milk, to say, "Eat lots of greens like mustard greens, and cut down on the milk." Another way of increasing calcium absorption is to have a glass of fruit juice after meals. Apple juice, for example, has been shown to be particularly effective in facilitating the absorption of calcium from food.[11]

While one may increase the absorption of calcium in the food he takes, it is unfortunately very difficult to calculate exactly how much calcium is really needed, despite the much publicized "Recommended Daily Allowances" (RDA). Not only is there a wide variation, as we have seen above, in individual requirements, but there is a lack of precise knowledge about how much of the calcium of various foods is in a form that can be absorbed. Fortunately, many population groups show an ability to tolerate rather low intakes of calcium. Children in Ceylon often maintain adequate growth and a positive calcium balance on intakes of about 200 mg of calcium a day. Similar observations have been made in Johannesburg, Mysore, Peru and in Africa. In fact, the Bantu, receiving no more than 300 mg a day, have not only a normal blood calcium but also normal amounts in their bones.[12]

Calcium requirements also vary markedly from one individual to another. Two apparently normal five year old children living together in the same environment and eating the same food were found to be quite different in the way they handled calcium. One retained just over 250 mg of the calcium eaten each day during a six week study, while the other retained nearly twice as much.[13] In studies done on nineteen healthy men, it was found that the amount of calcium required in the diet to prevent a net loss from the body varied from about 200 mg a day to just over 1,000. That is to say that the man at the upper extreme required nearly five times as much calcium as the man who had the lowest needs.[14]

Such differences may be partly due to adaptation. Intensive research was done on twenty-six Norwegian prisoners to see to what extent they would "learn" to tolerate diets low in calcium. The subjects were healthy men, and all but four adapted satisfactorily to a diet containing only 400 mg of calcium a day. This means that somehow their metabolism shifted to the point that the amount of calcium excreted in the urine and feces was approximately the same as what they took in.[15]   It is important to realize that all these men were apparently in good health. A study of people with obvious health problems might reveal much less ability to adapt to low calcium intakes and some persons with much greater requirements for calcium.

Though it is obviously impossible to establish a calcium intake that is suitable for everyone, official "average" requirements have been set which reflect trends for each age group. Whereas adult men and women are estimated to need only 800 mg of calcium a day, boys and girls between the ages of eleven and eighteen are said to need 1,200 mg, despite their smaller size, since they are busily building bones and teeth. Even infants require 360 to 540 mg of calcium a day because of their rapid growth. Pregnant and lactating women also should have a minimum of 1,200 mg. This is especially important during the last two months of pregnancy, since over half the calcium present in the baby's body at birth is deposited during that period.

CALCIUM IN MUSCLES AND NERVES

Though ninety-eight percent of the body's calcium is in the bones and one percent is in the teeth, the other one percent which is present in all the other tissues is essential for certain metabolic reactions such as the contraction of muscles. Calcium is one of the ions that acts between the muscle fibrils during the contraction process. If the muscle doesn't have enough calcium, the fibers are motionless and do not slide together and mesh. So the muscle cannot contract, or, once it has contracted, it will not relax. The result is a rather painful situation we call a "cramp."

One of the most common causes of cramping pains is calcium deficiency. Sometimes supplying calcium is a simple solution to a puzzling ailment as the following case illustrates:

> A forty-five year old woman came to the emergency room complaining of severe cramps in the lower abdomen, extending into the hips and legs, making it impossible for her to get about or even to tolerate the pain. A thorough examination showed no discernible pathology and so the nurse was asked to bring a vial of calcium gluconate, since that was all the typical emergency room stocked in the way of calcium preparations. Though it was supplied for intravenous or intramuscular injection, the vial was broken open, the solution was poured into a cup and, to the surprise of both patient and nurse, the patient was asked to drink it. Within five minutes her cramps were gone, she stood up and walked home feeling quite relieved after the importance of getting adequate calcium in the diet was explained to her.

Calcium has also been found to be helpful for some people who are troubled by anxiety and feel "like a bundle of nerves."[16] A cup of warm milk at bedtime not only supplies needed calcium during the critical hours when it can be lost, but it is also a traditional bit of folk wisdom that it promotes better sleep and relaxation, effects often attributed to the calcium it contains.

Calcium and magnesium often occur together. Unlike the salt sodium chloride or table salt, which is quite soluble in water, their compounds tend to be insoluble and form solid masses. Calcium and magnesium are thus called "the earth alkalis" since their compounds or "salts" are found in the earth's crust. Magnesium carbonate and calcium carbonate together form huge outcroppings in certain areas of the world such as the Dolomite range in Austria and northern Yugoslavia. This naturally occurring mineral combination called "dolomite" has come to be mined and marketed as a dietary supplement. It is not known, however, to what extent this mineral, taken directly from the earth, can serve as an alternative to the calcium and magnesium of foods which are complexed with plant or animal matter. Clearly, most of the minerals used by the body, including these, are normally taken in the form in which they occur in living protoplasm.

MAGNESIUM

In most diets, cereals and vegetables contribute two-thirds or more of the daily magnesium intake. Seeds and grains are rich in this mineral too, and green vegetables contain significant quantities because magnesium is an essential component of chlorophyll. In chlorophyll, it occupies a position very similar to that occupied by iron in hemoglobin. In the animal kingdom, however, magnesium is found along with calcium in the bones and serves, as does calcium, an important role in the transmission of the nerve impulse. In fact, high doses of magnesium can produce a sort of tranquilization or even a narcosis with loss of consciousness. But a magnesium stupor can be immediately interrupted by injecting calcium. This is fascinating when we consider that calcium is also capable of producing relaxation and is considered by many people a sort of tranquilizer. The solution to the paradox could involve the ratio between calcium and magnesium. When one exists in excess of the other, the functioning of the nervous system may be upset.

In any case, it was the search for a balanced supplement of calcium and magnesium, along with phosphorous and other minerals which occur in bones and teeth, that led many nutritionists to recommend "bone meal," the ground powder of animal bones. While this may seem preferable to dolomite, since it would seem to be in a more biologically compatible and usable form, it has not always been safe. Bones tend not only to concentrate useful minerals but to be a site where toxic metals are deposited too, perhaps to "get them out of the way" so they don't interfere with metabolic processes. Lead is a case in point and, especially in older animals who have been exposed to an environment containing significant amounts of lead, there will be high levels of it in the bones. When such animals are used as a source of bone meal, the results can be catastrophic.

In 1967 the career of a California actress ended because she was unable to walk without a cane. She had been ill for three years with fatigue, dizziness and ill-humor. Her auburn hair had turned dark brown, then black and finally had begun to fall out. Muscle weakness had progressed to near paralysis. A year later her blood count was so low she was hospitalized. It was thought at first she may have leukemia, but no diagnosis was confirmed. After seeing 22 doctors and having 340 X-rays, she was advised she must "learn to live with it."

Though too weak to walk, she had friends carry her to the library where she read everything she could find on conditions like hers. Descriptions of metal poisoning sounded a familiar note. After six years of illness, perhaps there was some hope of finding out what was wrong. A toxicologist agreed to do tests though she assured him that she had not been exposed to any chemicals nor was she taking any medicines other than a calcium supplement prescribed for her menstrual cramps.

But tests showed she had lead poisoning, and that her supplement, bone meal, contained 190 parts per million of lead. Two years later her urine was still carrying out ten times the usual amounts of the toxic metal.

Samplings of bone meal from health food stores in her area showed that all were contaminated. The product originated at a glue factory in England and was packaged for distribution locally. Three others who had also taken the bone meal were traced. One had become insane and was committed to a mental hospital where, off the supplement, she recovered. A second, in a trip to Paris, had finally been diagnosed as having lead poisoning. A third died before the patient made her discoveries.

After learning what was wrong and stopping the bone meal, the actress recovered some strength, but her health never returned to normal.[17]

Mechanically deboned meat is allowed to contain 4% of

bone fragments, which may contain lead. Powdered bone meal is often added to commercial baby foods, which may be why they are sometimes contaminated with lead. The FDA stipulates no limits for the amount of lead permitted in foods.

LEAD

There is little lead naturally occurring in the body or even on the surface of the earth. Lead is largely deposited deeply underground. It has been mined increasingly over the last two hundred years, and during the past fifty years it has been used in growing quantities as an "anti-knock" additive in automobile gasoline. In 1967, 247,000 tons of lead were released into the air as the result of automobile exhaust.[18] Thirty to fifty percent of the lead in inhaled air is absorbed into the body. As a result, those persons who are frequently around automobile exhaust often suffer from some degree of lead poisoning. Levels measured in several Japanese cities and Paris showed levels of lead pollution that would produce a definite toxic illness in anyone who lived in that area for more than ten years.[19] The degree of lead pollution is more severe at street level where automobile exhaust fumes settle and is reduced as one goes to a second or third story apartment. Children, who are more susceptible to the effects of lead anyway, suffer especially since they tend to play at the level of the street. In the average American city, one out of four children is estimated to be suffering from some degree of lead toxicity.[20] Some of this has been thought to come from eating lead paints which flake off walls. On rare occasions, this may be a serious problem since very toxic doses can be ingested in a few minutes. Though leaded paints are still used, there has been an increasing effort to take them off the market. Yet automobile exhaust is a more pervasive problem since it affects more people, is present on a larger scale, and the low levels of toxicity that result often go undetected, causing a variety of symptoms usually not connected with lead poisoning. Hyperactivity, temper tantrums, withdrawal, crying for no good reason, fearfulness, loss of affection, listlessness, refusal to play and other emotional and behavioral problems in children have been linked with lead toxicity.[21] There may also be a decreased resistance to infection. If exposure to lead continues long enough, there can be damage to the brain with decreased intelligence and a tendency to epilepsy and psychiatric problems. It has been estimated that nearly one hundred thousand American children who live and play in areas with heavy traffic are in need of treatment for lead poisoning.[22]

Nor are the small towns immune to this problem. A variety of cities of different sizes showed similar lead levels in the air.[23] Samples of the soil along roadsides show elevated lead, as do the soils all along the Eastern seaboard, though concentrations do tend to be higher in areas where traffic is more frequent. Apparently, airborne lead is also carried by winds far away from busy cities and seems especially prone to be deposited at higher altitudes. In the Western United States, deer killed by hunters in the early 1970's at 7,000 feet in the mountains showed as much as 250 parts per million of lead in their hair, as well as extremely high tissue levels.[24] This is six times the 45 parts per million of lead in hair that is normally considered an indication of toxicity. There has even been a sharp increase in the accumulation of lead in glacier ice laid down in Greenland since 1940 due to airborne lead. Fortunately, the sale of leaded gasoline has already been banned in some cities.

Because lead normally exists in only small quantities in the surface of the earth, biological systems seemed to have evolved no adequate means of handling it. Other metals such as iron, for example, which is 5,000 times more plentiful in the surface soil than lead, is not only non-toxic (except in extremely high doses) but actually plays a strategic part in the biochemistry of living matter. The cell has evolved around the iron, and using it as a component of important biological molecules, regards it as essential rather than toxic. Quite the opposite is true of lead, which is toxic in even relatively small amounts. When 400 subjects from America and around the world were tested for lead levels it was found that in America, lead accumulated in the body with increasing age, whereas in seventeen other countries it did not.[25]   In fact, comparison of the lead in the bones of skeletons from around the world show Americans to have higher levels than any other peoples, ancient or modern, with the possible exception of the ancient Romans, and it has been suggested that their use of water from lead vessels and pipes contributed to their downfall.

For those whose health is not good, the extra burden of borderline lead intoxication might be enough to push them into a serious crisis.   Awareness of such problems is increasing as laboratory methods for detecting mineral levels improve.   Diagnosis has been simplified by the discovery that the measurement of lead levels in the hair accurately reflect how much is in the body.[26]

Lead toxicity has been shown to be affected by the intake of a number of nutrients and is apparently more severe when the diet is poor.   For instance, if calcium is higher in the diet, then less lead will be absorbed.   The same is thought to be true of iron.[27]   In winter when vitamin D levels are low, children seem more susceptible to lead poisoning.   High doses of vitamin C have been said to help detoxify lead,[28] but an intravenous treatment with a chelating agent is the most rapid and effective method of removing lead from the body.

A chelating agent is, as we have seen, a large molecule which locks around the mineral and holds it.*   In some cases it is then carried out of the body.   The discovery that minerals can be managed better by such chelating molecules has opened doors to whole areas of new research.   It has been found, for example, that not only lead, but other toxic minerals as well, can be removed from the body in this way.

Toxic minerals owe their destructive effects to their

---

* See Chapter 2, The Soil.

ability to displace others that normally play a vital role in metabolism. Because of their weight and tenacity, the toxic minerals tend to displace a normal mineral from its proper position in, for example, an enzyme molecule rendering the enzyme ineffective. Yet the disabled molecule may remain in the cell, occupying the place that should be taken by a normally functioning enzyme. Thus important reactions are inhibited and vital steps in the metabolic process blocked.

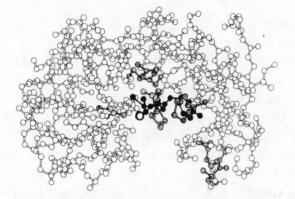

A model showing the importance of trace minerals in molecular interactions. The presence of a single zinc atom,O, is critical for the completion of the biochemical reaction between these two organic molecules, one represented by solid colored circles, and the other by the open and grey colored circles.

The tenacity of the toxic mineral, however, is very convenient during the process of chelation. The chelating molecule is put into the body, carrying, for instance, a calcium ion. The toxic metal, such as lead, promptly displaces the calcium, taking over its position in the chelating molecule and remaining there insistently. The chelating agent can then be excreted in the urine, carrying the lead with it.

If, of course, the chelating agent given is complexed with a weakly held mineral, it may turn it loose and latch onto some other mineral which is essential, carrying *it* out of the body. Thus, EDTA, the agent which is used in removing lead, can pick up calcium if it is introduced into the body as sodium EDTA, since calcium holds on more tightly than sodium and will displace it. Based on this rational, sodium EDTA has been given to people with advanced arteriosclerosis. It is thought to pull out calcium and help break down the plaques which have formed in the blood vessels.* Though such treatment is still very controversial, there is some evidence that it can be effective.[29]

CHROMIUM

Another trace element which has only recently been discovered to be essential is chromium, without which the body cannot produce an enzyme-like substance called "Glucose Tolerance Factor"—GTF. This substance is necessary for the proper production and utilization of insulin, and when it is not found in adequate amounts there may be elevated blood sugar and the condition known as diabetes mellitus.[30] When experimental animals were given a diet free of chromium they soon developed all the symptoms of diabetes, with sugar in the urine. When the chromium was replaced in the diet, the symptoms promptly cleared up. Other conditions also may result from chromium deficiency, though the mechanism has not yet been clarified; for example, animals placed on a chromium-free diet have developed arteriosclerosis with plaques in the arteries. Again, restoring a chromium-rich diet reverses the condition.[31]

To what extent such chromium deficiency may play a role in human arteriosclerosis is not yet clear. When a series of autopsies was done, it was found that none of the people who died from heart attacks had any detectable chromium in the body while those dying from other causes had small amounts.[32] Actually, Americans in general had extremely low levels of chromium when compared to a group of foreigners from around the world. Orientals had 4.5 times as much and other nationalities

---

* Of course it may also pull out other minerals which are essential, so such treatment should be carried out under careful medical supervision.

also had markedly more.[33] This is very interesting considering the unusually high rate of diabetes and arteriosclerosis that are found in America. It is even more intriguing when we learn that chromium deficiency seems to make one more susceptible to lead poisoning since we already know that Americans have the highest lead levels in the world.

The chromium content of food varies considerably, for example, from 0.02 parts per million (ppm) in refined sugar to more than ten times that amount in molasses. Raw sugar or sugar cane juice come "equipped with" an intermediate amount, which is not surprising since some chromium is apparently necessary to metabolize the sugar properly. Thus refined white sugar has been said to "deplete" body chromium since its use requires a great deal yet it contributes virtually none.[34]

In general, refined foods like white sugar and white flour are extremely low in chromium since it is lost in the refining process. Whole wheat contains about 0.4 ppm of chromium. Herbs and spices may contain significantly larger amounts. Black pepper, for example, has 10 ppm of chromium, five times as much as chicken (1.7 ppm) or milk (1.6 ppm). Meats range from .02 to .04, while brewers yeast contains 44.9 ppm.* Diets in which spices are used in significant quantities may be unusually rich in chromium.[36] Inorganic chromium, on the other hand, seems not to be assimilated by the body so that chromium salts are of little use as supplements.[37] Meanwhile, GTF remains more of a vitamin perhaps than a mineral, since the chromium must be complexed with a large organic molecule—in the same fashion as cobalt in vitamin B_{12}. Recently, there have been attempts to prepare chelated forms of chromium which would mimic those that occur naturally. If these turn out to be well absorbed and utilized, they may prove to be an important

---

* Other work, in which the biologically active chromium complex, GTF, was extracted using ethanol, also indicate that brewers yeast and black pepper contain the highest amount of that form of chromium.[35] However, in the case of other foods, the literature is not consistently in agreement on best dietary sources because of incomplete knowledge of possible forms and availability of chromium in foods.

weapon against arteriosclerosis and diabetes.

But as we shall see throughout this book, it is unlikely that any of the commonly occurring chronic degenerative conditions like diabetes and arteriosclerosis are produced anywhere, except in the laboratory, by the deficiency of a single nutrient. More often, there are a number of nutrients whose deficiency can be linked to a given disease, as well as other causal factors involving the psychological and emotional makeup of the person, his heredity and constitution and his environment. For example, diabetic-like conditions have also been produced in experimental animals by feeding their mothers manganese-deficient diets during pregnancy. Dietary supplementation of the diabetic animals with manganese was found to increase the number of insulin-producing cells.[38]

MANGANESE

At least one dramatic case has been recorded where a young man with severe diabetes who was unresponsive to insulin controlled his disease by drinking alfalfa tea. Since alfalfa contains high levels of manganese, a manganese supplement was given and found to produce the same results.[39] The manganese content of foods varies, and deficiencies in the soil have been recorded in twenty-five states, although it was found to be more available to plants when the soil was rich in humus.[40] Of course, manganese can be added to soluble chemical fertilizer preparations, but this requires careful determination of soil levels before the preparation of the fertilizer since too much manganese can also create problems. The same principle holds for other trace elements, and the advocates of artificial fertilization have proposed that the most suitable plan is to custom-make fertilizers for each field and application. The formulation of suitable soluble fertilizer preparations then becomes extremely complex and so prohibitively expensive that it seems unlikely it will ever be practical.[41]

Meanwhile, the use of soluble fertilizers which contain predominantly nitrates, phosphates, potash and sometimes calcium and magnesium continues, while the trace elements are gradually washed out of the soil. The problem of mineral loss is a big one. As we saw earlier, soil is leached of minerals by rain once it has lost its humus. Moreover, once this process reaches a certain point, the soil itself, which can to some extent correct imbalances, is also lost through erosion by wind and rainfall.

While the manganese content of a food will vary a great deal depending on the condition of the soil, those generally rich in it are whole grains, dried beans and peas and leafy green vegetables. Meat, milk and refined cereals tend to be poor sources. Though seeds such as grains and legumes may provide a continual, moderate supply of manganese, tea, by contrast, is extraordinarily rich in it and a cup of tea may contain as much as 1.3 mg, as much as is found in fifty loaves of whole wheat bread! Manganese requirements have not been established for humans, but the average diet contains 2 to 9 mg a day.

In experimental animals, manganese deficiencies produce bone deformities which do not seem to be due to a lack of calcium, since it is present in normal amounts, but rather to a failure of the bone to "stretch out" to its normal length and shape. Manganese is thought to have something to do with the connective tissue which provides the framework for the bone and promotes its lengthening, outward-moving tendency.[42] This mineral is present in all plant tissues but is particularly concentrated in the green leaves, the shoots and the seeds. Here again it seems to play some strategic role in the process of stretching and growing outward. Wheat, for example, is often considered a fairly rich source of manganese. It contains at most 49 parts per million. A deficiency (or an extreme excess) of manganese has been associated with poor reproductive capacity, schizophrenia and Parkinsonism.[43] All of these are, in a sense, a failure in "outward-movingness."

Manganese is among the least toxic of the minerals. Poisoning from too much manganese-rich foods and beverages has never been reported and is probably impossible except where there is industrial contamination of the food with the inorganic form of the mineral. Manganese poisoning has been seen among miners, for example, after prolonged working with manganese ore. It is characterized by a severe psychiatric disorder similar to schizophrenia and is followed by a permanently crippling neurological disease which is very similar to Parkinson's disease.[44] On the other hand, interestingly enough, the Parkinson-like syndrome that results from taking high doses of the more powerful tranquilizers has been reversed by giving manganese supplements.[45] To round out the paradox, schizophrenic patients have been treated using manganese supplements and have in some cases been definitely improved.[46] It would appear that either excessively high or excessively low levels of this mineral in the body can produce very similar symptom pictures that psychiatrically resemble schizophrenia and neurologically resemble Parkinson's disease. This principle has been recognized by homeopaths who produced Parkinson-like symptoms experimentally more than a century ago by giving repeated small doses of manganese acetate. On the basis of this data, they used homeopathic doses of the same compound to ameliorate the symptoms in those who presented clinically with Parkinson's syndrome.

It is the clinical impression of some physicians that certain patients with a tendency to exaggerated allergies respond well to manganese supplements. This has been borne out by the present writer's clinical experience with those patients who are manganese deficient. In schizophrenic patients, manganese helps to restore balance when histamine, the substance that is released during allergic reactions, is either too high or too low in the blood.[47] Furthermore, in those schizophrenic patients where serum copper is elevated, it has been reported that manganese along with zinc seems to lower the copper and promote its excretions in the urine which is followed by improvement of the psychosis.[48]

COPPER

In those schizophrenic patients whose copper levels are high, the zinc level is often found to be depressed. Zinc and copper often have an inverse relationship to one another and may act like a "see-saw," one going up as the other comes down. Both are closely related to the functioning of nervous tissue. When chronic doses of copper are given, seizures can be induced.[49] Prolonged overdosage with zinc is more likely to produce twitches but the resemblance is clear. (This information was collected through double blind studies, called "provings" and was summarized in, for example, Boericke's *Materia Medica.*[50]

In certain schizophrenic patients, a substance called kryptopyrole has been found in the urine. This is thought to combine with zinc, pulling it out of the body and permitting the elevation of copper levels. In many schizophrenics then, zinc produces an "anti-anxiety" effect that seems to be reflected by changes in brain waves. Urinary copper excretion is consistently less for schizophrenics than for normals.[51]

When the elements of the earth's surface are arranged in the order of their size, weight and number of electrons, protons and neutrons, they fall into definite groups. Those in each group have similar properties. Chemists have devised a chart which lists the lightest (hydrogen) all the way up to the heaviest of the elements. On the left we see magnesium (Mg) and calcium, (Ca) which are, as discussed earlier, very much related. On the far right, we see Helium (He), Neon, (Ne) and Argon, (Ar), the inert gases that have completed shells of electrons in their outer orbits and therefore do not tend to react chemically with anything. (Thus the safety of helium balloons as opposed to those filled with hydrogen, which is highly reactive and will explode.)

If we look at elements 29 and 30 on the periodic table, we see that these two, copper, (Cu) and zinc (Zn), are side by side.

Periodic Chart of the Elements

1 H Hydrogen																	2 He
3 Li	4 Be											5 B	6 C Carbon	7 N Nitrogen	8 O Oxygen	9 F Fluorine	10 Ne
11 Na Sodium	12 Mg Magnesium											13 Al	14 Si	15 P	16 S	17 Cl Chlorine	18 Ar
19 K Potassium	20 Ca Calcium	21 Sc	22 Ti	23 V	24 Cr Chromium	25 Mn Manganese	26 Fe Iron	27 Co	28 Ni	29 Cu Copper	30 Zn Zinc	31 Ga	32 Ge	33 As	34 Se	35 Br	36 Kr
37 Rb	38 Sr	39 Y	40 Zr	41 Nb	42 Mo	43 Tc	44 Ru	45 Rh	46 Pd	47 Ag Silver	48 Cd Cadmium	49 In	50 Sn	51 Sb	52 Te	53 I	54 Xe
55 Cs	56 Ba	57 *La	72 Hf	73 Ta	74 W	75 Re	76 Os	77 Ir Iridium	78 Pt	79 Au	80 Hg Mercury	81 Tl	82 Pb Lead	83 Bi	84 Po	85 At	86 Rn

Number at top is "Atomic Number" of each element and reflects the number of protons in the nucleus.

This explains in part their close relationship, their tendency to compete in the intestinal tract for absorption, and their ability to "trade places" metabolically. Also closely related to copper is silver (Ag) which comes immediately beneath it. While there is no evidence so far that silver is essential for any living organism, it does occur naturally in low concentrations in soils, plants and animal tissue. It can also enter in significant quantities from silver utensils, vessels and foils and, probably most significantly, from the breakdown of silver-mercury amalgam fillings in the teeth. Though it was previously thought that such fillings were inert, it has recently been found that significant amounts of mercury, and possibly silver as well, can be continuously released into the system through the breakdown of the alloy as it undergoes an electrolytic process in saliva.[52]

Silver is known to interact metabolically with copper also. Of all the known copper antagonists tested in experimental animals, silver turned out to be the strongest, even stronger than zinc. Silver toxicity in experimental animals has been found to be prevented by copper supplementation.[53] As metals, both copper and silver have the physical property of being extremely efficient conductors of electricity and heat. Perhaps this characteristic somehow provides a clue as to their role in the functioning of the nervous system.

An intriguing case which may throw some light on the interaction between silver and copper is seen in a patient who accidentally swallowed a silver coin which lodged in the intestinal tract and remained there for eighteen months. He had been epileptic but was cured by the end of this time.[54] Since copper has been known to produce seizures, we can at least postulate that the silver, by replacing copper in some strategic sites in the nervous system, might have decreased the tendency to seizures.

There is a curious thread of interrelatedness running through silver, copper, manganese, epilepsy and schizophrenia. Manganese has been successfully used to treat schizophrenia and is thought in some way to block the action of copper.

Not only has copper been found to be high in about one-third of schizophrenics[55] but it also tends to produce epileptic-type seizures. Historically it was observed that, among the insane, those who had seizures showed dramatic recovery. This led ultimately to the use of electro shock treatment (to induce seizures) as a treatment of schizophrenia. One might wonder if the copper were somehow "used up" during the seizure, allowing normal functioning of the nervous system to return. During the emotional disturbance that comes just before the menstrual period in women copper levels are often elevated,[56] a problem that can be aggravated by birth control pills.

To the extent that zinc levels rise, copper levels are lowered. While this seems to decrease the tendency to psychiatric illness, lowering the copper too much may make one susceptible to other problems. In a wide variety of experimental animals deficiency of copper has produced disease in the hearts and blood vessels such as occurs in some strokes and heart attacks.[57, 58]

All of these facts suggest that while excessive copper may lead to mental and emotional problems, too little may predispose to cardiovascular disease. Yet this may be even more so when zinc is also low. In fact, good results have followed the treatment of groups at a high risk for zinc and copper (along with other supplements).[59] Iron metabolism is very much dependent on copper, and the anemias which result from deficiencies of the two are hard to distinguish. High levels of vitamin C which tend to promote the absorption of iron can interfere with copper absorption.[60]

Green vegetables, some sea foods and liver are the primary sources of copper, providing twice as much as milk, meat and bread. There is no established daily requirement of copper for humans, but the average daily diet contains about two mg, which is apparently adequate since copper deficiencies seem to be rare. Problems from excess copper are more common, though they are probably not so much a result of diet as of the contamination of food and water with inorganic forms of copper. This may come in some cases from copper water pipes, but there is a danger too of taking multiple mineral supplements which provide too much copper and too little zinc.

ZINC

Zinc levels in the hair of patients admitted with arteriosclerosis have been found to be markedly lower than normal,[61] and it has been suggested that zinc may have some effect on the health of the lining of the arteries. It is certainly true that zinc is important for the health of another epithelial or surface tissue, and that is the skin. Veterinarians found that animals whose feed contained inadequate amounts of zinc developed red and cracked skin with loss of hair or wool as well as other problems that developed later. Zinc supplementation is a well-documented,[62] effective treatment for acne which is, if not the most widespread, certainly the most visible skin disorder in America.* Unfortunately, the success in treating acne with zinc in a large proportion of cases seems to be leading to its routine use, not only by physicians but by laymen who treat themselves. The dose customarily used, 135 mg a day, is near the range that can be toxic, at least in some persons.[63]

Zinc has also been effective in treating some cases of bed sores and other ulcers that are slow to heal. Some researchers have claimed that zinc speeds up the healing of any wound, but other research tends to indicate that it is only effective if the person happens to be deficient or somewhat low in zinc.[64] Massive wounds and injuries such as burns may require increased quantities of zinc since it is involved in certain enzymes which are important for the production of new cells and especially the formation of keratin, a substance which is present in hair and

---

* Again this might sometimes be related to the zinc-copper ratio since acne often is worse in young women before their menstrual period and it is at this time that copper levels rise.

nails as well as skin.

Wool fibers in sheep lose their crimp, become thin, are readily shed and stop growing until zinc is replaced in the diet when it has been deficient. Nails often reflect zinc status and may be either speckled with white spots or curbed, dented and misshapen.[65] In fact, in animals with horns, which are made up primarily of keratin, a zinc deficiency will result in the loss of the horn with a remaining short, spongy outgrowth that continually bleeds.[66]

By contrast, horns were said to have sprouted on the head of the satyr who was known for his sexual prowess, an interesting idea since we now know that adequate levels of zinc are required for the proper functioning of the sexual organs of the male. In fact, zinc is found in dramatically high concentrations in the prostate gland and the semen, and zinc supplements have been used to treat prostate problems as well as retarded development of the genital organs.[67] There is a popular, though as yet unproven, notion that increasing one's zinc intake will increase libido. Similarly, there is a persistent and widespread bit of folklore which insists that if one eats oysters he will "love longer," and oysters happen to be the richest source of zinc known, containing nearly 100 times as much as the average of other foods. Curiously, in the Southwest where steers were castrated wholesale and the testes became an article of diet, they were popularly called "prairie oysters" and prized by the local people for their nutritious qualities.*

A case history further attests to the concentration of zinc in oysters.

> Fran was adopted at two weeks of age. No evidence of
> difficulty was observed in her behavior until she started
> school when problems with her behavior and learning caused
> her to fail first grade. Psychological counseling did not help,

---

* In the Appalachians it is hogs that are so castrated, and the corresponding dish is called "mountain oysters."

and she was later diagnosed as having "minimal brain dysfunction" and "learning disabilities."   At thirteen, her
pediatrician, believing her erratic and irritable behavior to
be caused by low blood sugar, hospitalized her and placed
her on a sugar-free, high-protein diet. Her behavior suddenly
changed for the better, but once home, her cravings for
candy could not be controlled. Her parents noticed that
candy wrappers could usually be found in her room after one
of her destructive tantrums.   They also noticed that after
Fran had eaten fried oysters she was unusually alert and
cooperative and never had any tantrums.   So the family had
fried oysters very often.   Meanwhile through their own
reading, the parents discovered that oysters contain more
than twenty times as much zinc as the next richest food.
Having seen no significant improvement in Fran as the result
of megavitamin therapy, they decided to give her zinc.   She
showed marked improvement the day after her first dose.
Within two weeks, she obtained a driver's license, got her
first job and started taking a college course.   The parents
were amazed and very pleased at her change.   They continued zinc for three and a half months and then stopped to
see what would happen.   Three days later, Fran had a severe
temper tantrum, and the next day she had another.   The
parents resumed the zinc at 8:30 a.m., and by 6:00   that
night, she was once again a changed person.[68]

Properly controlled assertiveness and activity seem to be
somehow related to zinc. Studies have shown that dark, highly
active muscles located in one part of the body will contain four
times as much zinc as those lighter colored and less active
muscles from other areas.[69] A need for more or less zinc may
account for the strong food preferences of those who choose
light or dark cuts of meat. The zinc content of vegetable foods is
variable and may depend a great deal on the soil in which they
are grown, as well as on the type of agricultural practices that
were used. The additional conventional chemical fertilizers can
reduce available zinc in the soil by nearly half.[70] Where soils are
already low in zinc, as they are in many areas of the country, this
could have a critical effect on the nutritional value of food
crops.[71]

In fact, a study of college women showed an intake of 12 mg of zinc a day of which 6.6 was retained.[72] The recommended daily allowance, however, is 15 mg a day, more than twice this. On the basis of their clinical experience, some workers in the field of trace elements feel that zinc deficiency is very widespread and serious in the United States. That this may be having a serious impact on health was suggested by research done in Denver where it was discovered that low levels of zinc in the hair were found in nearly half of boys between three months and four years of age. Nearly ten percent had extremely low levels, and a majority of these had a history of poor appetite and failure to gain in height and weight. Their response to zinc supplementation was dramatic.[73] One of the symptoms noted among these boys was a loss of sense of taste. This tends to decrease appetite and the relish for food and leads to further malnutrition and failure to grow properly. In every case, the sense of taste was restored by taking zinc.

One example of how important zinc may be for normal growth in youngsters is in the formation of bones, which contain significant amounts of zinc. Zinc deficiency in animals produces shortened and thickened bones,[74] and zinc has been used successfully to speed up the healing of fractures.[75] The first and most dramatic cases of zinc deficiency in humans were dwarfs who were raised in areas of the Middle East where there was severe zinc deficiency. Part of the problem was felt to be the local tendency to use a whole wheat bread to which extra bran had been added and which had been prepared without being yeasted. It has been shown that the phytic acid present in bran can tie up zinc and interfere with its absorption, carrying it out through the intestinal tract in a way similar to what occurs with calcium.[76] With zinc, the problem may be particularly pronounced since phytase, the enzyme in the gut which normally destroys phytic acid, appears to be an enzyme containing zinc. Therefore a vicious circle ensues: the enzyme can't work, therefore the phytic acid is not broken down, therefore it ties up more zinc, and as a consequence less enzyme is present, etc.

Fermenting the bread with yeast to make it rise increases the availability of zinc in part, it seems, by producing enzymes that destroy some of the phytic acid.[77] Therefore, yeasted bread is less likely to lead to zinc deficiency than unleavened bread. This would be especially true if extra bran had been added to the bread. In India, where unleavened bread or chapatti is used widely, extra bran is never added to the bread. In fact, a small percentage of the bran, the outermost layer which is richest in phytate, is removed. But most of the other bran layers are kept in the flour, a wise step from the point of view of zinc intake, since they contain a large portion of the zinc, and the use of completely refined white flour can result in zinc deficiency.

Zinc bears an important relationship to cadmium, a toxic mineral which is, as we can see from the periodic table (see page 244), just below it, indicating that it is similar in shape and properties to zinc except that it is heavier and tends to replace it. The presence of a small amount of cadmium in food, then, greatly increases the need for adequate zinc since generous supplies of zinc must be present to prevent its displacement by cadmium.[78] Zinc, however, is concentrated in the germ and in the bran of grains. The milling process which produces white flour by removing the bran and the germ therefore removes much of the zinc. Whatever cadmium might be present due to pollution and other factors, is concentrated in the white part of the grain, however, and remains. Thus, whole wheat has a zinc to cadmium ratio of over 100 to 1, whereas white flour has a ratio of only 17 to 1.[79] The difference could be crucial for those whose diet is largely wheat since it is the ratio between cadmium and zinc that is most important both in terms of how much zinc is available and how toxic the cadmium can be.

CADMIUM

Millions of years ago, most of the cadmium in the crust of

the earth, like the lead, was locked away deep underground, but it has gradually and increasingly been brought to the surface by the mining of zinc. Even in the mineral deposits of the earth, cadmium and zinc are closely related and they occur together in natural deposits. Since they can't be separated underground, the bringing up of zinc from the mines also brings cadmium. Moreover, it often accompanies zinc in its industrial applications so that galvanized pipes, tires, batteries, paints, plated metals and many other materials contain cadmium as well as zinc.

Cadmium is virtually absent from the human body at birth but accumulates with age up to about 50 years. One might naturally wonder if this accumulation of cadmium could be another factor having something to do with the diseases that develop so characteristically around middle age, such as hardening of the arteries, high blood pressure, etc.

A few years ago it was discovered, in fact, that high blood pressure could be produced in rats by putting small amounts of cadmium in their drinking water.[80] Treatment with a chelating agent to remove the cadmium reversed the high blood pressure.[81] Studies of the blood and tissues, especially the kidneys, of some patients with high blood pessure, also showed elevated levels of cadmium.[82] Moreover, a correlation was found between the cadmium content and the air in different parts of North America and the incidence of death from high blood pressure and other cardiovascular disease.[83] Soft or acidic drinking water had also been correlated with high blood pressure and this was found to frequently contain higher levels of cadmium.[84] It was easy to conclude that cadmium, a widespread pollutant, was the cause of high blood pressure and many articles appeared in the popular press to this effect.

If this were true, there was cause for concern. Every year in the U.S. more than 2,000 tons of cadmium is lost into the air from zinc and cadmium processing plants and from the burning of coal and oil. Cigarette smoke and automobile exhaust also carry cadmium, and the percentage of inhaled cadmium that is retained is 10-40%. However, this turned out to add only a small part of the total cadmium burden of the body. Most of it enters through the food and water. Run-off water from mines and waste water from industry brings cadmium into the water supply, and further cadmium may be absorbed from the pipes. Galvanized pipes, of course, contribute cadmium, but the black plastic pipes that are currently being used also do this. Suddenly it became a commonplace assumption that plastic pipes caused high blood pressure. Most water systems were found to contain permissible levels of cadmium, and it is thought that only ten to twenty micrograms of cadmium per day is consumed by the average person from his water supply.[85]

As further research was done, there were other pieces of the puzzle too, that did not fit together so neatly as had been thought. Surprisingly, for instance, it was found that industrial workers exposed to high levels of cadmium did not have a higher than normal incidence of high blood pressure even though they came down with symptoms of cadmium toxicity.[86] Moreover, analysis of the cadmium in the kidneys of patients who had died from various diseases showed no correlation between cadmium levels and hypertension or any other disease of the arteries and heart. [87, 88] The situation has remained both controversial and puzzling.

Meanwhile, other disorders have been more firmly tied to cadmium as a causal agent. Emphysema, for example, seems to be due to a great extent to the cadmium inhaled by cigarette smokers.[89] Cadmium seems to have an affinity for testicular tissue, possibly because it replaces zinc. A single small injection of cadmium has been able to produce hemorrhage and destruction in rat testes. This can be prevented by zinc as well as selenium.[90] Industrial workers exposed to cadmium have a definitely higher incidence of cancer, and this is often cancer of the prostate.[91]

Whether or not such diseases can result from the cumulative effects of the low doses of cadmium to which the average person is exposed through air pollution and contamination of his food and water is not certain. Actually, in some cases the reverse may be true. It has been shown that exposure to very low levels of cadmium results in some sort of protection against later challenges with more toxic levels.[92]   This may be a sort of antibody response to the cadmium. There is even some evidence that there may be a cross immunity from one toxic metal to another, so that after exposure to mercury, for example, one would develop some tolerance to cadmium. This is intriguing and if it is true, it would lead one to wonder why those who become ill from exposure to lead or cadmium do not develop the usual immunity. It often happens that of several people living in the same environment, one will develop signs and symptoms of heavy metal poisoning while another does not.

In any event, the average person probably takes in levels of cadmium which he is able to handle. But there may be some cause for concern by those who are exposed to air that is a bit more polluted than usual, to water pipes that contain a bit more cadmium and to larger amounts of cigarette smoke, etc. They may find themselves with a daily intake of cadmium that is significantly higher than average. Moreover, the problem can be compounded by a concurrent exposure to lead, since research has shown that the effects of the two are addictive.[93] They also probably work synergistically with ozone or the free radicals carried by oils.* Cadmium and lead are thought to act as catalysts for such damaging oxidations.[94]   As mentioned above, however, those who are in good general health may be able to develop some resistance to the effects of these toxic metals, and an overall good diet may be the key to this. A diet rich in iron and zinc, a flour of moderately high extraction rate, plenty of vita-min C-containing foods and an adequate intake of milk protein can all help decrease the cadmium retention. Taking vitamin supplements may be trickier than simply improving the diet; high doses of vitamin B_6 for example, have increased susceptibility

* See Chapter 5, Fats.

to cadmium toxicity.[95]

Selenium also protects against many of the effects of cadmium,[96] as it does against other potentially harmful substances such as vegetable oils, etc. This is apparently owing to its antioxidant effects, and in this respect it works in a way similar to vitamin E, to which it has a close relationship. However, selenium is not without danger itself. Though selenium supplements have recently been marketed, it is not a mineral that should be taken carelessly. Compared to many of the other trace elements, it has a relatively narrow range between what is essential and what is toxic. In certain areas where selenium content of the soil is high, certain diseases seem to result from eating the local food. Dental cavities tend to go up,[97] and there may be an increase of degenerative diseases of the nervous system.[98]

IRON

An appreciation of the importance of iron in the diet goes back further than perhaps that of any other minerals. The ancients thought of it as a carrier, and it was identified with Mars, perhaps in part because of the distinctive redness of the planet Mars. The redness of iron comes from its tendency to oxidize or "rust," and, in fact, the word "rust" comes from an ancient Indo-European or Aryan root which means red. Its tendency to take up oxygen readily, changing its color to red, is the basis for its function in the blood where it is the carrier of oxygen to the tissues of the body. Its affinity for other substances and its tendency to take hold of and carry is demonstrated in its metallic form, too, by its ability to become magnetized and to attract and carry metal objects.

Iron has the curious ability to change valences. It can either have two or three electrical charges. This means it can, by altering itself from one state to the other, take up or let go an extra oxygen atom. At some primitive point, the evolving organism seized upon this unique quality of the iron atom and made it the center of its oxygen transport system, which is based on hemoglobin. Hemoglobin is a complex, giant molecule which contains, like a tiny jewel in the center of each of its four basic components, a single atom of iron. This iron in the center of the hemoglobin molecule accepts the oxygen and as it does so, develops the bright red color which differentiates oxygenated blood of the arteries from the dark red, bluish blood of the veins.

However, today on farmlands where the soils have been cultivated for some time, iron deficiency is thought to be the most commonly occurring of the mineral deficiencies in plants. Plants which are iron deficient are often marked by a pale mottling of the leaf.[99] Such bleached-out and faded leaves, which develop a yellowish color, can often be seen in commercial produce, and they serve as a convenient warning that the vegetables are not as rich in iron as they should be.

Not only is iron deficiency common in crops, it has also been called "the most prevalent deficiency state affecting human populations." Women are far and away most often affected. This is in part because during their childbearing years, they lose significant amounts of blood through menstruation. Iron loss in women is estimated to range between one-half and two milligrams a day, two to four times the amount that is needed by the average man who requires only about a milligram a day total. Moreover, during pregnancy the iron requirements are even higher for a woman since during the last four months of pregnancy a great deal of iron must go into building the blood volume of the infant. During these months, up to seven and a half milligrams a day are required. It is estimated that the average American diet contains about 14 to 20 mg a day. This would seem to be more than enough but often it isn't because only ten to twenty per cent of the iron eaten is actually absorbed. This may be the reason that it was found that a large number (15-58%) of women in their childbearing years had less than adequate iron stores in the body.[100]

Fortunately, one who is iron deficient has a tendency to absorb a larger percentage of the iron present in their food. Significant amounts of iron may also be absorbed from cooking utensils. Absorption can also be increased when iron-containing foods are taken along with foods that are high in fructose, such as fresh fruits and honey. Iron is increased in most dried fruits except for dried apples, but apple juice is said in North India to be an excellent source of available iron. After special preparation, it is used to treat anemia. Protein also promotes absorption since certain amino acids tend to chelate the iron and help carry it into the system.[101] It has been suggested that the phytic acid of grains and other plant foods can also impair the absorption of iron, but in this case it is probably not of much practical significance.[102] The iron complexed in hemoglobin is more efficiently absorbed than that of vegetable foods, one reason perhaps that those who were anemic from lack of iron were often advised to "eat more red meat." Medieval physicians even treated anemia by having the patient drink blood.

According to an eighteenth century English dispensatory, physicians had observed "that the excellent medicinal virtues of iron have their effects so long as the iron continued dissolved in a mild acid." Recent research has shown, in fact, that organic acids such as citric acid enhance iron absorption, as does ascorbic acid (vitamin C). Ascorbic acid has been shown to form a chelate with iron, helping it to carry it across the intestinal lining.[103] Studies have shown that iron which is free and unchelated tends to either react with other substances in the intestinal tract, forming an insoluble and inaccessible compound, or tends to attach itself to the intestinal lining because of its positive charge. The absorption of chelated forms of iron was more than three-fold that of the free ionic form.[104] This has led to a tendency to use chelated iron supplements in treating iron deficiency anemia, an approach which is often quite successful if the anemia is indeed due to a deficiency of iron.

Anemia, which is a decrease in red blood cells, usually

shows up as tiredness, fatigue, paleness and a tendency to dizziness on standing. Though a deficiency of iron is one of the most common causes of anemia, especially in women who are menstruating, there are many other substances that are necessary to build red blood cells, and deficiencies in any of them may result in anemia. Copper is also necessary for building blood, as is manganese, and adequate levels of protein, calcium, vitamin E, vitamin C and many of the B vitamins are also important. Simply taking iron for anemia may be not only ineffective but, in some cases, possibly harmful.

Though iron is generally considered one of the less toxic minerals, the body's ability to excrete it is limited. For this reason, it can build up if unnecessarily large doses are taken over a long period of time. Acute poisonings can also occur from iron salts such as ferrous sulfate, which has been customarily used as a supplement. Accidental poisoning in children with ferrous sulphate has sometimes been fatal. Long term heavy doses of dietary iron have been observed in the well-publicized Bantu who cook their meals and make their beer in huge iron pots. The native diet may supply 200 mg of iron a day, about ten times that contained in the most iron-rich American diet. In some malnourished Bantu, iron accumulation has produced a disease called siderosis which results from deposits of the mineral in tissues throughout the body. This has led to dire predictions about the dangerous effects of "iron overload" which is said to occur in America mostly in middle-aged men whose iron requirements have not been high but who have taken iron-containing tonics in patent medicines for many years.[105]

It would appear, however, that in those cases where the diet is otherwise well-balanced, contamination of the food with iron from cooking vessels is not likely to be dangerous. In Ethiopia, where the staple cereal not only has a high iron content but also becomes heavily contaminated with the mineral as a result of grinding, storing and cooking in iron pots, the intake, 470 mg of iron a day, is more than twice that of the Bantu.

In fact, the average Ethiopian consumes more than twenty times that in a good American diet.   In these people, who are not malnourished, however, siderosis is uncommon, and an examination of the iron storage of Ethiopians dying from accidents has shown no difference from levels in a comparable group of Swedes.[106] Apparently the siderosis or iron toxicity that occurs in the Bantu is due not merely to excessive doses of the mineral but to the fact that the body is malnourished in general, disabled and incapable of dealing with it properly.*   The small amounts of iron normally entering the food from cooking utensils is not only harmless, it may even be beneficial for someone who is iron deficient.   Compounds in the food, like ascorbic acid, may chelate the iron, causing it to be easily absorbed, and it is sometimes said that iron deficiency in women may have increased in recent years because of the move away from the use of the old-fashioned cast-iron utensils.

SODIUM AND POTASSIUM AND WATER

Sodium and potassium are the alkalis.   They have a single charge as opposed to the two electrical charges on most of the other minerals.   (See the periodic table on page 244.)   For this reason, they are less tenacious in their hold on other structures and tend to move readily through solutions, especially water.

In fact, the large bulk of the water covering the surface of the earth is essentially a sodium solution containing huge quantities of chloride, the combination of which is of course common table salt.   This is mostly what is responsible for making sea water "salty," and it is this saline solution which has remained the basis of living matter, long after the simple one-celled plants and animals which evolved in the ocean had finally reached the stage where they could emerge onto dry land.   Along with potassium, sodium plays an important part in the movement of

* See also Chapter 16, Cooking.

electrons through the water-based solution that makes up proto-plasm, and the two of them are termed "electrolytes." They exist in an important ratio and distribution on each side of the cell membrane. Potassium tends to be concentrated inside the membrane (inside the cell) whereas sodium tends to be higher in the fluid surrounding the cell. Taking an excess of sodium will lead to an accumulation of sodium outside the cells and may pull water, by virtue of its concentration, from the cells into the extracellular space, creating the feeling of puffiness or bloated-ness noticed by some people after they take too much salt. This concentration of potassium inside the cell with sodium outside reflects something of the basic nature of the two alkalis since sodium is concentrated on the earth's surface in the larger bodies of water (sea water), whereas potassium tends to be concentrated inside the plants, e.g., on land.

The high concentration of potassium inside the cell membrane and of sodium outside it establishes a sort of dynamic tension that is responsible for the ability of living cells to respond to a stimulus. In the case of a nerve cell, for example, stimula-tion or excitation results in a temporary "hole" in the cell membrane which allows sodium to rush in and potassium to rush out. As this process spreads down the cell membrane running the length of the nerve fiber, an electrical "impulse" is "conducted" down the nerve. Similar processes are responsible for conduction of impulses in the heart and other muscular tissue. Thus a de-pletion of either sodium or potassium would reduce the ability of a cell to respond.

Actually, one is unlikely to become deficient in sodium since daily requirements are extremely low. Patients on a thera-peutic diet for obesity, high blood pressure and kidney disease have been maintained for years on sodium intakes as low as 150 mg per day, equal to less than one-eighth teaspoon of salt.[107] In these cases, their overall health seemed to improve dramatically despite, or perhaps even because of, this low sodium intake. Meanwhile, it is estimated that the average person in America eats five to ten thousand mg of salt (between one and two tea-spoons) a day. Many diets, especially those which include large quantities of processed and "snack" foods, may contain more than four teaspoons. Apparently most people have an amazing capacity to rid the body of excesses of sodium, though if the amounts are very great it may be at the expense of a gradual but significant wear and tear on the body and its metabolic machinery.

By contrast, it is thought that one requires about 2,500 mg of dietary potassium each day. In a typical American diet, based on processed and convenience foods, this amount may be difficult to get. A cola soft drink for example, will contain about 7 mg of potassium, a slice of toast 20, a cup of coffee 40, twelve ounces of beer about 36, a mixed drink made of whiskey about 2 mg of potassium and a serving of ginger ale or Kool-aid only one each. During summer, when appetites lag, and the diet is largely limited to such foods as these, potassium intakes may be quite low. Yet it is a time-honored tradition to "take salt-tablets" when one is to be in extreme heat. This is done, despite the fact that after an initial period of adaptation, little sodium is lost through perspiration,[108] while larger quantities of potas-sium may be. It all adds up to a curious paradox whose solution, as we shall see later, is quite surprising.*

Salt (sodium chloride) was known by the Ayurvedic phy-sicians in ancient times to be a stimulant of *pita*, the digestive fire, and to greatly accentuate one's feeling of energy and aggres-siveness. In the Far East, it is one of the principle dietary condiments used to make food more yang, the yang principle again being that which is active, assertive and hot.

Clearly we must distinguish the pharmacologic and psy-chological effects of table salt from its purely nutritional value. While it may in some cases be desirable as a condiment for those people who need it but are not susceptible to its potentially

---

* See Chapter 20, The Philosophy of Nutrition.

harmful effects, the addition of inorganic sodium chloride to foods does not seem to be of nutritional value. It is acknowledged by academic nutritionists that "a separate supply of salt in addition to that present in the food is not essential for man."[109]   There are good records of primitive populations who use no salt at all beyond what is present in the food. Moreover, Sanskrit and its daughter languages have no common root word for salt, so it seems likely that the Indo-Europeans at the time that they first migrated into Europe had not formed the custom of using salt.

Nevertheless, the use of salt is not new. It was used by the ancient Greeks, and Homer called it "divine." The first known salt mines were found in the Austrian Tyrol and date from the late Bronze Age, about 1,000 BC. Since that time, salt has been highly prized and wars have even been fought over its sources. It was used in some cases as a form of currency, the "salaries" that are paid today having taken their name from the Latin root for salt (sal) ever since the days when Roman soldiers were paid in salt money.

Salt has long been used as an important means of preserving food, and salted meat is known the world over. Some American Indian tribes are said, however, to have soaked their salted meat in water, carefully removing the salt before they prepared it for eating. Nevertheless, the taste for salt was strong among others, and even animals have been said to walk long distances to find a "salt-lick." This does not mean that animals have an inherent need for added salt. In fact, most populations of wild and domesticated animals get along quite well with no salt added to the diet. It would appear that animals, like man, developed a salt habit and that this is an acquired taste which must be learned. One former cattleman tells of dripping salt onto the muzzle of a cow so it would lick its lips and taste the salt, gradually learning to like it. Once learned, however, the desire for salt may become quite strong.

SALT AND HIGH BLOOD PRESSURE

Some medical authorities feel that "salt appetite is determined by early dietary habits and has no relationship to salt needs." Though its use may depend on habit and taste, it can have serious repercussions. A high intake of salt in early childhood and infancy may set the stage for the later development of high blood pressure. It is certainly true that the populations of the world where high blood pressure is virtually unknown are those who have not adopted Western ways and who eat 500 mg or less of salt a day. Among these people, blood pressure often falls with advancing age rather than rising as it does in the West. Recent research done on various groups around the world in an attempt to find dietary factors correlated with high blood pressure revealed one item that seemed more important than any other factor or group of factors, and that was salt. In studying the Solomon Islanders, for example, it was found that the Lao tribe, which had retained in large part its native culture, nevertheless had the highest blood pressure at every age and in both sexes than any other tribe. However, there was one custom that set them apart from the others. They had long boiled their vegetables in sea water and had the highest sodium intake of any of the tribes, amounting to as much as 15,000 to 20,000 mg a day. It seems safe to say that "without exception, low blood pressure societies are low salt societies."[110] Animal studies have also demonstrated that salt feeding is related to blood pressure.[111]

Research has thrown some light on the way this may work. Four out of five rats develop high blood pressure on a high salt diet while the other one seems not to be affected by it. This may explain why an occasional person will scoff at the idea that too much salt will cause trouble, pointing out that he eats a lot of it and has normal blood pressure. There are clearly differences in individual susceptibility. For the 80% of the animals in the experiment who were susceptible, salt had a more powerful effect when they were young, though it took some time for it to show up. Once the blood pressure began to rise, however, it could not be brought back down to normal, even though the salt was taken out of the food. Drastic salt restriction did improve the blood pressure to some extent, however.[112]

Something similar apparently happens in man. It is well accepted that salt restriction lowers the blood pressure in many hypertensive patients, and many physicians feel that it is the most effective treatment for it.* But *preventing* high blood pressure probably requires much less restriction of salt intake than *treating* it. Thus keeping salt at a reasonable level in the diet of children and young people pays off more than eliminating salt completely later in life after blood pressure has already started rising. Other conditions which have responded to salt restriction are Meniere's disease (vertigo, hearing loss and ringing in the ears)[113] and swelling and puffiness such as may occur in the face or ankles.

It is sometimes said that, because of the dynamic tension that exists between sodium and potassium in the body, too much sodium drives out potassium.[114] Such a view is not current among conventional physicians since it is usually assumed that the body throws off excess sodium, keeping what potassium it needs. However, rats on a high salt regimen have lived seven to eight months longer when their diets were supplemented with extra potassium,[115] and it seems possible that sodium and potassium have the same sort of relationship to each other that we have seen earlier in the case of calcium and magnesium or in the case of zinc and copper. High intakes of one may to some extent depress the other.[116]

The concentration of high levels of potassium inside the cell is an accomplishment that came with advancing evolution. The more primitive forms of life that evolved in the salty ocean water existed in a medium with a higher concentration of sodium.

---

* If the kidneys have already been damaged by long-standing and severe high blood pressure, complete elimination of salt has been known to precipitate kidney failure.

Only gradually was this excluded by the cell membrane and potassium concentrated within.   The advantage of this advance was apparently to permit more advanced forms of biochemical reactions.   The lower forms of living matter that predominate in the sea are based on biochemical processes, such as fermentation, that can occur in the absence of oxygen. They are also typical of stagnant waters which are poorly aerated. One strain of bacteria has been shown to shift to anaerobic metabolism when sodium concentrations were raised, and back to oxygen-dependent functioning when sodium concentrations are lowered again.[117]

Perhaps by depleting potassium levels within the cell and allowing sodium concentrations to rise, the stage is set for a more primitive state of cell functioning.   Interestingly enough, it was shown nearly fifty years ago by Otto Warburg that anerobic glycolysis, the less efficient metabolism of carbohydrate that occurs in the absence of oxygen, predominates in tumor cells. It is now well accepted that malignant tissue is embryonic, more primitive, and less-differentiated.   It might be said then, that in cancer the tissue falls back into the anaerobic and more primitive mode of functioning. One of the factors which may, in some cases, promote this process is a depletion of potassium and an excess of sodium, though as we shall see later, this probably depends on more than diet.* In any case, encouraging improvements have sometimes been documented in cases of cancer where treatment included careful attention to potassium supplementation and sodium restriction.[118]

If future research turns up further evidence along these lines, it may be important to pay careful attention to the ratio of sodium to potassium in the diet.   Processed and prepared foods usually contain relatively high levels of sodium and diminished levels of potassium.   For instance, three and a half ounces of fresh raw peas contain 316 mg of potassium and only 2 mg of sodium, but by the time these same peas have been canned,

---

* See Part V.

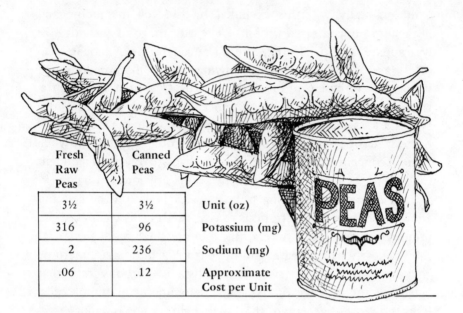

Fresh Raw Peas	Canned Peas	
3½	3½	Unit (oz)
316	96	Potassium (mg)
2	236	Sodium (mg)
.06	.12	Approximate Cost per Unit

the process which includes adding salt has run the sodim content up to 236 mg and somehow lowered the potassium value to 96. By contrast, fresh fruits and vegetables are high in potassium and usually quite low in sodium. For instance, a medium sized raw apple will contain over 100 mg of potassium to 1 of sodium. A half cup of steamed broccoli will contain over 250 mg to about 10 of sodium. Other foods very high in potassium are grapefruit, bananas, orange juice, spinach, lettuce, cantaloupes, etc. It is often said that meats, unlike fruits and vegetables contain "high amounts of sodium than potassium." In fact, the opposite is true. Most meats, fish, fowl, etc., contain much higher potassium to 75 of sodium. Similar figures hold for chicken, beef, pork, etc. This applies only for meat before salt is added, and the amount of salt added in the process of cooking will change the ratio of sodium to potassium accordingly. Unfortunately, most people salt not only their meat but also their vegetables, so the result is a reversed ratio of sodium to potassium in almost every food that's eaten.

That potassium is especially abundant in plants is evident even from the origins of the word itself. It was from the remains of burnt firewood that the earliest preparations of potassium were made. Early settlers in America took this "potash," put it in a wooden keg, and dripped water through it, collecting the resulting alkali solution to combine with animal fat to make "lye soap," a practice which continues today in the southern Appalachias.

According to the ancient teachings of the East, sodium chloride (table salt) is heavy and downward moving. In the Ayurvedic system it is also considered to be hot and stimulating, while in Chinese and Japanese terms it is more masculine or "yang." Potassium, on the other hand, tends in the other direction. It is more upward moving, and the life forms which have concentrated it have tended to move out of the water, up toward the sky, and toward more evolved and intelligent levels. One Western physician expressed it this way: "For my part, I always picture sodium as masculine, bold, uncomplicated, obeying simple laws and making his presence felt, whereas potassium is a lady—devious and difficult to understand, now advancing, now withdrawing and obeying her own whims."[119]

Though we actually use the term "salt" most often to refer to sodium chloride, in the context of chemistry it has a much broader meaning. Similar "salts" are formed by potassium and chloride or calcium and chloride, etc. Most all of the metals mentioned above, like magnesium, zinc, copper, etc., can and do form salts. Most of these, of course, are present in the ocean where life originated. In fact, though the ocean is somewhat more concentrated than the tissue fluids of man and other animals, the proportions of the various salts are in many respects similar. Calcium and magnesium are present in considerable amounts, for example, while zinc, copper, manganese and the other "trace elements" are present in only tiny amounts. When sea water is evaporated and the solid residue collected, it will not be pure sodium chloride. In fact, only about 75% by weight is sodium chloride while the rest, the other 25%, is a collection of other minerals. When the sodium chloride is removed, the remaining solids, (the "bitters") are the "salts" of other minerals in the sea water. This is a rich source of trace elements, as well as magnesium and calcium.* The Japanese traditionally use such a preparation which they call *nigari* to solidify soy bean curd or *tofu* by the traditional methods. It seems likely that the combination of the amino acids of the soy protein and the minerals from the sea forms a rich exchange resin, a sort of depot of minerals and trace elements in what is essentially a chelated form.

HARD WATERS VERSUS SOFT

Whereas potash or potassium combines with fats to form a soluble substance that can be used for sudsing and cleaning, the salts or other minerals such as calcium and magnesium will combine with the soap to form insoluble compounds that settle out and interfere with the cleansing process, leaving one's hair coated with an unflattering sediment and making an annoying ring around the bathtub. Thus water containing salts of calcium and magnesium is called "hard" water and may make not only the Saturday night bath but the Monday washday a trying experience. Modern technology has come up with an answer, however: the water softener. This is a device which exchanges the calcium and magnesium salts, which tend to form insoluble compounds, for sodium salts, which as we noted above are more soluble. Therefore, softened water is water which has had calcium and magnesium eliminated by replacing them with sodium. For those who use this water for drinking and cooking, it becomes yet another source of added sodium in the diet.

Though hard water may form deposits around the bathtub,

---

* If the water for making the salt is drawn from areas contaminated by industrial wastes, then there is a danger of including toxic minerals like mercury, cadmium and lead.

in the water pipes and even in your hair, it apparently does not do the same in your arteries. In fact, statistical studies have shown that deaths from heart disease are lower in areas where the drinking water is hard.[120]   It has been suggested that the calcium and magnesium in such water may have some protective effect against coronary heart disease.

Even though it may deprive one of the protective effects of the magnesium and calcium in hard water, artificially softened water is unlikely to significantly elevate the sodium intake in most people's diets, except for those people who are on very stringent salt restriction. The major danger of softened water is that it is more likely than hard water to dissolve the lining of pipes.[121]   In plastic and galvanized pipes, for example, there are significant amounts of cadmium, and though normally only negligible amounts enter the water, where softeners are used amounts may be large enough to be cause for concern. Lead pipes, of course, pose a serious threat, though they are no longer installed in new homes. Only several decades ago they still were, however, and in old houses which have not had their plumbing replaced, lead pipes may still sometimes be found. Most modern installations now use copper piping, but this can result in troublesome levels of copper in the water.

In many areas, municipal water processing plants soften the water to some extent and the consumer may be unaware of this. More often other chemicals are added in order to kill bacteria which may be present due to an impure water supply. Chlorine, of course, is the most commonly added disinfectant and chlorinated water is the rule rather than the exception in most metropolitan areas. About half the cities in America have also begun to add fluorides to the water, primarily in an effort to control tooth decay.

FLUORINE

The dispute over whether fluoride is either healthful or

harmful has been a highly debated issue for some years. The idea of adding a foreign chemical to drinking water has horrified some people who see it as unnatural, dangerous and foolhardy, but it has appealed to many others as a logical, scientific and sensible measure. Pro-fluoridationists and anti-fluoridationists have had it out in almost every city across America. Opponents of fluoridation range from those who see fluoride in any form as harmful, to those who claim that it is only sodium fluoride which is undesirable and that other fluoride compounds are more natural. One physician, for example, wrote to the Canadian Medical Journal describing his experience with two vitamin-mineral preparations containing fluoride. One was a syrup which contained 3 mg per dose of sodium fluoride and the other was a tablet which contained 25 mg per dose of calcium fluoride. He reported on nine cases to whom he had prescribed these preparations. Five who had taken the calcium fluoride had no side effects whatsoever and continued well thereafter. The four, however, who had taken the soluble sodium fluoride in the syrup became ill. One was told by her boss to see a doctor because she looked so bad. After having been on the supplement for six months, she had lost six pounds, her skin color was poor and her hair was falling out. Her physician was shocked by the change. She said she felt as bad as she looked, but a month after stopping the syrup, she had regained her weight and good health. The other three patients had similar adverse reactions. The physician felt that the soluble sodium fluoride, by forming a more stable calcium compound in the body, had robbed the blood and tissues of calcium, whereas calcium fluoride did not pick up calcium, having its full quota already.[122]

By contrast, Henry Schroeder, M.D., one of the best known authorities on trace elements, presents figures demonstrating that fluoride compounds are present in extremely high concentrations both in sea water and on the earth's crust. This fact, he says

shows the idiocy of the dogma pounded at our ears by anti-

fluoridationists over and over until it has become the Big
Lie: fluoride added to drinking water at one part per million
is toxic; sodium fluoride is the "unnatural form" of fluoride;
calcium fluoride is the "natural" form. The truth is that
almost all the fluoride in the sea is in the form of sodium
fluoride; that calcium fluoride is insoluble in water; that
there are 1.846 billion tons of sodium fluoride in the oceans;
that the seas are teeming with life of all kinds exposed constantly to 1.3 parts per million fluoride; that life began in
the presence of fluoride of which the earth's crust contains
700 parts per million.

He goes on to say "fluorine in the form of its most abundant
salt, sodium fluoride, is an element which promotes the strength
of bones and teeth, and marine vertebrates benefit from its
presence even if people living in low fluoride areas who don't
fluoridate their drinking water don't."[123]

And so the controversy rages. The pro- and anti-fluoridationists have been at war for many years, and so far, it seems that
the victories chalked up to one side are about equal to those of
the other. At present, approximately half of American cities
have fluoridated their water supplies while the other half have
refused to do so. The result is, of course, a large scale experiment, but the results are not yet all in. A recent statistical
analysis of the incidence of cancer in the fluoridated and un-
fluoridated cities reportedly found a higher incidence in those
cities where fluoride had been used for some time.[124] Unfortunately, the study was carried out by a researcher who had long
been publicly opposed to the use of fluoride, and his findings
brought a flurry of criticisms, counter-claims and reinterpreta-
tions of the data.

MINERAL WATERS

For those who find/their drinking water unacceptable,
either by virtue of what they know it contains or simply because
it tastes bad, one alternative is bottled spring water. If the water

is pure and comes from a good source and if it is bottled in glass, this may, despite its expense, sometimes be necessary. However, water that stands in a container loses something by virtue of being removed from the earth. It was observed many years ago that mineral waters rich in iron lost their medicinal properties after they were allowed to sit for some time.[125] Though this has not yet been investigated with newer laboratory techniques, it has been the custom the world over to come to famous mineral springs to "take the waters" directly as they gushed from the ground.

Famous mineral springs and waters have formed the basis of well-known spas since time immemorial. In eras past, when ill, one went to Baden-Baden or to Wiesbaden (in Germany) or to Aix-les-bains (in France) or to Hot Springs, Arkansas to drink and bathe in the mineral waters. Even today, many people still do so. A number of the best known American springs were used by the Indians before the Europeans came. While some found that they improved, at times even dramatically, others were made worse, and many persons report that even a bottle of "mineral water" of certain kinds is upsetting to them. Such water should be regarded with caution and respect. If it is indeed genuine mineral water, then it contains minerals, but which minerals it contains is crucial. If it happens to contain those needed, one's in luck. If not, it may have effects opposite from those desired.

Perhaps the most ideal water for drinking is the "organic water" squeezed from a fruit or vegetable. This juice has not only been "purified" by the plant, but it is also most likely to contain minerals in the organic (chelated) complexes which are best utilized by the body. If one must use ordinary water, however, it can usually be improved by boiling. This not only drives off some of the volatile substances like chlorine, but may inactivate and precipitate any minerals that would disagree. It also, of course, destroys bacteria and viruses. A diet high in natural juices, fresh fruits and vegetables, soups and dishes cooked in their own broths decreases the need for added water in the diet. Even though the water used in cooking may not be of the best quality, the boiling does improve it, and a number of studies have shown that pollutants, contaminants and toxic chemicals are less harmful to the body when they are taken along with natural fruits, grains, vegetables and so forth.[126, 127]

BACK TO THE SOIL

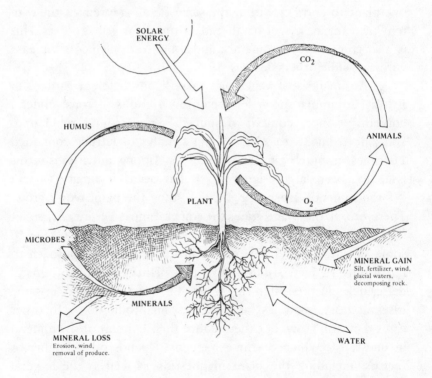

It is customary for nutritionists, in working with the vitamin, protein, carbohydrate and fat requirements of patients, to analyze various foods and construct food tables so that one may have access to information about the approximate amount of each nutrient that is contained in whatever food he might wish to serve. Though there are variations from one crop of corn to another as far as the amount of carbohydrate goes, for example, or from one sweet potato to another as far as the content of vitamin A goes, the variations are not major and one can still work in terms of averages.

Unfortunately, attempts to use the same approach with minerals has not been successful. This is especially true for the trace elements. The manganese content of alfalfa, for example, may vary not only from one variety to another but even from one plant to another within the same field. Moreover, the content of manganese will be altered as the plant grows older. This is also true of other minerals, and some trace elements increase with age while others decrease.

An analysis of vegetables taken from different gardens in British Columbia showed incredible variations in trace mineral content. Copper content of spinach varied from 3 to 11 ppm and zinc from 35 to 230! Some samples of lettuce contained 20 times as much zinc as others.[128] Among nutritionists this issue has been largely ignored. It has been customary to say, "If the minerals are not in the soil, then the plant won't grow. Therefore, if the plant grew, the mineral must be present, so let us not concern ourselves further." While this may be true to some extent, it has been proven inadequate as an approach to nutrition. In fact, studies show that plants respond to mineral deficiencies in the soil in two ways. First of all, they do, in some cases at least, grow less and decrease in production. In other cases they still grow, but they reduce their content of the mineral in question. Which of these happens depends on a number of factors, including the plant in question as well as the mineral involved. Therefore it is sometimes quite possible that a soil deficient in a certain mineral will produce a plant which, although plentiful in quantity, may be dangerously low in the concentration of that mineral. In fact, research has verified this.[129, 130] This should not come as a surprise since plant physiologists have long been trained to observe the signs and symptoms of mineral deficiency, although those deficiencies caused by some of the recently discovered trace elements are only now being catalogued by botanists and agronomists. Current studies are finding, for example, that the mineral content of grains has been steadily decreasing in the last few years.[131]

MINERALS: PILLS OR MEALS?

Such data has been used as a justification for using increasing quantities of mineral supplements, and many "multiple vitamins" have become "multi-vitamins and minerals," carrying a hodge-podge of trace elements. This is far from an ideal solution, however, since the intake of one mineral affects that of others. It has been said that trace minerals are like a spider web—if you tug at one thread the whole complex shifts. The results, of course, can be serious.

In any case, the breaking down of food into a carbohydrate fraction by removing sugar or refining flour, into a fat fraction by pressing out oils, into a protein fraction by making protein powders or liquids, and into a vitamin fraction by extracting the active compounds and making them into pills, is an absurdity. We have created a bizarre situation in which our food is fragmented and sold to us in bits and pieces so that we are faced with the impossible task of trying to reassemble what amounts to a biochemical Humpty-dumpty.

This does not mean that learning about vitamins and minerals is an exercise in futility. An understanding of which foods are rich in which of the known nutrients and which symptoms appear when these nutrients are deficient or absent may help us in the task of selecting the whole and natural foods that we need. Thus we have come to understand that a susceptibility to colds may result from a deficiency in vitamin C, and the regular use of freshly squeezed orange juice might have some benefit in preventing this. Acne is likely to mean zinc and vitamin A deficiencies, so a generous intake of sunflower seeds as well as fresh carrot juice may help. Sunshine is helpful for those who tend to have easily fractured bones, while one who sees poorly in the dark can benefit from more carrots in the diet. This minimizes to some extent the process of trial and error and enhances our instinctual sense of taste with a dimension of understanding when we are faced with the selection of foods.

Though one may have questions about the way that foods are grown and their mineral content, he need not resort to supplement tablets. Natural foods can provide generous quantities of minerals when handled properly. With skill and care, vegetable dishes can be prepared in such a way that the volume of the vegetables is condensed without destroying their value. This is accomplished by searing or stir frying at a high temperature with selected fats and seasonings, afterwards continuing the process so that the vegetables "shrink" yet retain their texture and flavor.* Thus one is able to eat and digest a larger quantity of vegetables than would otherwise be possible. Moreover, a number of different vegetables are used for this purpose, and in the U.S., this usually means they were grown in a wide variety of soils and have been shipped from all across the country. This ensures a compensatory affect. What one vegetable is deficient in another will likely contain.

Another way of getting more concentrated sources of naturally occurring minerals is through fresh fruit and vegetable juices. They are rapidly absorbed, and one can drink the juice of a pound of carrots, whereas he would be hard put to eat that many—cooked or raw! Fresh cheese, *(paneer)* made by boiling milk and adding lemon juice, is probably very rich in easily absorbed naturally chelated minerals. Such acid-treated preparations of milk protein, or casein, are considered superb sources of trace elements,[132] and casein-based livestock feeds have been found to improve zinc absorption and utilization.[133] Soybean curd or *tofu*, made in the traditional way with sea

---

* See Chapter 14, Cooked versus Raw.

Paneer
(Fresh Cheese)

The cottage cheese found in grocery stores usually contains additives and lacks freshness. The Italian version called ricotta is also slightly aged. Paneer, a homemade variety prepared in India with lemon juice tastes fresher and better and also gives one access to the whey, a very healthful beverage.

To make about one cup of such fresh cheese or paneer, simply bring one-half gallon skim or 2% milk to a foaming boil and add the juice of two lemons. Stir the milk and lemon juice together very briefly and allow the milk to boil for another few seconds until the milk curdles. Then leave the pot undisturbed so the curd separates from the whey. The liquid whey can often simply be poured off while holding the mass of curd with a large spoon. Otherwise it can be strained through a thin cloth draped over a collander. Using a cheesecloth allows one to squeeze out enough whey to create a tighter "cheese" which can be cubed and will not fall apart when cooked in vegetable dishes.

The following examples illustrate how paneer can be used.

Strain it dry and crumble it into fruit salad, green salad or cooked vegetables.

Cube firm paneer and add to stir-fried vegetables (see box p. 416).

Use it in any recipe instead of cottage, ricotta or cream cheese. Cheese cake, lasagne and sandwich spreads, for example, are delicious when made with paneer. It can also replace soy bean curd (tofu) in most recipes.

A rich and creamy dessert topping which is especially appealing on fruit salad can be made by whipping moist paneer in a blender with honey (see box p. 419) or it can be used to make a rich, high protein, non-fat, low calorie dressing for green salads (see box p. 411).

Blended with carob and a bit of honey, this also makes a superb "chocolatey, " unsugared frosting for a cake. (If blended and applied hot it will "set up" as it cools.)

water, *nigari*, should also be rich in trace elements.

Such preparations probably contain generous quantities of natural chelates, and this has the advantage of not only making needed minerals more available, but of protecting against over absorption of those which, like copper, are needed but can be harmful in amounts too large. There is a narrow margin between adequacy and toxicity when many such minerals are present as simple salts. Chelation, as we saw earlier, apparently widens this margin and protects against toxic overdosing by making the minerals more amenable to "selective absorption." Moreover, intelligent planning of meals further ensures that appropriate quantities of minerals, as well as carbohydrate, fat, protein and vitamins are provided.

Developing a Balanced Diet

9

While thousands of experiments have been done on everything from soil science to cooking fats, and the quantity of information on nutrition is overwhelming, the knowledge of how to put it together in such a way that it will be meaningful and helpful in the practical down-to-earth situation confronting one as he stands before a grocery shelf is a challenge that has not yet been met. Moreover, as we have seen earlier in the book, many very important, practical and relevant questions have not yet been asked, much less answered, in the laboratory.

To fill the gaps that are left in our knowledge and to help us ask the questions that are relevant and useful, it is very beneficial to take some hints from the traditional methods of selecting a balanced and healthful diet that have been time-tested throughout the world. This does not mean we can assume that all commonly practiced methods are reliable. For instance, in the 1930's, it became the practice in the Southeastern United States to subsist on cornbread and fat-pork, a diet which, as we have seen, led to the development of pellagra. Likewise in many areas of India, it has become the custom to take a diet comprised primarily of potatoes and wheat spiced with huge amounts of chilis. Not only does this diet lead to an irritated, inflamed intestinal wall that is very susceptible to dysentery, but it creates nutritional deficiencies as well.

In each of these cases, a more careful examination shows that these diets are not "traditional" in the true sense of the word, but that they actually represent an abandonment of tradition occurring out of economic necessity. Cornbread and fat-pork were indeed traditional food in the southeast of America even before the Europeans came to this country, but an integral part of the tradition was also the inclusion of leafy green vegetables and beans or peas. These were more expensive, though, and so were dropped from the diet during the depression when many people were too poor to purchase them. In a similar way, the traditional diet of India also includes dahl (dried beans and peas), vegetables and fruits which are now often eliminated primarily due to economic necessity. The addition of huge amounts of chili peppers was probably, in part, an attempt to supply the vitamin C that was missing and to preserve taste in a diet that included only starchy foods.*

When dietary practices are examined more closely, however, we increasingly discover that many of the rules of proper food selection are universal. Cross-cultural comparisons reveal certain food combinations that have been chosen independently in many cultures and that have sustained healthy, robust populations for many generations. We can feel confident in applying these rules to the selection of our own food, at least until we have the opportunity to utilize the methods of laboratory science to verify their validity.

TOWARD A UNIVERSAL DIET

There are many different types of diet in the world, each

---

* See also Chapter 15, Ayurvedic Nutrition.

being based on specific conditions, available foods and culturally developed tastes. Even within most countries, there is a vast difference between the diets of the common rural folk and the food selection practiced by urban dwellers. For the latter, meals are based primarily on industrialized agriculture, and as a result, the foodstuffs are often deficient in nutritional value.* In addition, the urban diets are greatly influenced by international fashion and lean heavily on refined and "convenience" foods which have lost much of their nutritive value during their processing and are often contaminated with chemicals.

By contrast, the food habits of more rural people show greater variation. This "peasant" diet is infinite in its variety and includes some of the most healthful and delicious foods known to man. After generations of growing a certain food and making it an important part of their diet, people develop a sensitivity to the ways in which it enhances their well-being. In cultures which have maintained their traditions and integrity for hundreds or even thousands of years, there has been an opportunity to develop a diet which is well-suited both to local conditions and to the maintenance of health and longevity.

When we look at what is considered healthful, wholesome, everyday fare by the traditional cooks in various cultures around the world, many similarities emerge. A comparison of these diets will guide us in developing nutritional norms for food selection. The basic East Indian diet, for example, is very simple and straight-forward. The one or two main meals of the day are comprised primarily of bread and/or rice (grain), a small amount of dahl (beans or peas), one dish of cooked vegetables, and lastly, a small serving of yogurt or in some cases, a bit of meat, fish or fowl. Frequently there is at least a small amount of something raw: radish, salad greens, fruit or sprouted beans. Though variations on this theme occur, the basic ingredients remain the same.

* See Chapter 2, The Soil.

Chinese and Japanese diets vary tremendously depending on the region involved and the basic foods grown there. Though it is difficult to generalize, it is probably safe to say that the most typical meal for this area consists of rice and vegetables with small amounts of soybean products and/or meat or fish. Rice is sometimes replaced by millet in certain areas of China, and in still others, wheat is the major grain. Nevertheless, the same basic ingredients which are found in East Indian cooking (grains, beans and vegetables) are usually present in some form or another in a Chinese meal, and in roughly the same proportions.

European diets show as much variety as those of China or India. It may not be inappropriate, however, to take the French diet as a sort of standard since it is highly regarded throughout most of the continent. A typical French meal consists of a vegetable and/or salad or soup, and a generous quantity of good French bread. Meat or cheese is usually present, though in smaller amounts than in an American diet. A fermented wine or beer is a common accompaniment and seems to replace the fermented milk (yogurt) or fermented soybean products (miso and tamari) of the Indian, Chinese and Japanese meals. While the legumes (beans and peas) may not be as ubiquitous in the French diet as they are in the diets of the Orient, a hearty country meal in a French wayside inn is likely to turn up a plate laden with bread, lentils and vegetables and topped by a small piece of meat.

The indigenous diet of North America is also hard to characterize since the natives were separated into many tribes at the time of arrival of the Europeans. The hunters and gatherers, of course, relied primarily on what was available locally, but the agrarian Indians of the Southeast and Southwest had evolved a fairly stable agriculture and cuisine. What remains of the traditional diet of the Southeastern Indians has been absorbed by the Europeans, and cornbread, leafy green vegetables and cooked beans and peas have become their tradition. Probably the only remaining intact example of the indigenous North American diet is found among the Indian tribes of the Southwest and Mexico. In those areas, the basic diet is tortillas (grain) and frijoles (beans). This is supplemented with cooked vegetables and occasionally small quantities of meat or dairy products. On the other side of the world, the Middle-Eastern diet includes more meat than the diets described thus far, but it is primarily based on the *pita*, a flat bread (grain), and on garbanzo beans. Some vegetables are served with the garbanzos, and various types of yogurt (laban) are not uncommon.

FIVE TRADITIONAL FOOD GROUPS

It is apparent, then, that when one looks beneath the more sophisticated veneer of urban food fashions and investigates the dietary practices of the most stable population groups in the world, certain recurrent patterns emerge. Whole grains constitute the bulk of most of these diets and are consumed in the largest quantities. The ever-present legume, which is taken in approximately half that quantity, complements the grains, and together they provide the proper proportions of the eight essential amino acids. This grain/legume combination is the core of the meal, but the vegetables give it flavor and vitality. The amount of fresh vegetables which are consumed varies according to availability, but in those areas where they can be obtained, they are usually included in sizable quantities. Generally, this means that they are taken in larger portions than the legume but in smaller portions than the grains. Green vegetables are the most highly prized, yielding larger percentages of vitamins and minerals and more protein than most other vegetables. They are often combined with or alternated with summer squash, carrots, green peas, okra, string beans, etc. Spinach and mustard green (gathered when young and tender) are very important, but potatoes and especially eggplant and cauliflower are considered in many traditions to be inferior.

In addition to this basic trio of grain, legume and vegetable, most traditional diets contain varying quantities of a fourth group of foods which includes dairy products, meat, eggs, fish, fowl and certain fermented bean preparations (such as tofu and miso).* This food group might be referred to as the B_{12} group since all the foods included in it contain this vitamin whereas foods in the other three groups do not. B_{12} may be absent in the other strictly vegetarian items on the menu, but since it is needed only in tiny amounts, the little contained in a small portion of some food from this group every few days is sufficient. A small daily serving of raw foods constitutes the fifth food group found in traditional diets. This may be fruits, though they are often regarded as a luxury. When in season they are generally taken separately, serving as a light breakfast or supper rather than a routine part of the meal. If they are absent, small amounts of some other raw food which can be easily digested is added to the daily menu. Such side dishes include grated radishes in Japan, a mint sprig in Lebanon and gram (bean) sprouts in the Punjab.

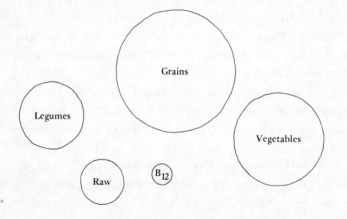

---

* Other fermented foods such as sauerkraut and wine may also contain B_{12} depending on the microorganisms which have grown in them. Unfortunately, detailed data is not generally available on exactly which fermented foods contain B_{12} and which do not, since this will often depend on the specific variety of bacteria, yeast, etc., which happen to be present in that particular batch. (See Chapter 15, Ayurvedic Nutrition.)

Although the average American school child is taught a diet based on daily selections from the "Four Basic Food Groups"—meat, milk, fruit/vegetable and grains—the trans-cultural comparison of food habits yields a five-fold food grouping with large quantities taken from the three major groups (grains, legumes and vegetables) and smaller quantities taken from the two other groups (B_{12} and raw foods). The development of diets based on these cross-culturally consistent food groups seems to be well validated by centuries of experiential experimentation, and it is on such firm ground that we can build some basic guidelines for the selection of a balanced and healthful diet.

THE MODERN AMERICAN DIET

Before describing these guidelines in more detail, however, it would be helpful to investigate how the modern American diet differs from these traditional diets. The most outstanding characteristic of standard traditional diets is that the foods the people eat are selected fresh from within their own natural eco-system and (with the exception of oils) are left intact in their whole, natural form. This is in marked contrast to the typical American diet. Foods currently considered to be "traditional American fare" such as hot dogs, coke, corn flakes, oreo cookies, cheese whiz and crisco were nowhere to be found in American kitchens at the turn of the century. New "traditions" spring fully grown almost daily from television advertisements and the most popular food items come from the supermarket rather than the garden. In modern urban settings, menus are generally constructed on the basis of fashion, convenience and taste rather than solid nutritional information or time-honored tradition. Although taste can in some cases be a good guide for food selection, the typical American menu depends for its appeal on meat, salt, sugar, fat and artificial additives. These liven up the taste of refined foods which would otherwise be bland. Traditional diets lean more on the flavor of natural seasonings, whole grains and legumes and depend for their liveliness on fresh vegetables. The zest of fresh vegetables is in no way approached by the comparatively dull taste of most canned or even frozen vegetables. The modern urban palate has become so acclimated to a barrage of brash tastes that it is no longer satisfied by the more subtle flavors of traditional cuisine.

The results of all these changes within the past century have been a marked shift in eating habits as well as in the types and amounts of nutrients consumed. The most obvious aberration that modern urban diets display is a dramatic reduction in the intake of complex carbohydrates with a concomitant increase in that of simple ones. Modern eating habits tend to reduce the intake of vitamins, minerals, essential amino acids, essential fatty acids and bulk. On the other hand, there is an excess of total calories, of empty calories, of total fat, saturated fat, cholesterol, refined sugar and salt.[1] As a result, the ratio of nutrients to calories is lower, explaining the common occurrence of mounting "nutritional debts." Subsequently, obesity and poor nutrition are national problems.

A closer examination of what the average American diet might contain and an analysis of the specific nutrients which comprise it will provide a clearer picture of the problem. The following menu includes all the food that a typical American who is relatively "careful about what he eats" might consume during one day. The nutritional value of the total input is then broken down to display the constituent calories, fats, carbohydrate, protein, vitamins and minerals.

As the chart indicates, this diet contains well over 3,000 calories, many of which are "empty." About 40% come from carbohydrate and 40% from fat with protein providing approximately 10% of the total caloric intake. Over half of the carbohydrate is simple carbohydrate, so sugar makes up over 20% of the caloric intake. (Since most people's calories are 20-25% sugar, this is about average.) The fat content at 40% is, if anything,

DIET I: A MODERN AMERICAN DIET

BREAKFAST

1 cup orange juice from
frozen concentrate
1 piece of white bread, toasted
with 1 pat margarine
2 eggs fried in margarine (over
light)
2 strips of bacon, fried
1 cup coffee with 1 tsp. non-
dairy creamer and 1 tsp.
white sugar

LUNCH

Sandwich:
  2 slices white bread
  1 tsp. mayonnaise
  2 slices bologna
  2 leaves iceberg lettuce
1 12 oz. coke
20 potato chips
1 apple

SUPPER

Salad:
  1/5 hd. iceberg lettuce
  ½ fresh tomato
  1 T. french dressing
2 dinner rolls, 2 pats
margarine
6 oz. ground beef, fried
15 pieces frozen french
fried potatoes
2 T. ketchup
½ c. canned green beans
½ c. canned corn
1 slice chocolate cake
with fudge icing
2 cups coffee (2 tsp.
non-dairy creamer, 2
tsp. white sugar)

MID-MORNING

1 cup coffee with 1 tsp. non-
dairy creamer and 1 tsp.
white sugar
1 doughnut

MID-AFTERNOON

1 12 oz. coke
1 2.6 oz. package of
peanuts, roasted in
oil (unsalted)

EVENING

3 chocolate chip
cookies
1 cup coffee with 1 tsp.
non-dairy creamer
and 1 tsp. white sugar

ANALYSIS OF TOTAL NUTRIENTS*

		MDR†
Calories	3733	1900-2700
Protein	119 g	70 g
Carbohydrate	394 g	
Fat	208 mg	
Iron	29 mg	10-18 mg
Calcium	760 mg	800 mg
Vitamin A	4423 IU	4000-5000 IU
Vitamin B$_1$	.30 mg	.8-1.4 mg
Vitamin B$_2$	.45 mg	1.2-1.6 mg
Niacin	22. mg	13-18 mg
Vitamin C	111. mg	45-70 mg

* Figures computed from *Let's Eat Right*[2] and *Nutrition Almanac*[3].
† Minimum Daily Requirements from Davidson, S.[4] and Davis, A.[5]

better than average (which runs close to 45%). Here over half of it comes from refined oils and almost all the rest from saturated animal fat. This not only piles up potentially dangerous stores of unused fat, but also crowds out other necessary nutrients from the diet. According to estimated average minimum daily requirements, this diet is deficient in vitamins B_1, B_2 and calcium and has a surplus of calories. The salt contained in these foods and the extra salt most people add to their food has not been included here, but it would be a large amount (at least 4,000 mg). The assorted artificial additives in the food have also not been calculated, and their total effect on the system is generally unknown.

This diet contains no alcohol, no candy, no chewing gum, no salty TV snacks, no "convenience foods," and no other foods which, although popular, are generally recognized to be of questionable nutritional value. Far from exaggerating American eating habits, it has been chosen as a better-than-average sample of how the typical person eats. If everyone ate this way, the overall nutritional status of the U.S. would actually improve. An even more typical diet for the average person would be likely to show only a sugared cereal with a bit of milk and juice for breakfast, a piece or two of candy or gum during the day, more "convenience foods," and a cocktail in the evening before dinner. It would probably also contain more salt and fewer vegetables. Teenagers, who are notorious for their poor eating habits, have diets which are probably representative of a large segment of American society, including many working people, housewives and school children. Such a diet, comprised of more ready-prepared foods and sweets, might look something like the following chart.

Although the teenager on this diet eats less than our previous American consumer, he also gets less since the nutrient content per calorie is even lower. This diet is deficient in calcium and vitamins A, B_2 and C. It is very high in simple carbohydrates, and as is the case with many urban diets, sweets have replaced

DIET II: TYPICAL TEENAGE DIET

BREAKFAST	LUNCH	SUPPER
2 glazed doughnuts	1 hot dog	3 oz. meatballs
	8 oz. carbonated	4 oz. spaghetti
	beverage	3 slices garlic bread
	1/6 apple pie	¾ cup green beans
		¾ cup tossed salad
		1 piece chocolate cake

MID-MORNING	MID-AFTERNOON	EVENING
1 sweet roll	1 candy bar	3 filled cookies

TOTAL NUTRITIONAL CONTENT[6]

Calories	3,000	Iron	12 mg	Vitamin B_2	1.2 mg
Protein	62 g	Calcium	246 mg.	Niacin	24 mg
Carbohydrate	388 g	Vitamin A	1640 IU	Vitamin C	22 mg
Fat	137 g	Vitamin B_1	1.2 mg		

much of the protein-containing food. Nonetheless, many people would consider this a "normal" diet, and many worried mothers would be pleased if they could get their teenage children to eat this well with at least one "solid meal" in the evening.

TOWARD A MORE HEALTHFUL DIET

A more ideal diet would contain much less fat, less carbohydrate and more fresh fruits and vegetables. Consequently, it would also be lower in calories. A healthful transition diet would eliminate many of the items characteristic of modern urban eating and would more closely resemble the traditional diet of many cultures. It could still, however, retain foods which are familiar and well-liked. A diet of this type might resemble the following.

DIETS III and IV
Based on Traditional Food Groups

	DIET III VEGETARIAN	DIET IV NON-VEGETARIAN

BREAKFAST:
8 oz. fresh squeezed orange juice
1½ slices whole wheat raisin toast
1½ pats butter, 2 tsp. honey

DIET III VEGETARIAN: 1/3 cup tofu (or) scrambled in ghee

DIET IV NON-VEGETARIAN: 1 large egg, soft boiled, butter

MID-MORNING:
1 cup 2% milk

LUNCH:
Fruit salad (1 apple, 1 banana,
¾ cup uncreamed cottage cheese,
4 tsp. roasted sunflower seeds,
1/8 cup raisins, 2 tsp. honey)

AFTERNOON:
8 oz. apple juice

DINNER:
Salad (4¼ oz. Romaine lettuce,
¼ carrot, 3½ oz. bean sprouts,
4 tsp. sunflower seeds, ¼ cup
yogurt dressing)

DIET III VEGETARIAN: 1¼ cup rice (or) ¾ cup split peas cooked with ghee and spices, soy sauce

DIET IV NON-VEGETARIAN: 1 large baked potato 2 pats butter, 4¼ oz. flounder filet, baked 1 oz. sour cream, tartar sauce

1 slice whole wheat bread, 1 pat
butter

NIGHT:
1 cup 2% milk

TOTAL NUTRITIONAL CONTENT[5]

	VEGETARIAN	NON-VEGETARIAN
Calories	2055	2037
Protein	94 g	93 g
Carbohydrate	321 g	270 g
Fat	48 g	62 g
Iron	18 mg	13.7 mg
Calcium	1339 mg	1227 mg
Vitamin A	13,470 IU	14,703 IU
Vitamin B_1	3.24 mg	1.76 mg
Vitamin B_2	1.35 mg	1.5 mg
Niacin	38 mg	15.67 mg
Vitamin C	269 mg	288.6 mg

These diets contain a balanced amount of all the essential nutrients, and yet they have only about 2,000 calories. This is an ample intake for the average person, but it can easily be modified for weight loss by reducing the portions and the amount of bread and milk products, for example.* Similarly, it can be geared to a person with a more active life-style by increasing the amounts served and by adding more bread. These diets supply abundant quantities of vitamins A and C and calcium. Interestingly, although the vegetarian option contains slightly less vitamin A and C than its non-vegetarian counterpart, it contains more protein, carbohydrate, iron, calcium, niacin and vitamin B_1. It also contains less fat. It would seem more than adequate for the average person to have somewhere around twenty percent of his caloric intake as protein.† These two diets include almost exactly that amount. The Modern American (Diet I) and Typical Teenage diets, (Diet II) however, have comparatively low levels of protein, only 13% and 8% respectively. This may seem surprising since they are the "red meat" diets, but when one considers the high levels of fat and sugar they contain, it becomes apparent that there simply is "not room" for large amounts of protein. When the content of protein, carbohydrate and fat in the diet is viewed from the percentage per total caloric intake rather than the number of grams consumed, the picture becomes much clearer.

PERCENTAGE OF CALORIES OF PROTEIN, CARBOHYDRATE AND FAT

DIETS	Protein	CHO	Fat
Preferred Ratio	20%	60%	20%
I Modern American	13%	43%	44%
II Typical Teenage	8%	51%	41%
III Vegetarian	18%	61%	21%
IV Non-Vegetarian	20%	57%	23%

* See Chapter 6, Protein.
† See Chapter 7, Vitamins.

Demonstrated in another way, it is easier to compare the nutrients one gets per calorie in each of the four diets. This is especially useful information for those who want to lose weight:

A Comparison of the Approximate Nutrition per 100 Calories in the Four Diets

	Protein (g)	CHO (g)	Fat (g)	Iron (mg)	Calcium (mg)
Modern American	30.6	96.6	53.3	9.7	253.5
Typical Teenage	20.6	129.3	45.6	4	82
Vegetarian	47	160	24	9	670
Non-Vegetarian	46	135	31	6.8	613

	A (IU)	B_1 (mg)	B_2 (mg)	Niacin (mg)	C (mg)
Modern American	1475.5	.1	.15	7.5	37
Typical Teenage	546.6	.4	.36	8.0	7.3
Vegetarian	6735	1.62	.67	19.0	134.5
Non-Vegetarian	7351	.88	.75	7.8	144.3

The improved diets contain significantly more protein, complex carbohydrate, calcium, vitamins A, B_1, B_2, Niacin and C as well as less calories, salt and fat. Almost across the board, then, the diets based on traditional cuisine (diets III and IV) contain more nutrients per calorie, and these are presented in balanced proportions. These diets supply nutrients in the proper amounts and ratios to support robust health while the diets consumed by most Americans do not. The guidelines used to develop these menus, however, can easily be superimposed on an American menu, thereby creating meals which are both highly nutritious and appealingly familiar.

GUIDELINES FOR IMPROVED NUTRITION

An essential criterion for improved nutrition is the selection of healthful foods, but locating and selecting good groceries is not always a simple matter. In recent decades, our supermarkets have become vast emporia, housing the by-products of the millions which are spent on advertising and packaging. They contain long isles lined with brilliantly designed items that dazzle the eye with their colors and the mind with clever slogans that imply a wholesomeness they don't possess, that appeal to the desire for youth and excitement, that tempt one with promises of pleasure and convenience, or that tug at nostalgic memories of happier times when food was country-fresh and homemade-simple. The most basic guideline for finding one's way through this labyrinth is to focus on obtaining foods which are as close as possible to their whole natural state. This means steering clear of those foods whose natural integrity has been disturbed.

In moving toward a whole foods diet, gradually substituting for unhealthy foods others which are more healthful but similar enough to seem familiar makes for a gentler transition. The good first step in this process is to change sweeteners. To alleviate some of the problems associated with refined sugar which have been previously discussed,* "raw sugar," raw honey, natural maple sugar, molasses, sorghum or date sugar can begin to be adopted. Which of these products is preferable depends on how it is being used, in what dish, etc. Frequently a "sweet tooth" can be satisfied by offering it fresh or dried fruit, and fruit juices make an excellent replacement for carbonated beverages. However, a very large intake of even natural sweets is not desirable.† Secondly, refined white flour should be omitted from the diet and replaced by a less refined flour. Breads made from less refined grains are not only more nutritious, but their earthier, richer flavor is often found to be more delicious. An increasing number of families prefer homemade bread from more natural flours, and bread making is becoming a popular and relaxing hobby. The third major change in diet would be replacing refined vegetable oils, shortening and

* See Chapter 4, Carbohydrate.
† See section on Hypoglycemia in Chapter 17, Interaction between Diet and Mind.

margarine with butterfat. The benefits of this have already been discussed,* although a word of caution must be mentioned about using excessive amounts. Considering the diseases associated with excessive use of either saturated or unsaturated fats, a maximum of two tablespoons of butter or ghee (clarified butter) per day is recommended. If butter is not available, sesame oil is probably the least detrimental vegetable oil, though it should be used in very small quantities.

Besides food items which contain white flour, white sugar and refined vegetable oils, others such as most canned, frozen, ready-prepared "convenience foods" and processed preparations like cheese spreads and hydrogenated peanut butter constitute the fourth category of foods which are best avoided altogether. Those which contain artificial preservatives, as well as excessive amounts of sugar and salt, also belong in this group. Many fruit juices, dried fruits, nuts, cheeses, frozen vegetables, and even some so-called "health foods" fall into this classification. The natural foods shopper is sometimes led astray by the growing array of such "health-food junk," and it would behoove him to read all labels, even if Mother Nature herself is depicted on the package. Claims such as "enriched" and "fortified" should also be regarded with suspicion as these additives would not be necessary had the product been left in its natural state.

Omitting refined white flour, white sugar, vegetable oils, processed foods and foods containing additives and preservatives from one's shopping list will simplify one's task of food selection remarkably. When one considers how pervasive these items are in currently popular foods such as mass-produced breads, pastries, cereals, crackers, pasta, candy, beverages, fried snacks and meat products, one might find himself limiting most of his supermarket shopping to the produce counter, dairy section and the shelves which hold dried beans, peas, rice and whole grain flours.

---

* See Chapter 5, Fats.

FRESH FOODS

The golden rule in food selection is to purchase foods which are as fresh as possible. These have the highest level of nutrients, especially if they are grown in rich, organic soil. The freshest foods, of course, are hand picked from one's own garden just before the meal. The next best are those procured daily from the local vegetable stand or farmer's market. The greater vitality and flavor of such produce has long been accepted, and the efficient farm to market system of central France, for example, is the secret of Parisian cuisine. The farm trucks arrive in Paris nightly, and by 4:00 a.m., the wholesalers have stocked their trucks and are headed for their distribution points, insuring the freshest selection of produce to discerning shoppers. Nothing is quite so exquisite as a good French meal, yet the returning tourist who enters his kitchen armed with a gourmet cookbook is usually disappointed by the results. He assumes the problem is that he is not a "trained chef." Little does he realize that the main obstacle to his creating French delicacies is his lack of the fresh, wholesome ingredients used by the French. Perhaps during his visit to Paris he didn't rouse himself early enough to see the morning appearance of the fresh produce. While the sun rises in Paris, a major intersection in each neighborhood is completely transformed into a bustling marketplace. The fresh fruits and vegetables brought into the city only a few hours before are piled high on movable stands. Housewives come out early to get the pick of the lot, but long before noon it is all sold out. Prices are lowered at the end of the morning to auction off the last odds and ends, and the stands are then whisked away until the following day.

In most of the modern Western world, transportation from farm to market is not so rapid as in Paris. Vegetables and fruits may stand many days in transit, often traveling thousands of miles in refrigerated trucks and reaching their destination after a long period. They then go to wholesalers, and it may be a day or two later before they reach the retail outlet. They are then put in the produce section on refrigerated display counters and may remain there another day or more before they are finally purchased. On arrival in the kitchen, the vegetables may then be shoved into the refrigerator by the shopper, only to be cooked another several days hence. It used to be said of the French that it was their inability to afford refrigerators and their consequent daily trips to the vegetable market that led them to produce delicious meals—an excellent example of making a virtue of necessity. In America, however, affluence has multiplied the number of days vegetables and fruits spend traveling from the field to the table, and has subtracted the virtues of nutrition and flavor from much American cuisine.

There are many other sources of fresh produce besides the supermarket, ranging from one's own garden to local farmers and roadside stands which sometimes sell wild nuts and berries and sometimes in-season fruits and leafy greens. An added bonus to buying local, in-season produce is that foods grown by small farmers for marketing in their own area are more likely to be varieties that are bred for their taste and nutritional content rather than for how well they hold up under shipping and storage, as is the case with most big business, one-crop farm produce. Unbeknownst to most people, many large cities have their own farmers' market where both local and shipped produce is brought in daily and is available in small enough quantities to be comfortably shared by two or three families.* In many cities, buyers' co-ops have sprung up which are formed by several families interested in purchasing as a group. Members take turns going once or twice a week to the wholesalers and distributing orders of fresh fruit or vegetables to each of the members. Not only are

---

* Such wholesale markets which may be privately operated do not advertize and do not encourage the business of small shoppers who will buy only a case or so of each vegetable. However, anyone is free to purchase from them and no institutional affiliation is required. They can often be located by looking in the yellow pages of the phone directory under "Fruits and Vegetables, Wholesale" or "Produce, Wholesale." A number of such businesses with addresses near to each other are especially likely to represent a center where much fresh produce comes in daily.

the foods fresher but, of course, prices are often dramatically lower.

Learning to use locally grown seasonal foods is an adventure in itself. It brings one back into a keener awareness of the shifting of the seasons and gives him an opportunity to experiment with foods which may be more likely to be suitable for the local conditions. Moreover, it throws the planning of meals into a new focus. If one is lucky enough to have a garden, he should walk outside and see what is ready to be gathered and plan a meal around it. This is likely to give interesting results. Perhaps this week all that is really plentiful is green peppers, for example, but they are superbly delicious. Who would ever think of stuffing peppers (or want to for that matter) when they are 50 cents apiece and taste like paper? But here is a great opportunity, and what would otherwise be an indifferent dish turns out to be a delicacy.

Of course, the most ideal source of fresh produce is still one's own backyard. A few tomato plants, a row each of spinach, lettuce, mustard and turnip greens, and a couple hills of squash will provide unending new stimuli for creating different dishes through the summer months. If one is not so lucky as to have his own backyard plot, then he should select the best foods at the produce counter before deciding what to have for dinner. Planning an appealing recipe from a cookbook and then going out to look for the ingredients is not likely to produce a very satisfactory meal. If one relies primarily on his own garden and locally grown produce when possible and resorts otherwise to what has been shipped, he will usually manage quite well. In a bind, he may have to make do with freshly frozen vegetables such as peas, but canned produce is a sad substitute for the real thing. Although canned and frozen foods are not totally devoid of food value, they are always inferior to that which is fresh. The first choice should always be to use what is fresh and in season. In the winter, one can rely more heavily on sprouts which can be freshly harvested from the kitchen window sill regardless of the season.

For non-perishables such as grains, beans and other dried products, however, one can well afford to be more discriminating. These foodstuffs, which store well and travel well, are available in good quality almost everywhere these days. Organically grown rice or whole wheat flour or beans and peas are no longer difficult to find, whereas organically grown produce may have to come too far or cost too much to be of practical value for the average consumer.

COMBINING NUTRITIOUS FOODS

In addition to revising one's diet to gradually include more and more of the whole, natural, pure, fresh and seasonal foods mentioned above, one must also learn to combine these in such a way to form a diet which is not only balanced, but also appealing. Adopting new and more healthful dietary norms involves more than simply selecting different foods. If one's diet has been based on the strong tastes of artificially processed foods or the bland tastes of refined breads and old produce, then he must re-sensitize his food preferences to the more subtle and vital flavors of natural foods. Through gradual changes, one is able to re-educate his taste buds, learn to appreciate taste experiences that were before unknown to him, and gradually come to find foods appealing and appetizing that before did not interest him. To select food in such a way that this change in food preference can take place gracefully is a tremendous challenge. It requires that the person planning the menu, as well as those for whom it is being planned, be sensitive, considerate and creative.

By making use of the five-fold food grouping compiled earlier from the cross-cultural comparison of healthful traditional cuisine, one can learn to create a variety of tempting and easily prepared menus. In learning how to combine foods to provide maximum taste appeal and nutrition, one can again turn to the cuisine of traditional cultures. This means making selections from the legume, grain, vegetable, B_{12}, and raw groups.

Using this framework as the basis for planning meals would probably involve a major revision in eating habits since the introduction of legumes would in itself constitute a big change in most people's diets.   However, if done gradually, the transition can be quite pleasant and filled with delicious experiences.*

When attempting to improve the nutritional value of a family's diet, it is good to begin by learning how to modify or revise old menus so that they gain in nutritional value and flavor.   For people who are suspicious of "strange new foods," nothing is more convincing than finding that a few minor changes in their old favorites produces an even tastier and "old-fashioned good" version of what they already like.   Meat dishes, for example, can be not only stretched but also made more nutritious and healthful by the addition of beans and peas. Stews, soups, meat loaves, etc., are ideal dishes for combining meats with beans, peas and sometimes seeds or even nuts.   This lends variety, enhances the flavor and reduces the percentage of animal food in the diet.   By decreasing one's quantity of meat consumption, one is also decreasing the amount of environmental toxins in one's food as well as lessening the chances of developing such degenerative diseases as hardening of the arteries and cancer. Making beans and peas a daily part of the meaty main course also permits the digestive system to adapt to their assimilation and use.   It then becomes easy to occasionally simply drop the meat, organizing the meal around a main dish based on beans and peas.

It may be encouraging for the busy cook who is trying to use the traditional food groups to know that he need not prepare four or five separate dishes to produce a balanced meal. As long as he includes something from each of the basic food groups in the meal, he may use all sorts of combinations. As a matter of fact, there is an almost endless array of delicious dishes which include several of the necessary elements of a balanced diet.

* See Chapter 6, Protein, and Chapter 11, Elimination.

These, when served with a side dish of the lacking food group, create satisfying and nutritious meals. Casseroles are the most obvious ways of combining foods as they usually include a vegetable (such as onion, zucchini and tomato) a grain, (rice or pasta) and some B_{12} food (milk, cheese or meat). Salads can house the entire family of food groups, having ample room for a variety of vegetables or fruits.* Beans and seeds such as cooked garbanzos, kidneys, black-eyed peas and roasted peanuts, sunflower seeds and sesame seeds are especially well suited to salads as are sprouts of all kinds. Bread with cheese or a creamy dressing complement these combinations very well. Soups made with vegetables, grains and legumes are another easy meal, and a raw fruit salad with paneer (milk curd—see milk section) topping completes the requirements for a balanced menu. Breads can be made with wheat and soy flour, toasted and served with steamed vegetables which are topped with yogurt, soy sauce or butter for a quick wholesome meal. A piece of raw fruit for dessert rounds it out. A sandwich can easily be made with tofu (soybean cheese), bread, sprouts and tomatoes. Taken with a leafy green salad and yogurt dressing, this is another time-saving but balanced meal. Nut loaves can contain both vegetables and corn meal or wheat flour. Served with a white sauce and salad they are delicious and complete. Even modern America's favorite meal can be revised to comply with the five-fold food groups. Soy burgers on whole wheat buns with lettuce, tomato and sprouts are familiar and "good-for-you" treats, especially with a steamed green vegetable or spinach salad on the side.

International cuisine yields a cornucopia of delicious food combinations based on the five-fold traditional food groups. A Chinese vegetable combination with tofu and bean sprouts over rice or noodles dashed with soy sauce is a meal in itself if some chopped raw scallions are sprinkled on the side. Indian kichari can be a one-pot meal consisting of mung beans, rice and assorted

* See Chapter 14, Cooked versus Raw.

SAMPLE MENUS BASED ON THE 5 TRADITIONAL FOOD GROUPS

Menu	Grain	Vegetable	Legume	Raw	B12
Casserole and Salad	whole wheat pasta	onion, zucchini, tomato	sprouts, seeds, nuts and beans in salad	green salad of romaine lettuce	cheese and/or meat, ghee (clarified butter)
Chinese Vegetables	rice	celery, bamboo shoots, broccoli, mushrooms	bean sprouts (and tofu)	scallion	bit of meat and/or soy sauce,* ghee
Indian Kicheri	rice, whole wheat toast	onion, broccoli, mushrooms, zucchini, tomatoes	mung beans	sliced cucumber	yogurt
Mexican Tostadas	tortilla	tomato, onion	refried pintos	lettuce	cheese
Middle Eastern Falafel	pita, bulgur (wheat flour)	onion, tomato, parsley, green leaves	humus: sesame seeds, garbanzo beans	sprig of mint, fruit	yogurt sauce

* Research on this is minimal, but it is possible that some soy sauce preparations contain B12 while others do not.

vegetables. Served with some raw cucumber sliced into a bit of yogurt, the meal is complete and easy to make. Mexican tostadas are comprised of refried kidney beans, corn tortillas, tomatoes, onions, cheese and raw lettuce—all the essential ingredients. The Italians combine spaghetti made of wheat pasta with tomato sauce made from peppers, onions and mushrooms. Beans such as pinto and garbanzo make a tasty substitute for meat in this. A raw salad with yogurt dressing or some cheese over the tomato sauce fulfills all the food requirements. An American variation of this is pizza, made by spreading the vegetable sauce over bread dough and topping it with cheese (or paneer or tofu). Many vegetables (such as broccoli, zucchini and water chestnuts) are delicious on top, and tofu makes a nutritious substitute for cheese. A raw salad or a piece of fruit completes the meal. A Middle Eastern falafel made of pita bread, humus (sesame seeds and garbanzo beans), several raw vegetables and yogurt sauce is delicious and balanced.

Once one understands which foods belong to each of the three major and two minor groups, he can creatively juggle ingredients to be appealing and complementary. Grains should constitute the bulk of the meal with vegetables and legumes in smaller quantities. Once a day, or at least every other day, some raw food and something containing B_{12} should be taken. Preparing these foods so they will maintain optimum flavor and vitality is an art and science which will be investigated in a later chapter. The selection and combination of foods, however, remain the basic steps in preparing a heathful meal.

III

The Physiology of Nutrition

Merely eating the right foods does not necessarily insure adequate nutrition. Once the food is in the digestive tract, it may or may not be absorbed. Absorption from the intestines is still not the final step since the nutrients, if they are to be used properly, must reach the cells where they are needed. A vast number of factors are involved in the digestion and absorption of food: how it is chewed, the secretion of enzymes and the condition of the lining of the digestive tract which the nutrients must cross.

Digestion and absorption, however, are only one half of the nutritive process. For nutrients to be properly used, there must at the same time be a continuous and effective process of elimination. This is true not only at the level of the intestinal tract, but also in the blood stream and in the cells themselves. Clearly, one cannot process a meal properly if the digestive system is unable to dispense with what was left from the last meal. Even the cells are unable to absorb and utilize important vitamins, minerals, fats, carbohydrates and protein if the inside of the cell is crowded with the by-products of metabolism.

Digestion and elimination are interdependent then, and one cannot proceed smoothly without the other. Timing of feedings and the tuning of the digestive physiology is an important part of the science of nutrition just as the rhythm and rate of breathing with a smooth coordination of inhalation and exhalation is crucial to a healthy respiration. An understanding of the digestive apparatus can greatly facilitate one's regulation of his diet and help establish a nutritional rhythm that is comparable to smooth breathing. Digestion is different, however, from breathing, which is unceasing and continuous. The intake of food can be stopped, and when it is, although there is an initial accentuation of the processes of elimination, this too eventually reaches a stage of completion. At this point, one's consciousness is not occupied with either digestion or elimination. It is this state we call "fasting."

The wealth of data available on the biochemistry of nutrition is much greater than that on the various physiological states of the digestive tract. This does not mean that gastrointestinal function is less important than the chemical makeup of the food. It simply means that it's easier to do research on the food than it is on the variable digestive functions of human beings each of whom is so unique and different. The digestive system is both the barrier nutrients must cross to reach the cells and a part of the person which is controlled and regulated by his autonomic nervous system. That in turn is powerfully influenced by mind and emotions.

At this juncture we enter a completely new realm of nutritional science: the individual makeup and the unique characteristics of the particular person who is eating. The digestive system and its function are very much a product of one's personality and constitution. One person secretes too much stomach acid and develops ulcers, another too little and cannot digest his food. The physiology of the digestive system is acknowledged in the East to be a central issue in medicine and nutrition and to be the major consideration in characterizing a person's uniqueness.

For this reason we will find it necessary to begin to move beyond the rather meager information available from laboratory research on individual variations in digestive physiology into the concepts and insights of Eastern medicine where there is a rich tradition based on lay experience. Moreover, the perspectives provided by this ancient science help us to select from among the scattered data so far accumulated in the laboratory, that which may be about to emerge as most important to the study of diet and nutrition.

Digestion

10

When we eat our food, we surround it. Though it is in the digestive tract, it is still not in the body proper. While some nutrients may penetrate the intestinal lining and enter the blood stream, others may travel the full length of the digestive tract without being absorbed. Two people eating the same diet may end up with dramatically different intakes of protein, carbohydrate or other nutrients. As we have seen, for example, in the case of calcium, this is to a certain extent a purposeful process, an opportunity for the digestive process to select what it needs, leaving the rest to be discarded with the feces. In other cases, however, that which is needed may not be absorbed, even though it is present in the intestine. Throughout the length of the digestive system, absorption hinges on the availability of enzymes, and if digestive juices are not secreted in adequate amounts, the food cannot be broken down and absorbed and will be lost.

All nutrients which are taken in from the digestive tract must cross the intestinal lining. Sometimes they do so passively. That is, the concentration of a sugar, for example, may be so high in the intestine as to force its movement across the intestinal wall. In other cases, the absorption is active, and special metabolic systems in the intestinal lining pull the nutrients from the intestinal tract, moving them into the blood stream. In either case, however, the process of absorption is dependent in a major way on the health and the condition of the intestinal lining. None of the processes proceed smoothly, of course, if the food does not remain long enough in contact with the intestinal wall. The speed with which it is propelled down the digestive tract is governed by the nervous system and is highly subject to influence by the mind and emotions.

Even after the nutrients travel to the blood stream, however, their journey is not ended, for they must be relayed to the cells in the appropriate form and at the appropriate time if they are to be used efficiently. The whole process, though lengthy and complicated, begins in the mouth where the food is ground into particles small enough to be handled easily by the rest of the digestive system.

THE MOUTH: THE FIRST STEP

The mouth is more than merely the opening into the alimentary canal. It performs an indispensable part of the digestive process. First of all, it is here that the food is chewed. Although most of us remember having been told as children to chew our food "properly," on the whole, we seldom give it a thought and really don't feel that it is particularly important. However, one need only picture large chunks of apple, cheese, carrots or meat lying in the stomach or intestine to realize that the digestive juices will only be able to work on the surface of such pieces of food and that the remainder will be left undigested. Chewing food until it is a paste breaks it down into tiny particles which can be easily attacked by digestive enzymes and decreases the likelihood of having difficulties with digestion. It often prevents much of the feeling of heaviness and discomfort which follows a meal that is improperly chewed.

The mouth also has its own digestive juice (saliva) that contains the enzyme ptyalin which is important in the digestion of starch. When starch is properly and thoroughly chewed, the salivary glands are stimulated to produce an alkaline, or basic secretion, which contains ptyalin. In this non-acid medium, the enzyme is able to begin the breakdown of the starch chain into shorter sub-chains by attacking certain links in it. However, saliva is not able to break certain links between sugar molecules, so some fibrous plant substances in the diet that are similar to starch are not accessible to man. One of these is cellulose which is the major component of plant cell walls and gives them rigidity. As the plant gets older, the amount of cellulose builds up. Wood is simply the cellulose skeleton of a mature plant whose cellular contents have dried up. Leafy vegetables that are picked too late accumulate too much cellulose in the cell walls so that they become fibrous or "woody," and the nutrients are locked away inside the indigestible cell wall.

Grass is of little use as food since its cell walls contain significant amounts of cellulose even when the plant is young. Its nutrients are unavailable unless it is squeezed, pressed or juiced. Cattle are able to live on grass not because they have enzymes to break down cellulose, but because they have "extra stomachs" which contain large numbers of the kinds of bacteria that are equipped to break down cellulose. Most animals, however, do not have this capacity and are limited to the use of starch.

No starch-digesting enzymes are present in the stomach, but when the food reaches the small intestine, an enzyme from the pancreas is added which completes the work begun in the mouth by the ptyalin. The pancreas also contributes additional enzymes which disconnect further linkages along the starch chain, breaking it down completely into simple sugar units. For this reason, it is often said that saliva isn't necessary for starch digestion since all the enzymes needed for it are present in the small bowel. Nonetheless, salivary digestion may be helpful. Even when ptyalin breaks only one tenth of one percent of the links in the starch chain, the particles of starch are reduced to a hundredth of their original size, and the starch paste can be more comfortably digested when it reaches the small intestine.

SALIVA AND THE TEETH

Moreover, salivary enzymes break down the starch particles that stick to the teeth after eating. This helps to dislodge and dissolve them. If starch is taken at the end of the meal, waiting for five to ten minutes before cleaning the teeth allows the enzyme-rich saliva, which has been stimulated, to act on these adherent particles so they are easily removed. If starch remains in the mouth, however, bacteria begin to grow in it. The calcium compounds which make up the enamel of the teeth will not dissolve in normal alkaline saliva, but they are soluble in acid. Where bacteria grow, they create an acid solution and the enamel begins to dissolve. This process can gradually eat away the teeth. Whether or not this happens depends on the saliva and its chemistry. When there is no saliva, the teeth quickly decay.[1] But the kind of starch eaten is also important. Gummy food, like the breads and desserts made from refined flour, are particularly prone to create problems. An experiment has shown that whole grain flours caused less decay in teeth than those which are refined.[2] This is similar to the marked tendency of refined sugar to cause tooth decay[3] which differs so from the effects of chewing the sugar cane itself.* It has even been suggested that the quality of the soil on which grain is grown may play a role.[4] One can often see for himself that a good quality of fresh whole grain bread leaves his teeth clean and smooth to the tongue while pastries and less fresh foods cause an unpleasant coating. Much depends on the chemistry of one's saliva. Some

---

* See Chapter 4, Carbohydrate, section on sugars.

persons secrete a saliva which tends to dissolve away any kind of food particle while an occasional person seems to collect deposits and plaque on the teeth regardless of what he eats. When such food deposits regularly remain around the teeth, one loses sensitivity to the acidity and bacterial growth. Not only decay of the teeth, but a recession of the gums and looseness of the teeth, called "periodontal disease" (or "trench mouth") will eventually follow. The common use of refined starches in the diet has resulted in a dramatic increase in periodontal disease. Most teenagers now have some degree of it, and by adulthood the incidence is near 90%. Eventually the nerve endings in the gums become damaged so that the acidity and tissue destruction create no sensation and the loss of gum tissue progresses without one's really being aware of it. The ultimate outcome of this is, of course, loss of the teeth. If the teeth are regularly cleaned, however, sensitivity returns to the gums. Then when acidity around the teeth occurs there is noticeable discomfort and one is reminded to attend to cleaning the teeth or making the appropriate changes in diet.

Acidity inactivates ptyalin, the enzyme in saliva, preventing starch digestion in the mouth. This means that as the bacteria begin to grow in pieces of starchy food left between the teeth, the particles become even more resistant to the action of the enzyme. It also means that taking an acid food, such as tomato, with a starch like bread will slow salivary digestion. If pancreatic secretions are weak, starch digestion will need all the help it can get from saliva, so this can be an important consideration. Persons who also have little acid secretion from the stomach may fail to sterilize the food, and bacteria will grow more readily in the digestive system. Then starch which is poorly digested in the mouth and stomach because of the acidity of tomato (as in spaghetti) or orange juice (as happens with a breakfast of toast and orange juice taken together) may lie uncomfortably in the stomach and breed bacteria and gas.

Digestive enzymes are the keys that unlock the complex

molecules of food, breaking them down into their components which can pass through the wall of the intestine. Different enzymes are secreted at different points along the digestive tract. Many of them must act if a food is to be properly broken down and digested. Bread, for example, contains both starch and protein (as well as small amounts of fat). Salivary ptyalin, working in an alkaline medium, starts the breakdown of starch, then the whole mass of food must be made acid if the protein digesting enzymes of the stomach are to work. Further steps are also necessary to complete the process. For a food to be properly handled, to "burn clean" and leave no troublesome residues or interfere with the smooth functioning of metabolic processes in the biochemical environment, each enzyme and digestive juice must be secreted in the right amounts at the right time.

Here's where the sense of taste becomes important. If one is not hungry, has no appetite, or if the food does not taste good to him, the digestive juices will not flow properly, and the food will be poorly digested.

THE SENSE OF TASTE

It is taste, along with sight and smell, which seems to "program" the digestive system for a certain sequence of enzyme secretions that are suited to the particular food eaten. For this reason if one has been having digestive problems it is helpful to eat foods in a simple form so that the gastro-intestinal tract can be set up properly for what's about to arrive. When this is done habitually, the body not only digests more efficiently, but it can learn to discriminate. If on the other hand, a huge conglomeration of different foods, each with sauces, chemical preservatives, flavorings and colorings is eaten along with great quantities of flavored and colored beverages, the digestive system is confused. Even if something had been taken in that was needed, the body wouldn't know which smell and taste to connect it with. If on the other hand, something causes pain or a toxic or harmful effect, the system doesn't know what to attribute that to either. But if foods are eaten in a relatively simple form and in simple combination, one can learn to appreciate the effects and value of each food. Then it becomes possible to recognize and select that which one needs and can handle and to pass up what he doesn't need or tolerates poorly.

Technically, taste involves only the taste buds of the tongue. These are able to register saltiness, bitterness, sourness and sweetness. The finer shades of what we ordinarily refer to as "taste" are a result of the sense of smell. Odors and aromas must pass backward between the soft palate and the rear wall of the throat to float upward into the nasal area and reach the nerve endings there.

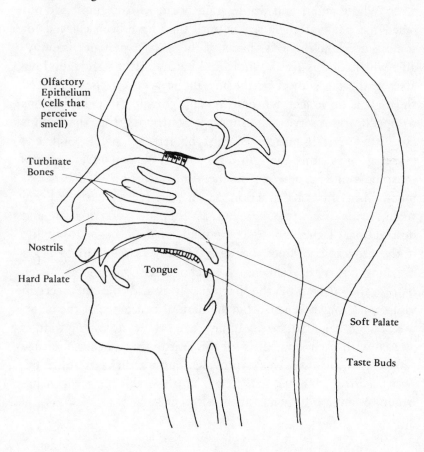

Olfactory Epithelium (cells that perceive smell)

Turbinate Bones

Nostrils

Hard Palate

Tongue

Soft Palate

Taste Buds

When one has a cold and his nasal passages are congested, the air will not pass freely from the back of the mouth and throat into the nasal area, so there is no experience of the aroma and more subtle taste of food. Everything is either bitter, salty, sweet or sour, or some combination of those four, and food loses much of its appeal. (This may be one way our bodies have of telling us that we don't need to eat at that time.)

As any accomplished cook can tell you, experiencing the taste, aroma and savor of food is a complex matter. There is an initial taste which is experienced as food is taken into the mouth, but as the bite is chewed, the particles are crushed and different aromas are released. As one master chef has noted, "The taste of every bite of food has a beginning, a middle and an end."

Whole grains and whole grain breads, for example, do not reach the peak of their flavor until they have been chewed for some time. Each of the phases of the taste experience is enjoyable when food is fresh, whole and natural. If it stands too long after gathering, however, the metabolic gears of the plant cell shift. It is no longer synthesizing and growing; instead it begins to operate on reserves. Its supply of nutrients from the earth is cut off. Certain processes must be left off, while only the essential ones continue. In an effort to sustain life, nutrients must be pulled from one biochemical operation to another as metabolism shifts to function on an "emergency basis." Eventually, cells begin to die, and as they do so oxidation and destruction of the various compounds in them begins. Finally, if the process continues, bacterial scavengers move in to begin breaking down the remains, "recycling" its constituents. Even before the arrival of the bacteria, it is possible that certain viruses, no longer repelled by the natural resistance of the plant, are able to begin to grow. In any case, the taste of the food is altered with each step. It is for this reason that a head of lettuce refrigerated for two weeks provides quite a different taste experience from one just gathered from the field. One which has begun to develop brown spots is different still.

Foods which are processed, of course, are partially destroyed during the processing and their taste is drastically altered. Chemical preservatives are currently added to many processed foods in order to prevent the oxidation that alters taste and to discourage the growth of bacteria in the food. This does retard some aspects of spoilage, and it may slow down the process of degeneration. However, these chemicals not only cause problems of their own, as described in Chapter 13, but they also usually have an unnatural and unpleasant taste. This is usually more prominent as the food is chewed and may linger as an "after-taste." For this reason, one might find himself eating such processed foods with the uvula and soft palate pushed backward against the rear wall of the throat. This prevents odors passing upward into the nasal area and is often done unconsciously to avoid the objectionable effects of chemical additives and of processed food that has been bereft of its freshness and appeal.

CHEWING AND FOOD TEXTURES

Highly processed food is, of course, usually soft and requires very little chewing. One is thus led to enjoy the initial taste of the food (which is enhanced by artificial flavoring) to swallow the bite, quickly by-passing the off-flavors, and to rapidly get another mouthful of food. In this manner a large number of calories are eaten in a short period of time, but one experiences little of the satisfaction that should come from normal chewing and tasting. Not feeling satisfied, he is tempted to continue eating far beyond his needs or capacity. People are sometimes heard to say, as they push away a box of processed tidbits which they have just half-emptied, "These things are habit forming." Persons accustomed to eating such foods may at first experience difficulty when they experiment with more natural foods. Trying to eat a piece of whole wheat bread at their regular pace, they will find it "tasteless," or complain that "the more you chew it the bigger it gets." When, however, one learns to open the pharynx, chew thoroughly, and experience the whole spectrum of taste and aroma, he often begins to find that he is enjoying his meals more, yet eating less! As has been mentioned, taste is potentially one of the most valuable guides that man has in selecting his diet. One's tastes are not there to deceive him nor to be struggled against. By working properly with the sense of taste, one can arrive at a pleasant and healthful diet.

If, for example, he feels his morning eggs and oatmeal somehow intolerable without the presence of bacon, yet he realizes that for a number of reasons he should reduce his intake of pork, animal fats, and the chemical additives which may be in the bacon, he can experiment to see what else might satisfy his taste. For example, sunflower seeds roasted slightly and sprinkled on the scrambled eggs or the cooked cereal give the taste and consistency of crisp bacon. While nutritionally similar in some respects to the bacon, these also have other quite opposite effects: the oil is both polyunsaturated and fresh since it has not been squeezed out and allowed to stand in the air, and it has been suggested that sunflower seeds are able to maintain the secretion of the endocrine glands in a meat-free diet.[5] Beyond this, however, there may be other similarities between the crisp roasted bacon and the crisp roasted sunflower seeds. The taste which is being satisfied may be for some nutrient which they have in common and which is needed. One's taste should never be ignored. If he offers himself only the best foods and satisfies his appetite from this selection, then he is likely to get the nutrients he needs.

TASTE PHYSIOLOGY: ANCIENT AND MODERN

The appeal of food is based primarily on its aroma or, technically speaking, its odor, and the sense of smell registers extremely tiny concentrations of molecules that float away from solid materials. These are mostly fat-soluble. Taste in the strict sense, by contrast, detects substances that can dissolve in water.

Since most of the body's tissues are water-based, compounds which can be tasted may be more simply and directly related to the body's biochemical balance.

In the physiological system of ancient Indian medicine, there are said to be six rather than merely four basic tastes. The first four are the same as those which are found to be mapped on the tongue in any modern anatomy book: salty, bitter, sweet and sour. But there are two others also mentioned in the traditional Eastern system. One of these is the pungent taste which is experienced on eating chili peppers, black pepper or other extremely spicy foods. In Western terms, this is not considered a "taste" but rather a sort of chemical sensation since it does not involve distinct and identifiable taste buds. The Eastern perspective, however, is not based on microscopic study of anatomical structures. It is more practical and operational. Pungency is a taste because it gives you information about the food you are eating. That information can be crucially important, as anyone will attest who has unwisely eaten a dish of hot Mexican peppers. The same is true of the sixth taste enumerated in the Ayurvedic system. It is astringency. Food is astringent when it creates a feeling in the mouth as though it will pucker or draw closed. Alum has this taste and is used in dill pickles to give them that hint of astringency which is considered appealing. Other aluminum compounds, similar to common alum, are used in deodorants for the same reason—they draw the pores closed, preventing perspiration. It is considered important to identify astringency in the food since it tells something of its properties. Such a food will have the tendency to draw together and pull shut. From the Ayurvedic point of view, it is to this astringent quality that such old-fashioned remedies as blackberry root or a blackberry cordial owe their ability to stop diarrhea. Their astringency tends to draw closed and dry up the loose bowels. Taste, as we shall see later, is, according to the traditional wisdom of India, more than simply a matter of pleasure and temptation. It is considered, in fact, the most reliable index of the properties of the food. A highly systematized and refined science of taste enumerating sixty-four basic taste qualities forms the foundation of ancient Indian pharmacology and medical science.

THE STOMACH

The stomach actually has six different sets of glands in its wall. The most important of the substances secreted by them are hydrochloric acid and the enzymes which begin the digestion of protein. Since pepsin and the other enzymes which digest protein require an acid environment to break amino acid linkages, gastric acid is perhaps the most strategic secretion of the stomach wall. When a concentrated protein, such as a piece of cheese or handful of nuts, is chewed, the stomach begins to react to the sight and taste of it by secreting hydrochloric acid and pepsin. When the protein reaches the stomach, digestion can begin immediately and may proceed for as long as several hours since protein digestion is relatively slow. The resulting product, which is partly digested protein, will then be passed on to the small intestine where other special enzymes may complete its breakdown into amino acids.

When a starchy food such as a baked potato is taken and properly chewed and ensalivated in the mouth, the stomach is not stimulated to secrete a high concentration of acid. As long as the starchy mass can maintain its alkaline condition, the salivary enzyme ptyalin can continue to act, and a major part of the digestion may occur in the stomach. Sixty to seventy percent of a starch or potato meal will ordinarily be digested here before the meal is emptied into the duodenum. In this case, it is mainly a solution of short starch chains and sugars that is forwarded to the small intestine, and the completion of the process can be effected easily. Though the complexities of digesting complicated mixtures of foods is little understood, it has been known for some time what happens when one whole food is taken alone, even though that food may contain both some starch and some protein.

Experiments done by Pavlov on dogs indicate that when bread, which contains both starch and a small amount of protein, is eaten alone and properly chewed, it is digested in the stomach through a special "schedule" of gastric secretion.[6] During the first hour or so, a gastric juice is secreted which contains very little acid but a great deal of pepsin. The absence of acid allows the ptyalin to continue to work on the starch, meanwhile small amounts of pepsin are reaching the protein. At the end of this time, as starch digestion nears completion, a much more acidic juice is secreted which rapidly accelerates the digestion of the protein. With an unambiguous signal or a "whole food," the stomach is able to manage both starch and protein digestion.

When more than one food is taken, the order in which one eats them may be important too. It has been known for many years that the succeeding portions of a meal are arranged in corresponding layers in the stomach. Though the whole mass is churned, what one eats first is largely kept separate from what is eaten later in the same meal. For the most part, large lumps of poorly chewed food are held longer in the stomach, and if they reach the juncture of the stomach and small intestine, they are squirted back for further digestion. Though the whole of the stomach's contents is squeezed and churned, in general, the food remains in the layers that were formed during the meal, and this is not disrupted by the motion of the stomach. Even liquid drunk while there is food in the stomach simply passes around the solid mass and enters the small intestine.

HOW LONG IS THE STOMACH FULL?

Liquids normally leave the stomach within a few minutes of the time when they entered. This is not true, of course, of heavier and more complex liquids like milk shakes, thick soups, etc. Next to clear liquids, fruits are emptied most rapidly and their digestion may be completed within an hour or two from the time they were eaten. The amount consumed is important, of course, as well as the thoroughness of chewing, the type of fruit and so forth. Vegetables are processed only a bit more slowly than fruits, though the time required for their digestion will be increased when they are served with fats or oils, sauces, etc. Starchy foods like grains will require a bit more time than simple steamed vegetables, and grain/legume combinations, which are higher in protein take even longer since protein digestion must be delayed while the starch is processed.

While protein foods may require a considerable time in the stomach and small intestine and give a meal a solid, "stick to your ribs" quality, it is fat that slows digestion most. Fats and oil delay the emptying of the stomach more than any other food, and this may be one reason that fats are so coveted. To "live off the fat of the land" is a proverbial luxury, and one feels especially content after he has filled his stomach with a meal rich in butter or oil or animal fat.

While fats with a meal slow gastric emptying, stimulants like tea, coffee and spices tend to accelerate the emptying of stomach contents into the small intestine since they stimulate gastrointestinal churning. They can also interfere with gastric digestion through the irritation of the stomach walls. In addition, the stomach can be irritated by certain food additives such as salt. The Japanese, who have a low incidence of vascular disease probably in part because their diet is very low in fat, have a high incidence of stomach cancer probably because they season their food instead with large amounts of salt.[7] Chronic irritation from very salty foods may be one of the causes of stomach cancer though improperly and carelessly prepared* miso which could contain molds that are potent cancer-producing agents (aflatoxins) may also play a role.

---

* Commercially prepared miso, made from a starter that is fermented with pure cultures of the proper fungus, have not been found to be so contaminated with aflatoxins.

Gastric acid, which is hydrochloric acid, is powerful enough to make one wonder why the lining of the stomach would not itself be digested. In fact, the cells of the stomach's lining are made up of protein, at least to a great extent, and the hydrochloric acid along with the protein-digesting enzymes that are being secreted by the same stomach lining should provide a perfect situation for eating away the stomach itself. The reason this does not occur is because there is another set of cells in the stomach wall that are busily secreting mucus. This mucus, constantly flowing across the surface of the stomach's lining, protects it from the action of acids and enzymes. Even so, much of the mucus, along with some of the cells from the stomach walls, is digested. It is estimated that for every 30 to 40 grams of protein digested and absorbed from food, another 39 to 50 comes from the protein of the digestive enzymes themselves along with cells and mucus from the lining of the digestive tract.[8] It is easy to see why diarrhea, a condition where the contents of the digestive tract exit suddenly without absorption of nutrients, can cause such weakness. Especially if it occurs frequently, the body not only loses the food, but it can be depleted of even greater amounts of fluids, minerals and the vital protein that it secreted in the form of mucus and enzyme-rich digestive juices.

MUCUS AND THE STOMACH

Normally, however, the secretion of mucus is responsible for maintaining a balance so that the concentration of acid and enzymes is sufficient to digest the food but not enough to corrode the walls of the stomach. When gastric acid overbalances mucus and becomes excessive, we find irritation of the stomach and sometimes ulceration. But mucus secretion can also become excessive, and though this is not a subject currently given much attention by medical scientists, the physicians of a century ago frequently talked about "gastric catarrh." The exact consequences of an overbalanced mucus production by the stomach

walls remains to be clarified by modern laboratory research. It
may have something to do with an increase in bacterial growth.
In any case, we do know that a deficiency in gastric acid is associated with severe disorders such as pernicious anemia and that
a low level of stomach acid is not a terribly uncommon condition. It occurs, according to some surveys, in up to 47% of the
general population, the highest incidence being found in older
people.[9]

It is the gastric acid, as we shall see, that is primarily
responsible for keeping the intestinal tract free from bacterial
growth. In the medical systems of India and Tibet, mucus
production by the stomach is considered important, and the
stomach is, in fact, looked upon as the primary factor responsible
for permitting or preventing the accumulation of excessive
mucus. It is called the "home," the site of residence and point of
origin of mucus in the body. This may be due, in part, to the
fact that mucus produced in the lungs and bronchi exits upwards
whereupon it is swallowed. Because of the influence of gravity,
most of this can happen only at night while the body is horizontal, and by morning, the stomach may be filled with a mucus
accumulation of impressive proportions.

The stomach lies at the left of the upper abdomen under
the ribs in the hollow created by the left side of the dome-shaped
diaphragm. Actually, it is only the diaphragm, a relatively thin
muscular sheet, that separates the stomach from the heart, which
lies atop the diaphragmatic dome. It is for this reason that pain
or gas in the stomach is experienced as occurring almost in the
left chest and often is mistaken as "heart" pain. The lower end
of the stomach lies to the right of the upper abdomen and here
is where the small intestine begins.

THE SMALL INTESTINE

When food leaves the stomach, it empties through a valve
into the first part of the small intestine which is called the

"duodenum." This might be called the fulcrum or "hub" of the gastrointestinal system. It receives not only the food from the stomach, but also a flow of enzyme-rich juice from the pancreas, as well as bile, the liver's contribution to the digestion. This is where the major events of the digestive process are focused, and the complex of autonomic nerves that supply the digestive organs of this area have sometimes been referred to as the "solar plexus." In a sense, as we have seen earlier, this is where the breakdown of the carbohydrate fuel derived from plants begins, making possible the release of the sun's energy which had been stored therein. This area of the body, often designated by a flame in Eastern symbology, is considered in Ayurvedic medicine to be the primary focus of the fiery aspects of a person's physiology as well as of his emotions and mentality.

The lower part of the small intestine, which makes up most of its twenty or so feet, is devoted primarily to the absorption of food molecules, many of which are being disassembled as they move down the tract. The surface area available for absorption is enormous. The inside of the small intestine can be seen with the naked eye to be lined with millions of tiny finger-like projections or "villi" that give it a furry appearance. Each of these villi in turn is covered by its own microscopically fine processes called "microvilli" which further multiply the surface area available for absorption.* This huge expanse of surface is extremely valuable for increasing contact of the food with the lining which it must cross, but it is also a potential liability since it constitutes a huge portal of entry for environmental pollutants, microbes and other unwanted miscellanea. Normally, however, it is an effective barrier. If digestion occasionally goes awry, the lining of the small intestine will usually function as a "filter," preventing undesirable materials from entering the blood stream while permitting nutrients to pass through. This may be weakened and disrupted if there is continual irritation

---

* See Chapter 11, Elimination.

from stimulants, harsh spices, drugs, pesticides and herbicides in the food supply, or from the by-products of undesirable bacterial growth occurring in the intestinal contents.

THE PANCREAS

The pancreas is a wedge or triangle-shaped organ that lies, fish-like, with its head buried in the curve formed by the duodenum and its tail pointing up toward the left side. It lies in the very center of the digestive system and, in fact, it lies near the center of the abdomen, for its location is roughly in the area of the solar plexus. Whereas the other organs of digestion serve to transport food or process it, the pancreas does not do so. Nothing flows *through* the pancreas. Rather, it is strictly an organ of secretion. It manufactures three kinds of enzymes and secretes them in varying proportions according to what has been eaten.[10] These enzymes are those which break down proteins, those which act on fats, and those which act on carbohydrates. Unlike the pepsin of the stomach, the proteolytic enzymes in the small intestine are not dependent on acid for their function but operate best in an alkaline situation. The pancreatic juice itself is mildly alkaline, and when the food mass coming from the stomach is strongly acid, the pancreas is stimulated to secrete an extra large supply of digestive juice.[11] The gall bladder (which secretes bile alkaline) is also stimulated by acidity in the food coming from the stomach. It also helps to change the mass of food from the stomach, which contained hydrochloric acid, to an alkaline condition so that intestinal digestion can begin.

The pancreas works hand in hand with the stomach to digest protein: the stomach secreting pepsin which begins the protein digestion, and the pancreas secreting enzymes which complete it. It also works in unison with bile from the gall bladder and liver to process and break down fat, which can then be absorbed through the intestinal wall and enter the lymphatic circulation. Finally, the pancreas works in conjunction with the small intestine as well as with the salivary glands to digest starch and break it down into sugar, which then enters the blood and moves to the liver where it is stored.

THE LIVER: BIOCHEMICAL MASTERMIND

The liver is the central clearing-house for all unabsorbed nutrients and the mastermind of many of the body's metabolic processes. It is one of the most complex and indispensable organs of the body. In certain ancient civilizations, it was said to be the center of the soul. It's certainly true that vibrant health of mind and body are not possible if the liver is not functioning properly.

When food is absorbed through the intestinal walls, it doesn't go directly to the cells of the body. Actually none of the nutrients entering go directly into the systemic circulation. Instead, everything is channeled into a special vein called the "portal vein." All other large veins go to the heart from where their contents are pumped all over the body. Not so the portal vein. Instead, it goes to the liver where it breaks up into a bed of tiny capillaries. By means of an ingenious arrangement, the blood is allowed to pass around and through the liver cells and then is collected again into another large vein (the vena cava), which finally empties into the heart. The liver cells filter out of this blood most of the nutrients which have been absorbed by the gastro-intestinal tract, and they process them so that they may be properly used or stored. In some cases they hold them back, waiting to release them into the bloodstream until they are needed.

For instance, the liver takes the various sugars, which have come directly from sugar in the diet or which have been broken off starch chains and absorbed across the intestinal wall, and hooks them together to create a huge storage molecule (glycogen) that is in some ways similar to starch. When the liver is healthy, it can take a fairly large dose of sugar from the intestinal blood and convert it into glycogen to be slowly released later when there is no sugar coming in. It thus prevents the blood and the general circulation from being deluged with sugar (glucose). When it is sick or has been depleted and it is unable to perform this duty, the sugar is not filtered out of the blood and passes into the bloodstream where it is distributed throughout the body. When one experiences a jolt of energy from eating a large candy bar, it may mean that the liver has been overwhelmed—either because it is weak or because the dose of sugar was very high.

As mentioned before, when sugar floods the circulation, it stimulates the pancreas to release more insulin in order to bring the blood sugar down to its level. When this insulin is released, the permeability of cell membranes to sugar is increased and the sugar passes into the body cells. Some of it is used up immediately, giving on the feeling of warmth and energy. That which cannot be used, however, is converted into fat for storage. If insulin release is not properly modulated and too much is released, the excess insulin has soon caused so much sugar to pass from the bloodstream into the cells that the blood level of sugar begins to sink, and one begins to feel weak, tremulous and irritable. This is the state of low blood sugar called "hypoglycemia." The sugar which was converted to fat for storage is not changed back to sugar.* If the debilitated liver has little stored glycogen to break down and offer the bloodstream, the blood sugar remains low. One feels compelled to eat more sweets in order to relieve the situation and so the cycle continues. With each turn of the screw, the fat builds up and eventually one is sadly overweight.

The liver also plays a major role in the processing of protein. It takes the individual amino acid units which have

---

* The fat itself, of course, can be burned as fuel, but when it is burned in the absence of sugar, residues called "ketone" bodies collect, and this adds to the body's discomfort by creating an acid situation.

been absorbed by the small intestine and reassembles them to form various proteins.   The most important of these newly assembled proteins is albumin (similar to that of egg white). Much of the protein that comes in is put into this form and released into the blood. The albumin in the blood helps to pull fluids from tissues when it is low. During starvation, for example, the blood may lose this ability, so that there is swelling and fluid accumulation.   During starvation, body cells break themselves down to supply enough protein to keep the blood level of albumin steady and to furnish amino acids for use as fuel.   In this way the blood sugar can be kept high enough to ensure the survival of vital cells such as those of the heart and brain. Under normal circumstances, however, some of the amino acids are passed on by the liver to the rest of the body where they are rearranged into whatever particular protein molecule the cell happens to need.

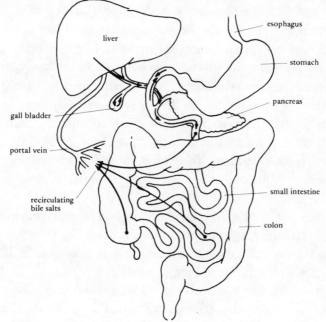

Recirculation of Cholesterol

THE LIVER, BILE AND CHOLESTEROL

The liver also plays a role in fat digestion since the intestinal breakdown and absorption of fat depends on the presence of bile, which is another product of the liver. The bile disperses fat globules throughout the solution so that the pancreatic enzyme lipase can get at the fat molecules and break them down into the fatty acids which pass through the intestine walls. Creation of this substance, bile or "gall," is a very ingenious process which serves two purposes at once.

Bile salts are formed in the liver from cholesterol. These substances pass into the gall bladder where they are stored until food enters the duodenum. When the food reaches the small intestine, the gall bladder is stimulated to squirt out the bile to assist in the digestion of fats. After the bile salts act on the fats, they are carried out of the body with the feces and give the stool its typical yellowish-brown color. It is thought that a more rapid transit time for the bowel contents increases the proportion of the cholesterol that is carried out of the body as bile salts. If the contents of the bowels move more slowly, there is more time for the cholesterol to be reabsorbed and reenter the circulation. Bacterial action also plays some part since it is the conversion of bile salts from one form to another that allows them to move from the digestive tract back into the bloodstream.[12] Though certain strains of bacteria in the intestine may cause cholesterol to go up, others seem to promote its removal from the body.[13]

When the bile contains very high concentrations of cholesterol, it begins to precipitate out, much as salt crystals begin to form in water when too much salt is dissolved in it. The result is the formation of large crystals or "stones" in the gall bladder where the bile is stored. These stones can obstruct the flow of bile from the gall bladder into the intestine. This also slows the excretion of bile from the body, and as a result, blood cholesterol levels may go up. When the bile ducts become completely blocked with a stone, the bile backs up, causing the gall bladder to become full, tight and painful. The result is often an attack of severe colic with vomiting that may land one on the operating table where the gall bladder, stones and all, is removed.

Normal bile is clear yellow, strongly alkaline and bitter, hence the expression "bitter as gall" (arising no doubt from the unpleasant experience of vomiting up bile or gall which has been forced from the duodenum into the stomach).

POLLUTION: EXTERNAL AND INTERNAL

Since everything coming from the intestines must go through the liver, it can be swamped with work. Overload interferes with its function. This can be a result of eating too much or of passing into the liver too heavy a load of chemicals and contaminants. Not only must it process needed nutrients, it must pull out all toxic compounds like insecticides, food additives, etc., and detoxify them. If the food it receives is refined, lacking in the many minerals, vitamins and similar substances which are necessary for their processing, then the liver cells are hard put to do their work. Poisoned by the toxins piling up waiting for detoxification, short of essential nutrients, and overburdened with work anyhow, they will begin to break down. The bloodstream is flooded with undetoxified chemicals, unprocessed sugars and amino acids. This condition, when full blown, is called "liver failure" and is cause for grave concern. It is often the last stage in a terminal illness.

Long before the liver has become debilitated enough for one to develop such an extreme condition whose signs and symptoms are likely to be observed by a physician, however, it may be struggling with a daily overload and a lack of nutrients which result from a habitually bad diet. In such circumstances, it cannot keep the blood properly filtered and cleansed, and its own functioning is disturbed and deranged. This gives rise to a whole host of symptoms such as sensitivity to certain foods which must be avoided, excess gas, constipation, diarrhea, headache and difficulty awakening in the morning, with puffy eyelids, stiff hands and feet and aching joints. The urine is dark in the morning but becomes increasingly clear and copious during the day. In the evening such a person has a great deal of nervous energy and difficulty going to sleep. There is often mild aching and a feeling of heaviness and fullness in the upper right part of the abdomen.

In France where the recognition of these symptoms is part and parcel of traditional folk wisdom, such an episode is called a "liver crisis." The French, who give particular attention to the quality of food, its preparation and the digestive tract, are sometimes ridiculed for their talk about liver crises, and today, even in France, the up-to-date medical doctor is likely to consider the condition "a myth." Whereas in the traditional Oriental systems of medicine, liver dysfunction is discussed in detail and given much attention, in conventional modern medicine disorders of the liver are considered to exist only when an acute or catastrophic disease has occurred, such as hepatitis or cancer of the liver. Though the symptoms of mild but significant liver disorder are widespread among Americans, the problems are usually attributed by the layman to "dyspepsia," "stomach ulcers," or "a touch of the flu." Conventional physicians do not think along the lines of liver dysfunction either, since most of their diagnostic decisions are based on laboratory tests. Unfortunately, a large amount of liver tissue must be damaged or destroyed before the customary tests of liver function reveal abnormality.

As a result, many physicians become frustrated with the liver patient, his multitude of odd complaints, and his consistently negative laboratory tests. Any pain he may experience will usually be in the vicinity of the liver on the right side under the ribs, an area termed, anatomically, the hypochondrium. Intriguingly enough, it is often the liver patient whom the busy and baffled doctor is likely to call a "hypochondriac," revealing the diagnosis without realizing it! In all fairness to the belea-guered physician, however, it should be added that liver patients do frequently suffer from emotional problems, both as a con-sequence of and a cause of the disordered liver.*

Another factor often contributing to liver problems is disorder in the colon or in the small intestine. Since all the blood coming from the intestinal tract is channeled first through the liver, disorders or imbalances involving the lining of the intestinal tract will have the most impact on the liver. This may be especially true of the colon where a huge quantity of bacteria, fungi, yeast and other microbes grow. If the delicate relationship between the microbes and the intestinal wall is disrupted, this can result in either a growth of undesirable micro-organisms in the intestine, such as is seen in certain diseases like dysentery, or it can result in a breakdown of the barrier provided by the lining of the intestine. The colon then is more than a mere receptable for wastes.

* See Chapter 17, Interaction between Diet and Mind.

Elimination

11

In the lower right hand side of the abdomen where the appendix is located, the small intestine ends and the large intestine begins. There is a sort of valve there, "the ileocecal valve" which keeps the two separate since their functions are quite different. The upper part of the digestive system—the mouth, the stomach and the small intestine—are designed for absorption, while the lower part—the colon or large intestine—is for elimination. But the colon is more than a conduit for refuse. It contains a thriving population of micro-organisms whose metabolism is active and variable. When we consider that the number of microbes in the intestinal tract equals or exceeds the cells of the body we begin to realize that the large intestine is an organ worthy of study and that its "guests" can be considered an organ in their own right.

THE LARGE INTESTINE: "CULTURE PLATE OF THE BODY"

By the time the food passes from the small intestine to the colon or large bowel, most of the nutrients have been removed.

What remains is a semi-liquid mass that contains a fairly large percentage of fiber, that is, the indigestible portion of the food. In the large intestine, water is absorbed from this mass, causing it to become more solidified. At the same time, bacteria which inhabit the colon begin to grow in what remains from the food, breaking it down further and helping to convert it into a substance which can be passed as feces. Thirty to fifty percent of the dry weight of the feces is made up of these bacteria. They are not only important in creating the proper texture of the stool, but they normally maintain conditions that are suitable for the intestinal wall.[1] Though we usually speak of the "bacteria" that inhabit the large intestine (colon), more than just bacteria grow there. The microbiologist finds an amazing array of fungi, yeasts and viruses as well as bacteria. Since the delicate lining of the large intestine is constantly in contact with this huge mass of microbes, their metabolic activities can either provide a suitable environment for the wall or provide a constant irritation.*

It is said that ideally, there should be very few bacteria moving through the upper part of the digestive tract. If the food is reasonably clean (free of the microbes which come with the food from the soil, or settle into the cooked food from the air, or enter it through poor sanitation) and the digestive juices are secreted in plentiful amounts, then most of the bacteria present in the food will be "digested" along with everything else. In the large intestine, however, the situation is different. Here bacteria *must* grow in large quantities. The last stages of digestion depend on it. For the proper accomplishment of this job, only certain strains of bacteria are suitable. But exactly which bacteria happen to grow depends to a great extent on what we eat.

To understand how this works, we need to look in on the typical bacteriological laboratory. When the doctor swabs a throat and sends the specimen to the laboratory for a "culture,"

---

* In fact, a mild degree of inflammation may be common.[2]

the technician has no way of knowing what bacteria are in it, though he may have some hunch. For example, he might be especially suspicious that the organism growing in your throat is streptococcus. To find out he selects several small dishes of "agar." Each of these contains a gelatin-like material that is brewed by a different recipe, each recipe being designed to feed a specific strain of bacteria. The swab from the throat is smeared across the surface of the gelatin in each dish, and then the little dishes are kept warm at approximately body temperature. If one of the plates of culture medium grows large number of bacteria, it's a sure bet which bacterial strain was in the throat since the agar was prepared so that it could support only the growth of that particular one.

In a similar way, the food we eat, along with the "cooking" it gets in our intestines, prepares a sort of "meal" for the bacteria in the colon. In this way, the "culture medium" that we create inside the large intestine determines to a great extent the strain of bacteria which will grow there.[3] The importance of this becomes apparent when we consider the enormous number of bacteria present in the colon. There are over three pounds of them. They are constantly breaking down fiber or other residues, producing at the same time their own wastes and by-products. Some of these by-products are probably very helpful while others can be harmful.[4] In certain animals, the bacteria of the colon produce vitamins which are a very important source of nutrition. The extent to which this is true in man is not yet known, although there is good evidence that in certain populations on certain diets, the production of B vitamins by intestinal bacteria is an important source.* There are probably many other functions performed by the microflora of the colon of which we are still not aware.[5]

* See Chapter 7, discussion on B vitamins.

NEW DISCOVERIES

In any case, the metabolism and physiology of the intestinal bacteria is quite complex and has only recently begun to be studied adequately. Up until a few years ago it was thought by bacteriologists that the bulk of intestinal bacteria were able to grow in the presence of oxygen ("aerobic"). These aerobic bacteria were cultured and identified, and medical textbooks confidently asserted that one of them, *Escherichia coli*, was the major constituent of the bacteria of the colon. More recently, however, it has been discovered that the bulk of intestinal bacteria die in the presence of air, not being able to tolerate a high level of oxygen. These "anaerobic" bacteria have, in the last few years, been extensively studied by culturing them on agar plates which are placed in specially designed chambers where no air can reach them. As a result, our knowledge of the intestinal bacteriology has increased enormously, and the facts which have emerged are quite surprising. It turns out that anaerobic bacteria constitute more than ninety-nine percent of the bacteria of the colon in most persons. *E. coli*, synonymous with colon bacteria for generations of medical students, turns out to be only a fraction of one percent.[6]

A great deal of research has gone into studying the anaerobic, or non-oxygen-tolerating bacteria that inhabit the intestinal tract and in trying to discover which bacteria are related to which disease. For a while it looked as though the presence of certain species might lead to cancer. It turns out, however, that the picture is probably not so simple. It's unlikely that one type of intestinal bacteria is related to one disease. Most people have an incredible variety of bacteria growing in the intestine. The average number of species in one person's large intestine exceeds four hundred.[7] Moreover, the bacteria present in his neighbor, or even for that matter someone else in his family, may be made up of a completely different selection. The difficulties encountered in isolating one particular species of bacteria, culturing it, and determining what products it manufactures and what effects it might have on the colon in the body is a major undertaking. Studying four hundred different species in this way is more than one can imagine. When the problem is compounded by the fact that not only does each person have a different selection of bacteria but there are also probably various interactions between them, the problem becomes truly staggering.

The magnitude of the problems involved in studying the gastro-intestinal bacteria does not in any way detract from the fact that this is a very important subject. The nature of the metabolic activities of the colon microbes and their effects on the body will certainly depend on the varieties that grow there. It has become increasingly evident that certain strains of bacteria can produce substances that not only have no constructive role in the body's economy but may actually be harmful. Some microbial enzymes, for example, break down normally non-toxic compounds into by-products that are damaging.[8] When it is appreciated that the microbes constantly growing and carrying on metabolic processes in the abdomen outnumber the cells in the body,[9] the importance of their metabolic operations and by-products and their possible effects on the body becomes highlighted. Their constant output of materials whose effects are not known will be a subject for research over many years to come.

On the other hand, certain of the bacteria are being discovered to carry out important protective functions. For instance, some strains of bacteria have the capacity to break down and destroy toxic chemicals which might have been ingested with the diet.[10] It is possible that the absence of such bacteria in certain people may explain why they absorb a greater than normal amount of environmental toxins and contaminants such as pesticides, heavy metals, food preservatives, etc. Thus a diet that encourages the growth of such bacteria may indirectly provide protection against such common pollutants.

Certain intestinal bacteria such as those in the cow's "extra stomachs" also have the ability to break down plant fiber or cellulose into fragments called "volatile fatty acids." (VFA's). These are absorbed through the intestinal wall and can be burned to provide energy. In rabbits, for instance, this supplies twenty-two percent of the basal energy requirements. In man, the contribution to energy supplied by absorbed fiber products is generally small, but it may reach significant proportions where dietary fiber intake is high.[11] It cannot, however, be considered a desirable source of energy since the VFA's are irritating to the bowel wall and cause much of the gas and pain that many people suffer if they take large doses of bran (which is primarily cellulose).

HOSTILE GUESTS?

The relationship between man "the host" and his colon "guests" is one of symbiosis. The bacteria are provided with a home and nourishment, and in return they process fiber and wastes in the colon and probably serve many functions which we have not yet identified. It was an authority in the field of intestinal bacteriology who stated, "The colonic bacteria are worthy of consideration as an 'organ' of the body in their own right."[12] We might think of this "organ" being "sick" when undesirable strains of bacteria take hold and multiply, invading and causing infections or manufacturing by-products that are irritating or toxic. The intestine becomes inflamed, and chronic diarrhea, or diarrhea alternating with constipation, may result.

Spasms resulting from such inflammation can add cramps and pain to the picture, and this is the basis of many "stomach aches." The large intestine is horseshoe-shaped, running from the lower right, up, and across the top of the abdomen, overlying the stomach and descending on the left to the rectum. Discomfort in it may be confused with problems arising from the stomach itself. The more extreme forms of this are called "dysentery," and some of the bacteria (and amoebae) which can

The Position of the Colon

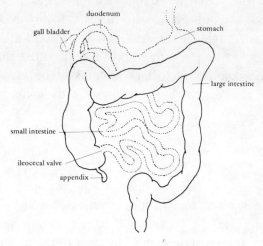

cause this have been identified. But as we learn more about intestinal bacteriology, it seems increasingly likely that what we call "irritable bowel syndrome" or "mucous colitis" may be milder and more chronic forms of a similar situation.[13]

Of course, the idea that the bacteria growing in the colon could have a harmful effect on the body is not a new one. In the 1920's it was fashionable to attribute many problems to this, and the situation was called "auto-intoxication." In its heyday auto-intoxication was regarded as the prime cause of all disease— a sort of bubbling cauldron of evil humors brewing in the belly of everyman. Constipation was the root of all this, since it prevented the free movement of the mass out of the body and its stagnation and "putrefaction" was the reason for the discomfort suffered as well as the diseases that were thought to follow. Later experiments demonstrated, however, that discomfort much like that of constipation could be simulated by stuffing the lower colon with inert material or inflating it with a balloon. When this mass was removed, the symptoms rapidly disappeared. It was concluded that the unpleasant effects of constipation and fecal retention were mechanical and that concern with any

harmful effects of the colonic contents was based on superstition and a repulsion toward feces.[14] More recent research,
however, is bringing back into view the importance of bacterial
microbes, and one research worker has admitted that, "The true
role of the colonic microflora remains to be assessed," adding
that "The colon is therefore an organ with uncharted metabolic
activities."[15]

THE GAS STORY

Apparently the reaction to the sweeping statements of
those who wanted to attribute all disease to "fermentation and
putrefaction" in the bowels, led to a rejection not only of the
"theory of auto-intoxication" but even to the idea that bloating,
belching and upper gastro-intestinal gas were produced by the
action of bacteria. While it is certainly compatible with common
sense to assume that food which is improperly chewed or
digested and confined in a dark, moist place with bacteria would
begin to serve as a culture medium, this idea was abandoned.
Physiology texts asserted that the upper bowel was free of
microbes and that bacterial growth was confined to the colon.
Moreover, experiments showed that much of the gas coming
from the gastro-intestinal tract contained a large percentage of
nitrogen, as does air, and it was therefore assumed that it came
primarily from swallowed air. More recently it has been shown
that gas produced by fermentation, being free of nitrogen, causes
nitrogen to move in from the tissues, reestablishing an equilibrium.[16] Though it was recognized that foul-smelling gas passed
from the rectum as a result of the fermentative action of the
bacteria that inhabit the large intestine, the possibility of the
importance of bacterial growth in the upper part of the gut was
ignored for many decades. Yet much of the gas experienced is
upper gastro-intestinal rather than lower.
Only recently has solid evidence emerged that often
bacteria *do* grow in the upper gastro-intestinal tract, creating

fermentation of food and the production of much of the gas that is experienced as bloating and belching.[17]   It is thought by many researchers that this results when bacteria move upward from the colon invading the small intestine,[18, 19, 20] producing gas, competing for nutrients and flooding the more permeable wall of the small intestine with their "unwanted metabolic products.[21] There is good evidence, for example, that invading bacteria from below compete with the intestinal lining for vitamin B_{12}, explaining in part, perhaps, why the bloated, gassy dyspeptic individual is also likely to be weak and tired. Some writers feel that the main purpose of the valve-like structure at the juncture of the small intestine and colon is to prevent such reflux.[22] In any case, intestinal peristalsis, the presence of bile, and especially the acid secreted by the stomach serve to maintain conditions in the small intestine so that the overgrowth of bacteria is prevented.[23] If there is too little acid and bile or if the propulsion of food through the tract is blocked and the intestine becomes inactive, then bacterial growth can begin.

Actually, if "invasion" from the large bowel does occur, it is probably not involved in many cases where the small intestine becomes overgrown with microbes. It is not known that large numbers of microbes are embedded in the mucous coating of the small intestine lining, even though they normally are not found in the food moving through this part of the intestinal tract. Rather, they are almost a part of the lining of the intestine, both structurally and functionally. As soon as inhibiting factors like bile, acid, etc., are reduced, however, these bacteria begin to multiply rapidly, reaching concentrations 100,000 times what is normal.[24] We might then think of the situation as an "infection," even though the microbes didn't come from outside. As long as they are properly regulated, however, the bacteria of the small intestine cause no dramatic problems; they can have a tremendous impact on digestion because of their close contact with the inner surface of the intestinal wall. They may physically by sheer number, for example, limit the area available for absorption of needed nutrients,[25] while in other cases they may significantly assist in the process. Some microbes in the small intestine may synthesize vitamins such as B_{12} that can be used, while others may compete with their host for the same vitamin. In some people it is even thought that bacteria in the digestive tract synthesize strategic amino acids which are used by their hosts who are then able to live on a diet that would otherwise be protein-deficient.[26]

The magnitude of the interaction between the intestinal bacteria and the host becomes understandable when we note the area potentially involved. The surface inside the twenty odd feet of small intestine is already nearly four times that of one's skin. Moreover, since the *microvilli*, tiny projections of the intestinal epithelial cells, increase the surface area of the lining of the intestine six hundred times, the total absorptive area of the inside wall of the small intestine of an average person is about the same as a standard football field! When we realize that every square inch of this surface is covered with mucus in which are imbedded and growing bacteria,[27] then we can understand what a great impact must be made by even slight changes in the strain of bacteria and their interplay with both the food being digested and the cells lining the intestine.

It becomes clear why, in Eastern traditions, the production of intestinal gas is regarded less as a humorous matter than as a significant indication of physiological functioning. This is in line, of course, with recent research which has made it clear that the widespread bacteria imbedded in the mucus coating of the intestinal linings can quickly ferment undigested food resulting in the immediate production of gas, and giving a nearly instantaneous indication of the status of food, digestive juices, intestinal mucus and bacterial growth.[28] Of course, eating habits play a role here, too. As we saw earlier, combining an acid with a starch will inactivate the salivary enzyme so that starch digestion cannot begin until arrival in the duodenum. For those with a meager supply of pancreatic juice, this may tip the balance just far enough so that undigested food remains for bacterial growth to begin.   There are other combinations which are troublesome for some people.   For instance, though it is not known why, melons will often cause gas if they are taken with anything besides other low acid fresh fruits such as blueberries, though they are usually handled if taken alone.   Milk is also best taken alone, or at least 20 to 30 minutes before or after a meal, since it is a complex food.   Perhaps its digestion requires a special schedule of enzyme secretions since during the time when it is naturally taken, in infancy, it is taken alone.

INTESTINAL ECOLOGY

The intestinal lining, then, serves as an interface of immense proportions between man and his "internal environment."   This interface is both a barrier and the portal of entry for all nutrients.   Yet the bacterial-mucus coating is in constant flux, as are the cells of the lining, which are completely cast off and rebuilt every twenty-four to forty-eight hours.   As a result, the mucosal "terrain" and its "vegetation" are at any given point in time a momentary reflection of some highly dynamic and constantly shifting equilibrium [29] between the microbes and man.

Since it is the gastric juice that is primarily responsible for maintaining the relative asepsis of the bowel, it is very important that gastric acid not be exceeded by the amount of food taken in.   If the proper measure is consumed, then enough acid is produced both to digest the food and to kill the bacteria. The same thing of course is true for the other digestive juices; the amount of food consumed should be proportional to the amount of them that can be produced.   Food which is in excess of this cannot be properly digested, nor will the digestive juice be sufficient to keep in check those bacteria which are embedded in the linings of the intestine, and to digest those bacteria the food contains.   As soon as the digestive juice is exceeded by the food, the balance shifts and bacteria quickly begin to grow.   It is also very important, for much the same reason, that sufficient time be allowed between meals so that one portion of food is thoroughly digested and a cleansing flow of digestive juice re-established before a new meal is introduced into the intestinal tract. If this clean-up time is not permitted then the chances of permitting an over-growth of bacteria are increased.

It also turns out that there is a significant difference between the bacteria which grow in the central part of the intestinal tube or *lumen* and those which grow directly in contact with the mucosa or lining.[30] The mucosal bacteria seem to feed more on the mucus produced by the lining than on the food which is moving through the intestinal tract. For this particular portion of the microbes in the intestine, the kind of mucus secreted will determine to a great extent the species which will grow.[31] Here we see even more dramatically the intricate interrelationship that exists between the microbes and the intestine. That is, the mucus secreted by the intestine determines the kind of bacteria, but the bacteria in turn effect the lining of the intestine, either irritating it or promoting its health, thereby providing one of the factors influencing the kind of mucus produced. This interrelationship can be affected by either one of the participants, but over the long haul, one very important factor in determining the kind of mucus produced is the diet. It is only as the biochemistry of the body changes as a result of an alteration in diet that the chemistry of the mucus secreted by the lining of the intestine also changes, and a different variety of bacteria is encouraged to grow. This is a gradual process, of course, and it has been estimated that more than a year on a new diet is required before the intestinal bacteria are measurably altered.[32]

FROM MIND TO MICROBES

Emotions play a role in determining the amounts of enzymes that are produced, the quality and quantity of bile, the activity of the intestine and the mucus secretion [33] of its walls.

For this reason, the emotional state of the person also has an almost direct effect on the kind of bacteria that grow in the gut. The ancient physicians of India and Tibet placed a great deal of emphasis on the interrelationship between nervousness and emotional illness on the one hand, and difficulties with a poorly regulated production of gas from the colon on the other. In view of our recent appreciation of the relationship between emotions, bacterial growth and gas production, it is interesting to find such an association made thousands of years ago between gas or *vayu* (wind) and nervous instability. A "jumpiness" was thought to result when the gas or "wind" was not properly regulated, because as it became overpronounced, it "moved up" from the large intestine to influence adversely the rest of the body and mind.

What we see, then, is that the micro-organisms growing in the intestinal tract are a point of interaction for the major factors involved in a person's functioning: physiological, dietary, environmental, emotional and mental. As noted earlier, the intestine contains not only the four to five hundred varieties of bacteria, but many species of fungi and yeast which have not been well studied, as well as possibly innumerable kinds of viruses which have not even yet been investigated. The different bacteria, fungi, yeast and viruses may well interact in significant ways. Moreover, not only is the population of micro-organisms inhabiting the center of the canal of the intestine different from those growing in the lining, but those that inhabit the right side of the colon are different from those that inhabit the left! There are even different "communities" of microbes growing at different levels along the villi and down into the "valleys" between them. This extremely complex growth pattern of microbes in the intestine is related to the complexity of the personality of the host, since each of his qualities—emotional, physiological, hereditary, environmental, dietary, etc.—play into producing it. What results is probably much more intricate and individual than a fingerprint and certainly much more indicative of the basic characteristics of the person. We might say that the microbial culture created in our intestinal tract reflects the totality of our personality and our physical/mental being. It in turn affects us in certain definite ways, perpetuating our continuance as the same kind of functioning system and having either certain definite beneficial or certain definite detrimental effects, depending on the bacteria involved. As our living habits, diet, or emotional patterns shift, then the flora of the intestinal tract will likewise shift to reflect this.

This can be for better or for worse. If one is constantly angry, for example, the quality of the mucus secreted in the intestinal tract changes and may begin to grow a less desirable breed of bacteria. A highly synthetic diet is not likely to cultivate healthy microbes either. The fact that some bacteria compete with their host for certain vitamins suggests that taking high doses of vitamins over a long period of time could promote their growth. This leads one to wonder whether once they were established such microbes might deplete one of vitamins from food or require that high doses of them be taken indefinitely to prevent this.

Many factors that have not yet been clearly defined probably enter into the determination of which microbes grow in the bowels and in what proportions. This varies tremendously from person to person. In the industrialized countries, highly processed diets, ubiquitous pollutants, the frequent use of drugs such as antibiotics and an emotionally unsettling way of life all contribute to creating a highly variable and rapidly changing population of microbes in the average person's intestinal tract. Where more natural and consistant diets are consumed, only two or three species of bacteria tend to predominate, and these tend to be stable.[34] It has been shown in experimental animals that there are profound differences between those that have one type of intestinal microbes and those which have another. One group had a lower infant mortality rate, more rapid weight gain, less resistance to infection and the ability to thrive on diets that would ordinarily be considered deficient in important nutrients.[35] It has been shown in humans that the microbes of the intestinal tract are significantly different in older people who are senile.[36] Such differences are probably established at birth. Babies who are breast fed have a characteristic population of bacteria that differs from those bottle fed.[37] It is even thought that some of the early establishment of microbes comes from the mother's body before birth while others enter the intestinal tract from the environment during infancy.[38]

As this picture emerged, the editor of a well known medical journal commented wryly: "The fact that certain of our physiologic and immunologic make-up may not be dependent upon centuries of genetic heritage but simply upon what bug resides in our lower gut is somehow disconcerting."[39] Disconcerting? Perhaps. Humbling? More likely, but basically encouraging. We may not be able to change "centuries of genetic heritage," but there is every reason to think that by following a diet that is consistently simple, largely unrefined and predominately whole grains, beans, vegetables and fruits with, perhaps, small amounts of milk products and butter fat,[40] we can gradually alter the balance of microbes present in the intestinal tract. The result is that, in turn, these "internal guests" return the favor by exerting an increasingly beneficial effect on our health.

YOGURT AND MISO

One of the ways that has been traditionally used to encourage a healthier and more desirable growth of intestinal bacteria has been through the use of fermented foods. In Japan, and in China to some extent, the fermented products of soybeans have been used for hundreds of years. The best known of these are shoyu (soy sauce) and miso. These are produced by a long process during which the soybean mash is left to grow local strains of bacteria and other micro-organisms. Though much of these products are now mass-produced under factory conditions, traditionally the fermenting material is kept for many months and sometimes even years at a fairly constant temperature somewhere in the home of those who use it. In this way it takes on and cultivates the various micro-organisms that are part and parcel of the ecological system in which it is produced. It reflects the microflora of those who grow it and is thought in turn to recreate within them an intestinal flora that is compatible with and in harmony with the ecology of which they are a part. Though miso is a rather concentrated culture of microbes, in Japan the average daily consumption is about one ounce, (approximately two tablespoons) and it forms an integral part of the traditional diet. Research has shown that Japanese-Americans living on a traditional diet have a significantly different population of microbes in the intestine than those on a Western diet.[41] How much of this is due to miso is not known.

In a rural setting where the ecological balance has been little disturbed and there is a harmonious interplay between the micro-organisms that inhabit the intestinal tract and those that are present in the outside world, it is possible that fermented soybean products play an integral role in the maintenance of good health. The soybean mash would naturally grow the bacteria which were present in the air, and the use of this culture by the household as food would insure a stable and consistent population of microbes in the intestinal tract. This would act as a flywheel, maintaining a steady influence on physiological processes and helping to keep the internal environment functioning in a regular pattern. Research suggests that in those populations where bacterial flora is simpler and more consistent, there is a lower risk of certain diseases such as cancer of the colon.[42]

However, where the ecological balance has been disrupted by such factors as pollution and a very mobile life style, then the home production of miso is not likely to be as simple or as healthful. The varieties of bacteria, yeast and other microbes that grow in an unstable isituation are likely to be very unpredictable and difficult to control.   The result could be a fermented food containing organisms that would be undesirable in the intestinal tract.   In fact, it has been suggested that some of the cultures of the fungus used in preparing fermented soy products may be contaminated with a near relative, *Aspergillis flavus*, which produces aflatoxins, the most potent cancer-causing agents known to man.*[43]   Where miso and other such products are produced commercially, there is less likelihood of contamination with dangerous organisms, but the results lack the unique suitability to one's own physiology and environment.

In India, the Near East and Eastern Europe, similar use has been made for thousands of years of fermented milk products. The result, one example of which is yogurt, has traditionally been prized for its beneficial effects on the digestive system. Again we find that certain bacteria which enter from the atmosphere in these local surroundings grow in the milk and produce a fermented culture that is suited to the individual living in that area. Traditionally yogurt is made by adding culture from the previous day to milk which has been sterilized or by simply taking the raw milk and allowing it to ferment as it will.   In each case, the bacteria and other micro-organisms which grow in the milk are determined by the local conditions and are considered in turn to be most suitable for the people of that area.   As one authority on the gastro-intestinal tract has pointed out, the inside of the gastro-intestinal tract is in a sense "outside the body," part of the *milieu exterieur*, or external environment—"like the hole in the doughnut."[45]

Of course, as in the case with miso, if the ecology of the surroundings has been disrupted, then the resulting culture may be of unpredictable quality, of questionable value and even of dubious safety.   For this reason, most yogurt is produced by

---

*   For example, it has been shown that antibodies to aflatoxins were found much more frequently in patients who had leukemia, suggesting that they were exposed to them and that this might play a role in the production of the disease.[44]

boiling the milk first and then adding an innoculant of selected bacteria. Much of the yogurt which is commercially produced is made with strains of bacteria* selected because of their ability to produce a stable, easily marketed product and may differ from the more complex cultures of many different microbes evolved in the near East and prized for their healthful properties.

YOGURT: "ALL IT'S CRACKED UP TO BE?"

Yogurt has gone through several cycles of being acclaimed as a boon to health and subsequently being denounced as a fad. The predominant organism in most yogurts is *Lactobacillus bulgaricus*, the species first identified in the fermented milk produced in Bulgaria. It was so highly regarded there as a treatment of digestive upsets, especially chronic diarrhea, that it came to the attention of researchers in western Europe and physicians in America where "Bulgarian milk" was a popular therapy in the early 1900's.

It was assumed that this bacterial culture was able to put a stop to diarrhea by displacing and replacing disease-causing microbes. Some years later, however, research showed that although large feedings of yogurt could change the composition of the feces so that *L. bulgaricus* was found in increasing quantities, the effect was temporary. As soon as the yogurt was stopped, the yogurt bacteria disappeared. *L. bulgaricus* could *not* be "implanted" after all, and yogurt lost much of its reputation in medical circles, though those who cared more for results than for theory continued to use it.

In the last couple of decades, it has been shown that *Lactobacillus acidophilus,* another milk-fermenting bacterium and a close cousin of the Bulgarian variety, *does* colonize the intestine and can remain permanently. This has led to a proliferation of fermented milk products containing *L. acidophilus.*

* Most commonly *Streptococcus thermophilus* and *Lactobacillus bulgaricus.*

Yogurt

Place a quart of milk over a medium flame, stirring as often as necessary to prevent its scorching. Adding a couple of tablespoons of non-fat dry milk just before the milk boils makes a thicker, creamier yogurt. After the milk has foamed up into a rolling boil (thus killing all the existing bacteria), allow it to cool for about half an hour, until it reaches a temperature of 105° to 115°. If the milk is too hot (over 120°) it will kill the culture; if it is not hot enough, the culture won't grow. An easy way to test for temperature is to place a clean finger in the milk. If it doesn't hurt when you keep it still but is painful when you swish it around, then the milk is at exactly the right temperature.

A powdered Bulgarian culture from a health food store is best for beginning the first batch of yogurt. Its flavor and quality make it well worth the higher initial investment (about $2.50). If treated properly, it will last for quite a long while. Traditionally, the same culture was used and cared for by generations of families. Dissolve the powder into a little of the cooled milk and gently stir this into the pot of milk until it is thoroughly blended. For subsequent batches, approximately two tablespoons of starter from the previous batch may be used instead. Though one need not be exact, much too much starter crowds the bacteria while too little will not make the milk gel. Pour the mixture into a covered glass or earthen container (metal may be eroded by the acidity), wrap it in a towel, and set it in a warm place such as over a pilot light or inside a gas oven kept warm by a pilot light or an electric oven set on the lowest possible temperature. The inside of the oven, or the surface on which the container is set should be almost, but not quite too hot to rest the hand on comfortably.

Check the yogurt at intervals by gently tilting the container. When the yogurt has thickened enough to lean away from the side, then it is ready to be placed in the refrigerator where it will gel as it cools. The first batch from a powdered culture may take from four to fifteen hours to "make" but subsequent batches may need as little as two. Be careful not to let it stand too long after ready as it will become too tart and lower in beneficial bacteria. Refrigerating it earlier results in a sweeter, mellower yogurt. It is better, however, if it is allowed to "ripen" in the refrigerator for at least six to eight hours. If whey gathers on the top of the yogurt, simply pour it off or stir it in. Traditionally, enough yogurt for the day's use was made fresh every morning, being sure to save enough to start the next day's batch. This keeps the yogurt at the peak of its taste and nutritional value and is still a good practice. Old yogurt makes less effective starter as it may be contaminated with undesirable bacteria.

Unfortunately, it does not produce the custardy, appealing dish we call yogurt, and its taste is rather sour. Nevertheless, many people have found the effervescent bottled acidophilus culture sold in health food stores very helpful for their intestinal upsets, and some dairies are including the bacteria in milk, cooling it before they can grow and then marketing it. Its taste is essentially that of regular milk. For those who don't like milk at all, anyway, acidophilus is sold in tablet form, though there is some doubt about how well the bacteria will grow without a supply of milk, since they are considered lactose dependent.

More recently it has been clearly established that the bacteria of yogurt are normally unable to grow or even survive in the intestinal tract of man because of their inability to tolerate bile or stomach acid and their requirement for a warmer temperature than that of the body. This does not mean that yogurt is unable to do what the Bulgarians as well as people of dairying cultures around the world have always known it could do. But apparently it works in another way, without actually growing in the intestinal tract. It has been shown that the bacteria growing in yogurt are able to produce antibiotic substances[46] and these are probably what is responsible for regulating bowel microbes. When yogurt is eaten in quantity, its bacteria may not grow in the intestine, but the antibiotics contained in the yogurt itself are apparently able to subdue undesirable microbes that would otherwise continue to grow. Apparently some fermented soybean products have this same property.[47] This is not surprising since many microbes are able to survive only by producing substances that inhibit the growth of their competitors.

This may be the correct explanation of the tolerance of yogurt shown by those who don't handle lactose well. Actually, yogurt contains large amounts of lactose, but it may be that its antibiotic content regulates bowel bacteria so that the usual explosive fermentation of the lactose which causes such discomfort is avoided. Whatever the mechanism, properly prepared yogurt continues to be soothing to the digestive tract, and even modern surgeons sometimes use it post-operatively to reduce intestinal complications.

In northern and western Europe, where temperatures are less conducive to the production of yogurt, one finds aged cheeses and sauerkraut which are also fermented foods. Fermented grains and fruits have also long been used to make the rich, flavorful beers and wines of France and Germany. These are prized for their nutritional value and their aid to digestion and are probably quite different from modern commercially produced beers and wines which use only a simple yeast for fermentation and are in any case, after the pasteurization which is used to stop the fermenting process, no longer "alive."

By contrast, local beers and wines were, and in many cases, still are, live cultures of various micro-organisms and it is perhaps some indication of the public awareness of the impact of this on the digestive system and the person as a whole that the preparation of these beverages was entrusted to the priests. Even today in the small towns of Germany, the thick, dark beers favored by the people are made in the monasteries where they were drunk. Small amounts of similar fermented beverages are used in the treatment of digestive problems in India and Tibet, but in Europe they have been used in quantity, possibly because the controlled fermentation and perhaps even natural antibiotics afforded some protection against contamination by undesirable microbes. The result is beneficial for the intestinal tract and assures the liquid intake required by the kidneys, but it brings along enough alcohol to be burdensome for the liver.

POLLUTION OF INTESTINAL ECOLOGY

Another important effect on the bacteria in the intestinal tract comes from the chemicals we ingest. Those which do not pass through the walls of the intestine may continue to the colon, poisoning desirable bacteria and creating a situation where only unnatural strains can grow. This is seen in a dramatic way when one takes certain antibiotics since the chemical agent is, in this case, selected precisely because it is toxic to bacteria. Some antibiotics are more toxic to intestinal bacteria than others. Penicillin, which is effective for most streptococcus, gonnococcus, etc., seems to have little effect on intestinal microbes. "Broad spectrum" antibiotics which are often given when no culture has been done to determine exactly what bacteria have caused an infection have a wider range and disrupt the ecology of the gut in a more profound way. Antibiotic-treated animals have higher blood cholesterol levels, for example, since apparently those bacteria which help rid the body of it are killed by the drug.[48] Moreover, by killing the usual microbes, such medications leave the surface of the intestinal walls exposed to irritants and the unprocessed components of foods so that it becomes raw and inflamed. The irritated bowel then contracts rapidly and jerkily, and the contents pass through quickly without having the water properly removed—a condition known as diarrhea. If the antibiotic is continued for a long time, different (and other undesirable) strains of bacteria which are resistant to the antibiotics may begin to grow.

On the other hand, the destruction of certain bacteria can be helpful—especially when they are causing trouble. This is the case, for example, in colitis, where the inflammation of the bowel is treated by giving sulfa antibiotics, which seem to eliminate some of the bacteria that contribute to the inflammation. The diarrhea then slows down, at least temporarily. In other cases, alteration of the intestinal bacteria may have more subtle effects. Chicks, for example, when given regular small doses of antibiotics, grow larger than those who aren't. If, however, both are raised in a germ-free environment, feeding with antibiotics has no effect.[49] Apparently there are, under usual poultry raising conditions, certain bacteria in the gut that interfere with growth. That such a shift in microbes can increase total growth bears witness to their importance.

The fact that giving antibiotics may on occasion produce

some symptomatic improvement does not mean that antibiotic use is the answer to the regulation of the delicate and complex balance between the hundreds of species of microbes and the intestinal wall. To use them for such a purpose is much like trying to fix a fine watch by banging it with a sledge hammer. While on rare occasions this may jolt it back into working order, the results will more often be disastrous. In the same way, antibiotic use will, as a rule, wreak havoc in the intestinal ecology.[50]

While antibiotics are designed to kill bacteria and would be expected to alter the microbes in the intestine in a major way, a more subtle effect may be produced by the residues of insecticides, which are left on foods as a result of agricultural methods, or by such chemicals as preservatives, which are added to food because of their ability to interfere with the bacterial growth involved in food spoilage. Anything which irritates the large or small intestine speeds up transit time through the bowels. This is true of harsh spices such as hot chili peppers, and it is through such chemical irritation that most laxatives work. To a certain extent this is true even of "herbal laxatives," though they are generally less harsh and might be considered more natural. But being "natural" does not guarantee against harshness. Castor oil is an oil squeezed from the seed of a tropical plant. It might be considered herbal as well as natural, but the ancient Indian medical writings classify it as a dangerously powerful purgative. Interestingly enough, some of the old-fashioned herbal laxatives like cascara are effective only because intestinal microbes break them down into constituents that irritate the bowel and cause it to move.[51] This is a very ingenious arrangement, since normally there are not enough bacteria in the small intestine to change much of the laxative into an active form. When it reaches the colon, though, the many bacteria immediately convert it to an effective laxative.

Of course, this works well only as long as the bacteria are mainly accumulated in the colon. If bacterial growth has moved up into the small intestine, then the laxative would begin to work there, irritating and inflaming the intestinal walls and interfering with digestion. The results could be unfortunate. It is fascinating to find that the medical scriptures of ancient India and Tibet warn against the use of such laxatives when the colon is not "ripe" (full) and when the solar fire is low, which would mean decreased gastric acid.

THE FIBER STORY

One of the most important influences on the microbes growing in the intestinal tract is the amount of fiber contained in the diet. For most of man's existence, having fiber in the diet was not a question since his foods were whole and natural and each morsel contained its own fiber as well as the other nutrients which he needed. Constipation and its various complications can often be avoided when the diet contains adequate fiber, which is the case when one eats primarily whole grains, beans and peas, green vegetables, and fresh fruits. Nevertheless, man has always had a certain proclivity for that which is tasty, light, highly refined and with an immediate impact on the appetite mechanisms.

The fiber is largely removed in the processing of many foods such as white flour or sugar. When very little or no fiber is in the diet, the residue that reaches the colon is not easily moved along. Instead of an easily managed mass, there is only a small amount of pasty material. The remains of such low residue diets pass through the intestine much more slowly, and constipation is likely to become a constant problem. One elderly lady studied in England who ate only pastries, sweets, and refined foods, was found to require more than a week for the small amount of residue from her food to pass out in the stool. Seventy-two hours or less is more normal and less stressful to the gastro-intestinal tract. In countries where the people eat only unrefined foods, transit time of the food through the intestinal tract may be as short as four to six hours.

When there is chronic constipation, hardened feces may cling to the walls of the large bowel, creating areas where conditions are altered so that unnatural bacteria breed. It is possible that these could inflame the patch of wall underlying the plaque, leading to the weakening and outpocketing we call "diverticuli." When such pockets in the walls of the large intestine become inflamed, the condition is known as "diverticulitis." This is a common disorder among middle-aged Americans who have made a habit of taking a poor diet of refined foods for many years. It is virtually unknown among people who eat no processed foods and have a bulkier, faster-moving stool that keeps the colon "swept clean." While officers in the British navy and their wives had stools that ranged in weight from 39 to 223 grams (from about 2 tablespoons up to a tea cup in volume), British vegetarians, like the vegetarian natives of Uganda, had stools weighing from 178 up to 980 grams (the average being twice that of the naval officers.)[52]

It is estimated that the dietary fiber intake of the average person in the industrialized West is only one-fifth what it was a hundred years ago.[53] This is primarily because of the drop in consumption of grains from 350 pounds per year per person to less than 150, and the fact that an increasing proportion of these grains have been refined. The use of fruits and vegetables, also rich in fiber, has decreased, too, but the use of refined sugars, which bring calories but no fiber, has more than doubled.

In the last few years, it has been realized that certain diseases that plague Western man, like cancer of the colon, were very infrequent in the people subsisting on a native traditional diet of whole foods, e.g., the African bushman. It was found that bile could be modified by certain bacteria to produce substances that can cause cancer of the bowel. The types of bacteria that do this are less common in the intestines of those who eat high fiber foods and no meat.[54] It was hypothesized that the higher content of fiber in the diet of the Africans was responsible for keeping the intestinal contents moving through faster and thereby reduced the amount of time available for irritating by-products of bacterial metabolism to affect the wall of the gut. Actually, as it turns out, excess fat in the diet is probably the major cause of the problem* and there is a growing suspicion that meat fat, especially that of beef [55] may be particularly important in bowel cancer.[56, 57] There followed a great rush of speculation that many diseases were due to a lack of fiber in the diet, and a rather hasty tendency to add large quantities of bran began. This has led to a flurry of popular "high fiber" diets. These are based on the usual refined and unnatural foods with the simple addition of huge amounts of wheat bran.

Unfortunately, adding quantities of bran to the diet is not without its danger. As pointed out earlier, bran contains phytic acid and when more of it is added than is naturally contained in the whole grain, it can chelate or bind minerals during the digestive process, removing them from the body and producing a deficiency of calcium, zinc, etc. Moreover, experiments have shown that at least some of the benefits of whole, fiber-rich foods cannot be gained by taking the fiber separately. Adding rice bran for example, to a starchy diet reduced blood cholesterol from 348 to 255. But when the whole grain was used the level dropped much further, to 165. This was true even when the bran was added to the starch diet in quantities twice that which was present in the whole grain.[58] Of course there are other important constituents of whole grains besides bran and starch, protein being one of them. There is evidence that vegetable protein helps lower cholesterol and prevent arteriosclerosis whereas animal protein has the opposite effect.[59] There are also other indigestible natural plant substances besides the fiber of bran that seem to be of equal or greater importance in lowering serum cholesterol.[60, 61]

* See Chapter 5, Fats.

Difference between Crude Fiber and Dietary Fiber

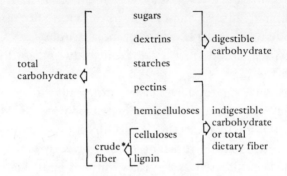

*With some methods of testing this includes small amounts of hemicellulose as well.

ALL FIBER IS NOT THE SAME

Unfortunately, much of the research that has been done to establish the benefit of fiber in the diet has relied on measurements of crude fiber. Crude fiber is the coarsest of the indigestible substances in food. It includes cellulose, the major structural material providing support for green plants and the chief component of such plant products as paper and cotton. It also includes lignin, another substance formed in the cell wall of plants. Lignin is a very tough material and is found primarily in plants that have become woody and hard. It is not made up of a chain of sugar molecules like cellulose and most of the other indigestible substances in plants which are technically carbohydrates even though the digestive enzymes cannot break them down. "Crude fiber" is actually defined by how it's measured. It is that which is left in food after it has been dissolved with first an alkali and then an acid. Besides lignin and cellulose, it will also include variable amounts of other substances similar to cellulose ("hemi-celluloses") which are a bit less indestructible and may dissolve during the test procedure or be broken down by intestinal bacteria. As we have seen, cellulose is also broken down in the intestine to some extent by bacterial action to produce gaseous substances (volatile fatty acids) [62] which are irritating to the bowel wall and cause an increase in its activity. Because bran is largely crude fiber, it is a laxative for most people.

But such crude fiber is not the only indigestible plant material in the diet. There are also a number of softer and more gentle substances in food which are not really "fibrous" at all, though they are usually included when one speaks of dietary fiber. One of these is pectin, a carbohydrate chain which dissolves in water, but is resistant to digestive enzymes. It jells when cooled and is used as the basis for jams and jellies. Pectins are found in the edible parts of most fruits and many vegetables but are especially plentiful in apples. Because they take up water inside the warmth of the body, they help make the stool bulky and soft. It has also been recently discovered that pectins were especially powerful in protecting against the toxic effects of certain chemicals in the diet such as cyclamates.[63] Whether they absorb such chemicals carrying them safely out of the body, or work in some other fashion is not known, but it is clear that an apple (or two) a day may very well "keep the doctor away."

The sum total of the tough, crude fiber and the softer fibrous compounds is called "total dietary fiber." Many of the softer substances such as pectins, gums and mucilages are broken down easily by acids and alkalis. In the laboratory, then, it is easy to test for crude fiber, whereas measuring the total of indigestible materials in the food is more difficult. Yet the semi-fibrous and non-fibrous substances like pectin that are so common in fruits, vegetables, grains and legumes may be more important and valuable than the coarser cellulose and lignin or "crude fiber." Estimates of the total indigestible materials usually termed "total dietary fiber" are therefore important. Though most of the popular books on fiber in the diet have simply used measurements of crude fiber for the figures in their tables and discussions, actually total dietary fiber may vary from this tremendously.   Nevertheless, authors generally either merely write in terms of crude fiber or else multiply it by a factor of four, for example, to arrive at an estimate of total dietary fiber. Often this is not accurate, however, since the two are not present in any consistent ratio.   For example, there is sometimes a great deal of total fiber with only a small percentage of it coarse, as is the case with young spinach which is picked when the leaves are very small and tender. By contrast, crude fiber content will be very high in tough, woody vegetables which have grown past the point of maturity.   Most of the tender fiber and substances like pectin will have already been replaced by cellulose and lignin. It is sometimes embarrassing to see to what lengths we must go in order to rediscover what common sense already dictates. Any rural grandmother, fussing over greens in her garden would be quick to cast off the coarsest and toughest, regarding them unfit to eat, and select only the youngest and tenderest for her family. That they are nutritionally superior she would regard as self-evident.   Of course, it is reassuring to have laboratory data to help us separate superstition from intuition.

Insufficient research has been done on the harmful effects of an excess of crude fiber or on the relative benefits of other dietary fiber as opposed to crude fiber.   It is quite likely that the softer and more gentle types of fiber are more beneficial to the intestinal tract, especially in those cases where there have been chronic problems with the digestive system. Mucilaginous foods like psyllium or flaxseed, for example, can soften and lubricate the stool in a non-irritating way and will often help in relieving constipation. They can be chewed plain, ground fresh, or soaked whole in a little warm water.* The husks of the psyllium seed are probably the best for this purpose. They contain a very soothing indigestible substance with little crude fiber. Not only are they the principle ingredient in many popular prescription and over-the-counter stool softeners, but they are a

* One to two tablespoons can be taken once or twice a day if necessary.

traditional Asian remedy for both constipation and diarrhea since they take up water from a loose stool and add moisture when it is dry and hard. Fresh fruits and vegetables also often help constipation, partly because of the bulk they provide. But even their juices have a cleansing or "purging" effect on the digestive tract and create less irritation than most laxatives. Yet they can be irritating to an inflamed bowel. Persons with acute intestinal illness should not take raw fruit and vegetable juices, though a diluted, cooked vegetable broth may be tolerated and is often found to be mild and soothing.

BODY RHYTHMS AND MEAL SCHEDULES

The human being might be thought of as having a dual capacity. First, he can actively engage himself in the external world, focusing his energies on issues of survival, sexual gratification, the search for food, etc. The second option is to suspend his involvement with the world around him, relax in a quiet place and devote himself to the internal processes of secretion, digestion and elimination.

The processes of digestion (eating, assimilation and excretion) cannot move along comfortably while the body is occupied with strenuous external activity. A full meal doesn't sit well when one is busy fighting off an attacking lion. The tuning of the body's physiological processes is done largely by the autonomic nervous system which is divided into two functional units, the sympathetic and the parasympathetic. The sympathetic nervous system activates muscles, adrenal glands, heart and lungs for dealing with the outside world (the issues of flight, fight, fright and sexual activities) while the parasympathetic nervous system activates the secretion of saliva and other digestive juices, the movement of the intestines, and the functioning of the kidneys, liver, etc. When the parasympathetic nervous system predominates, the functions having to do with digestion and the processing of food are accentuated. During this time, the sympathetic nervous system becomes inactive. The two tend to maintain a seesaw-like arrangement where one is relatively active while the other is more or less at rest. There is a natural tendency to rest while digesting one's food and to avoid eating on the run. If one is upset, anxious, or physically active, and the sympathetic system is dominant, the body has more difficulty digesting food. Food taken at such a time tends to sit in the stomach and provoke the overgrowth of bacteria. Even when such a meal is properly selected and prepared, it may not be handled well because the nervous system hasn't "geared" the body to digest it.

In India it is said that one should rest for at least ten minutes before a meal and one-half hour afterwards. It is thought that lying with the left side down and right side up is most conducive to digesting food since the right side of the body is considered to be more involved with active processes, both in the mental sphere and the physiological.[64, 65] The left side, by contrast, is more passive. According to yogic tradition, lying on the left side opens the right nostril and serves to stimulate the active processes of digestion and secretion. It also prepares the body to chew and ingest food, another active process. On the other hand, if one were about to drink a glass of liquid, a more passive matter, it would be more appropriate to reverse the position and accentuate the opposite aspects of the body's physiology.

One's emotional state can also have a marked effect on his digestive system. Anxiety and over-involvement and an identification with the details of worldly matters can lead to chronic tension and poorly regulated digestion. This can show up as overactivity, for example, an excess secretion of acid leading to ulcers, or hyperactive movements of the intestine and diarrhea, or even a tense, retentive constipation. On the other hand, indulging oneself in feelings of hopelessness and laziness can leave the digestive system underactive and sluggish.

Taking the largest meal of the day near noon is probably

ideal since in most people the body's physiological capacities are at a peak at this time. However, since it is also very important to be able to relax properly after eating a heavy meal, one may find it necessary to do this in the evening when the work day is over and leisure is available. Digestion and elimination are more efficient if sufficient time is allowed between feedings. The length of time required for a meal to be processed varies according to what it is made up of and how much is taken. Even with a relatively light meal, however, it is best to allow three hours before eating anything else. Some people contend that man is by nature a "nibbler," and advocate eating every hour or two. Though one can adapt to such a schedule to some extent, it has definite disadvantages. A genuine appetite is rarely allowed to develop, and so digestion is not as vigorous. Moreover, one's thoughts and activities become so constantly preoccupied with food that it is difficult to be productively engaged in other matters. There is also a certain kind of alertness that comes when food has not been taken for some time. As we shall see later, this experience may be unpleasant for those unaccustomed to it * and many people depend for a sense of well-being on having a constant input of food. Otherwise, a morning with only juice, which requires little digestion and has a cleansing effect, can be a very refreshing and peaceful experience for one who is not engaged in strenuous physical work.

Though activity in the outside world and internal processes are two major spheres of activity, the human being is not limited to these two. There is a third possibility. He has the potential for the exercise of mental awareness and altered or "slightly-different-from-the-ordinary" states of consciousness. Activities of this third category may range from daydreaming and dreaming sleep to the higher states of consciousness developed during advanced meditation. Generally, one of these three activities

---

* See Chapter 12, Fasting, and Chapter 17, Interaction between Diet and Mind.

cannot proceed smoothly if another of them is attempted simul-taneously. The goal of personal development in many traditions, from the yogic meditation of India to the spiritual disciplines of the Christian monk, was to reach a state where a higher con-sciousness was maintained, regardless of the activity with which one may have been involved at the moment. Until such advanced states are attained, however, it has been universally recognized that man is limited to the ability to deal effectively in only one of these three areas at a time. Therefore, guidelines have been laid down for accentuating clarity of consciousness by minimizing involvement in the other two spheres of activity—action in the external world and the processing of food. Such practices are found in many traditions and include techniques of cleansing and, of course, fasting.

Fasting and the Principles of Cleansing

12

While one's energies and attention can be turned outward for activity in the world or inward for the metabolic processes involved in digestion and elimination, there is also a third possibility. Most of one's energy can be freed from either of these jobs and turned toward the exercise of mental awareness and alternate states of consciousness such as dreaming, sleep or meditation. It is for this reason that fasting has been traditionally considered a spiritual practice.

The extent to which fasting is an uplifting experience, and one that enhances alertness and awareness depends in part on how it is done. Depriving the body of all nutrition when it is already deficient or nearly so can be dangerous and destructive. The effects of a fast will also depend on the condition of the body. When the intake of food comes to a halt and digestion stops, elimination is, as we have seen, promoted. First, of course, this means emptying the bowels. But once this is completed, the body may seize the opportunity to carry out a more extensive process of elimination. This can have far-reaching effects and probably involves the mobilizing and throwing off of wastes from throughout the body. Though contemporary medical scientists have not studied this subject, it is an almost universal experience that fasting is accompanied initially by a strong-smelling urine, a coated tongue, or an offensive breath or skin odor.[1, 2] This process of elimination seems often to involve, in some way, the production and discharge of mucus secretions.

WASTES AND CLEANSING

In Western physiology, mucus is usually considered to be simply a bodily secretion whose purpose is to protect sensitive surfaces of the linings of different parts of the body. Mucus is known to be made up of a combination of protein and sugar-like molecules. Little research, however, has been done on variations in mucus composition and how it might change in various states of health and disease. In the East, by contrast, according to the ancient writings on traditional medicine in India and Tibet, mucus plays an important role in nutrition and in the basic functioning of the body. In fact, mucus is considered but one form of *kaph*, a term which has a much broader significance than mere mucus secretion and has no simple equivalent in English. *Kaph* includes everything about the system which is substantial, solid and heavy and is one of three basic factors that are the foundation of Indian and Tibetan medicine. It is said that foods which lend the body solidity are predominantly *kaphic*. When this heavy, material substance is poorly assimilated, it is thrown off as waste. This waste is also called *kaph* and corresponds to the mucus with which we are familiar. Mucus in the nose, throat or lungs, or even in the stool, is considered an unassimilated form of *kaph*. It is that which could not be digested or integrated into the body's structure and was therefore discarded. It would make sense then, to expect that when food is of poor quality, that is, when a large proportion of it is of no nutritional value and must be thrown off, that the production of mucus would increase. Though from the point of view of Western medical research, this may all sound bizarre, from the perspective of traditional Eastern physiology, it is merely common sense. Poor food or bad digestion, and especially a combination of the two, will compromise one's ability to use the food to yield energy and build tissue and will therefore create an increased mucus flow. It is important to remove this.

There are very effective and time-honored yogic cleansing processes which remove mucus secretions and wastes that are contained in the body. One of these is a nasal wash which consists of pouring warm salt water in one nostril, with a specially designed pitcher, and allowing it to run out the other. This process is then reversed, and the mucus is forcefully expelled from the nose through rapid, short exhalations. The stomach can be cleaned by a similar wash, and one will find that in certain villages in India, part of the morning toilet is the drinking of a pitcher of water which is immediately thrown up, bringing with it the mucus that had accumulated in the stomach during the course of the night.* This not only removes all of the mucus which had drained from the nasal passages, sinus and bronchi during the night and then been swallowed, but it also, through the pressure of regurgitation, forces out that mucus which is found in the bronchial tubes at that time. Moreover, the more complicated cleansing processes for removing mucus which include difficult maneuvers allow the advanced yogis who have mastered them to draw up water into the bladder or colon, churn it around and then expel it. This is most often done while squatting in a river, without the aid of any instruments. Though it requires exquisite muscular control, it is very effective in cleaning out the accumulated toxins from the bowel and urinary tract.

People sometimes wonder why yogis, who have detailed manuals on pure and healthful diets, would need such elaborate

---

* Normally when this practice is used for health purposes, it is done daily for only a short while, and then under the supervision of a professional.

cleansing exercises. However, most persons who practice yoga intensely live in remote regions such as the mountains or jungle and do not have access to a good selection of fruits and vegetables. Moreover, many such students take vows of poverty and depend for their subsistence on that food which is given them. It would appear that an appreciation of the inability to secure the ideal diet under such circumstances has lead the yogic tradition to devise the effective cleansing processes which are so ingeniously designed to remove from the body the wastes that accumulate due to a less than ideal diet. It is also possible that the effects of heredity, constitution and early training take their toll on the body and digestive system so that even the most ideal diet may leave some wastes to accumulate in the body. If this is true, then it is only through the combined use of both cleansing processes and a very good diet that one will be able to reach his maximal level of physical health and an unclouded consciousness.

The most recent research on the microflora of the intestinal tract also throws a new light on traditional cleansing practices. When we recall that the huge surface of the small intestine is covered and imbedded with various microbes such as bacteria, yeast, fungi and spirochetes that are nourished primarily by the mucus secreted from the intestinal lining, then we can understand how a daily washing of this area might have a profound effect on the total functioning of the person. Imagine if you will, brush in hand, scrubbing down a floor the size of a football field, and you have a picture of the possible effects of a wash that cleans the entire intestinal tract. This will be especially true if we find, as the Eastern tradition suggests, that this mucus coat contains physiological wastes. Research has shown that the characteristics of the mucus are important in determining which varieties of bacteria grow. Some species, it has been noted, can become invasive and destructive if conditions are altered in the wrong way.[3, 4] This will, of course, affect the integrity of the intestinal lining, not only allowing things to go through that shouldn't, but also crippling the intestine's ability to absorb important nutrients.[5]

THE STOMACH AS "HOME" OF THE MUCUS PRINCIPLE (KAPH)

Where the question of mucus is concerned, its balance with stomach acid, as we have seen, is probably very important. In those cases where mucus production is excessive or unhealthy and undesirable bacteria are being cultivated, a restoration of a healthy flow of gastric acid can help restore a cleaner and better functioning intestinal tract. Interestingly enough, it has been shown that the stomach wash increases acid production so that in some people its daily practice could be an important technique for restoring the health of the intestine. When gastric acid is low, stray bacteria that are not of the type which can live harmoniously in the intestinal linings are allowed to proliferate. This in itself, along with the irritation it creates, could well cause an increase in mucus production throughout the intestinal tract. It is interesting, therefore, that excess mucus in the stomach, when correlated with decreased acid, can be a sign of increased mucus throughout. Yet, the stomach is, in fact, as we have seen, the place where a heavy protective coating of mucus is crucial. If the balance of acid and mucus is proper, the whole digestive tract is better able to function well, efficiently absorbing food for the building of tissues, adding "substance" (*kaph*) to the body. Mucus belongs in the stomach, yet if it is excessive there, according to Ayurvedic concepts, it "spreads through the system," decreasing digestive power and compromising the ability to assimilate food, and therefore further increasing the production of mucus. The stomach then, is called the home or special dwelling place of *kaph*.

IS EXHALATION LESS IMPORTANT THAN INHALATION?

While the removal of mucus is important in Ayurvedic nutrition, it is considered just one aspect of cleansing. Nutrition is seen as a two-fold process; one is putting nutrients in, and the other is taking wastes out. It is, in a sense, comparable to respiration, in which inhalation is no more important than exhalation. One cannot proceed without the other. Unless the stale air is removed from the lungs, it is quite impossible to bring in fresh. Though again it appeals to common sense, such a perspective has not been a part of Western thinking on the subject of nutrition. It stands to reason, however, that the biochemical milieu can only be maintained in smooth working order if there is not only the presence of the substances needed, but also the removal of those which are not. A growing awareness of how protoplasm is actually an intricate intermingling of complex molecules makes it clear that biochemical reactions cannot proceed properly if the field is crowded with inappropriate molecules. This is something quite apart from questions of "toxicity," for here we are not speaking of substances which have a destructive effect, but rather of those which, while "neutral," serve no useful purpose and simply "get in the way."

In the past, Western research methodology has been based on the isolation and identification of biochemical compounds that either serve strategic, constructive ends or have definite toxic and destructive properties. It is only now, as our research instruments have become more refined, allowing us to "peek into the cell," so to speak, by means of such devices as the electron microscope, that our understanding has become more sophisticated. We are beginning to get some perspective on the internal ecology of the cell, how chemicals or even harmless compounds cannot be thoughtlessly tossed into the biochemical field with no consideration of how they might crowd it and cause gradual but perhaps progressive disability. It is possible that our attention may now shift to the "expiratory" phase of nutrition, and elimination of wastes will be seen as an integral part of the subject.

In ancient systems of medicine and nutrition of the East, attention was given to all the routes of excretion, the kidneys, skin, lungs and the mucus membranes of the respiratory tract, as well as the digestive system itself.   The lungs, for example, were considered to play a significant role in ridding the body of wastes.   A traditional yoga practice, classified as one of the six basic cleansing exercises *(shat kriyas),* consists of rapid inhalation and exhalation, speeding up the removal of volatile substances from the blood.   Modern research has shown that certain wastes, such as the breakdown products from overheated oils in the diet, are often excreted with exhaled air. The same is true of such foods as garlic. The odor of this substance on the breath does not necessarily mean that it is present in the mouth. When a garlic solution was given by enema to a group of experimental subjects, the characteristic odor appeared in the breath within seconds, even though they had eaten no food containing garlic.[6]

DIET AND BODY ODOR

Care is therefore taken not to obstruct any of the excretory routes.   Advanced practitioners of yoga are trained in breathing exercises which not only result in the elimination of metabolic by-products through breath, forcing them through the alveolar membranes into the expelled air, but which also accelerate perspiration.   Some of these practices, which are especially designed to eliminate secretions by the skin, are said to produce such an accelerated process of elimination that visible flecks of material can be observed on the surface of the skin in less than an hour's practice.

The skin has been recognized in the West as an important organ of elimination and is sometimes called the "third kidney." It is known to produce enough solid matter to "frost" the skin when kidney function is poor. The skin also provides one of the most sensitive and easily observed sources of information about what is going on with the body chemistry and the nutritional situations. This is the body odor.

Just as there are normally bacteria in the intestines, there are certain bacteria which normally grow on the skin. While our knowledge about them is limited, it is thought that they serve some role in the maintenance of the health of the skin and thereby indirectly the health of the body. However, just as the kind and number of bacteria that grow on a culture plate is easily influenced by slight changes in the chemical compositions of the medium, similarly, the kind of bacteria and their number that grow on the skin is readily influenced by the wastes excreted by the skin as it eliminates them from the inside of the body. A particular strain of bacteria which is encouraged to grow by the particular substance excreted will produce a characteristic odor. In this fashion, the odor of the skin serves as a sort of "feedback" mechanism relating information about the chemical situation inside the body and thus reflecting the failure of the digestive system to comfortably handle certain foods.

But body odor is also influenced by other factors such as one's emotional state, the amount of oxygen available (a function of whether one is wearing loose or tight clothing), and by the application of chemicals to the skin such as soaps, antiseptics, cosmetics, etc. Soaps, especially the "deodorant soaps," which destroy the normal bacteria of the skin, are able to eliminate body odor. By using such soaps, a person who is suffering from a severe overload of wastes in the body can hide the fact from himself and, without the unpleasant body odor that would otherwise remind him that he has eaten improperly, he remains unaware of the dilemma. Among medical doctors, there has been some interest in a computerized device which might diagnose common diseases through a careful analysis of the body odor. Such research promises to throw more light on the relationship between the eliminative aspect of nutrition and the development of disease.

Ancient scriptures warn of the danger of ignoring such simple and basic urges as that for urination or defecation. Certainly it would not surprise a traditional physician of the ancient Ayurvedic school to find chronic disease (even though the diet may be fairly good) developing among people where constipation is common because of highly refined foods which provide no bulk, where anti-perspirants are used to prevent the throwing off of wastes through the skin, where posture is poor and the lungs function inadequately as a route of excretion, and where one hasn't even time to urinate!

THE COLON—WHERE VAYU (WIND) RESIDES

In Ayurvedic nutrition, foods are selected not only in terms of the nutrition that they offer, but often also because of their ability to promote excretion through one route or another. Whey, for example, which is advocated by many health food enthusiasts in the West, is also respected in the East as a nutritional drink, but it is valued particularly for its ability to promote a cleansing flow of urine. Great emphasis is placed in Ayurvedic medicine on saunas and steam baths, and particular attention is given to the promotion of good elimination through the bowels. Feces and gas are said to be carried downward by a special energy vector *(apana vayu)* that plays the primary role in the elimination of wastes from the body. When this fails to work properly, then the gas, or flatus, forming in the colon is said to move upward, affecting the rest of the body and causing mental and emotional disturbance. While from a Western perspective, this sounds like, at best, an interesting figure of speech, it is really quite compatible with what we are learning about physiology.

During a state of constipation, which is the failure of the colon contents to move downward properly, more of the cellulose in the food is broken down into volatile fatty acids which have an irritating quality. Moreover, when there is stasis of the stool, the growth of bacteria increases in the colon and begins to move up into the small bowel, where food is fermented more and digested less, causing an increase in gas. Moreover, we have also learned that when the bowel functions best, the stool is soft and well-formed. The softness comes from an even mixture of the solids with the gases which are carried out with it.[7]

The association of "wind moving up" with emotional disturbance might not be so strange as it sounds either. Constipation is often a result of uncertainty, insecurity or fear as almost anyone who has travelled a lot will know. Moreover, bacterial overgrowth is not only a result of a spread upward of the microbes of the colon, it is also a result of a decrease or inadequacy of the bile and digestive enzymes whose secretion is greatly dependent on emotional factors. Such factors also are responsible to a great extent for the quality and quantity of mucus secreted on the huge surface of the intestinal lining—the "culture medium" whose quantity and composition determine what kind of microbes grow and how fast they multiply. Moreover, blood supply to the intestines as well as the antibodies against various strains of bacteria that it might carry are both important here[8] and both are also under control of the autonomic nervous system and hence closely tied to the emotions and the mind. On the whole then, it is not difficult to see how the emotions and intestinal microbes and gas are so intimately interrelated that neither can be said to be the "cause" of the other. Even the conventionally trained physician will see patients who complain of gas which they cannot pass and which causes nervousness and irritability. Such gas is one aspect of *vayu*.

The traditional Ayurvedic physician thinks of the colon as the place of residence of *vayu* or wind, though this "wind" is more than simply intestinal gas. *Vayu* is a broader concept that includes all the motivating, energizing forces in the human being. While these forces have their normal role to play, such as animating bodily movements and activating creative thoughts, they do sometimes go awry on a more mundane level. It is this which is related to the intestinal gas that "moves upward," causing nervous instability instead of remaining well-regulated in its proper place of residence, the colon.

Digestive Functioning as an Intersection of Many Factors

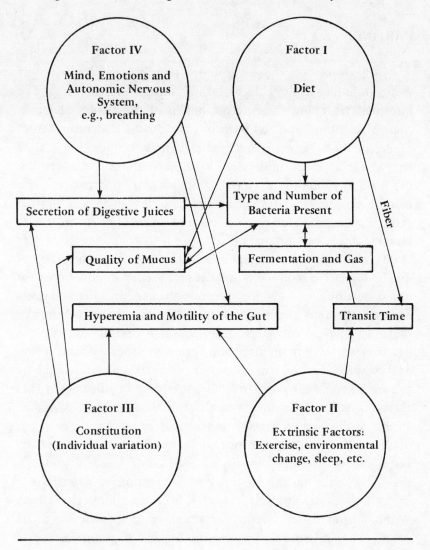

For each person there will be a certain degree of mucus accumulation, a specific microbial population, and a characteristic capacity to absorb in each segment of the digestive tract. In each case the digestive tract reflects the person's total functioning and serves to maintain him as a unique individual. For this reason, in Ayurvedic medicine, the three major sections of the digestive tract are considered the "home" (*kosht*) of the three dynamic forces (*doshas*) that underlie and shape one's experience.

FASTING

Cleansing, of course, is more than simply throwing off waste products through feces, urine, mucus, and so forth. The intestinal tract and the internal milieu of the tissues and cells themselves need time to "burn out the dross" that results from taking in food. Our biochemical machinery requires some time to sort through the molecules, sifting out those which are unneeded and should be excreted. Without this opportunity, there of necessity accumulates within the tissues, and even within the cells, a growing burden of useless and sometimes harmful substances.

In the nutritional teachings of the East, the scheduling of meals is given considerable importance. One should never eat unless he's hungry. Fasting increases the digestive fire and one's ability to secrete ample amounts of digestive juices. The solar plexus, which is considered the central focus of not only the digestive flame, but the fiery and aggressive aspects of the person as a whole, can, in some cases, be stoked and stimulated by fasting. From this point of view, it is easy to understand that there might be some times when fasting would not be advisable. In the traditional writings, it is said that in most cases of fever, one should not fast. The system is already overheated, and by fasting, one increases the fire of the body. Unfortunately, in the West, while fasting has enjoyed something of a renaissance in the last several years, it has often been used indiscriminately. Without properly evaluating the situation to see whether a fast would be advisable or not, some laymen's groups advocate fasting with blind enthusiasm as a cure for everything.

Very little research has been done in the West that would help one understand how to select those patients for whom fasting would be most beneficial. In the Indian/Tibetan tradition, however, fasting is used for those who show an excess of *kaph*, that is to say, those who are overweight or who accumulated a great deal of mucus. This will normally be people who have eaten excessively, especially those who have eaten foods which are sweet or starchy and thereby tend to create *kaph*.

When the fiery aspects of a person, which are subsumed under the term *pita*, are overactive, the result can be peptic ulcers, for example, and the traditional physician, like his modern counterpart, advises ulcer patients to avoid fasting and to take regular feedings of soothing foods. When this fiery principle escapes its home at the solar plexus, invading the other parts of the system, it is said to produce such disorders as irritability, a flaring temper, absent-mindedness and high blood pressure.

In the West, following somewhat similar lines of thinking, fasting has become popular as a treatment of obesity. Unfortunately, the situation in the modern West is quite different from that of Central Asia a thousand or more years ago. The ancient Indian who was overweight reached that condition by eating an excess of foods which, though fattening, were nevertheless largely whole foods that contained, besides starch and sugar, at least some protein, vitamins, minerals and fiber. The processing of foods was largely unheard of. The modern American who is obese, on the other hand, has most likely reached that condition by quite a different route. The average intake of refined oils, fats and sugars is, as we have seen, about 65% of the diet in America today. For the person who is overweight, it is likely to be even higher. When this is true, it means that one has been subsisting for some time on a diet which is made up primarily of empty calories. As a consequence, he has usually developed significant deficiencies of protein, vitamins, minerals and virtually every nutrient except poor quality oil and carbohydrate. This person is typified by the furtive, pasty fat lady who can be spotted in any supermarket, stuffing her shopping basket with candies as she glances about to see if anyone is watching before she samples them. She is quite likely to be not only overweight, but a nervous wreck, and is apt to be suffering from a whole host of more or less ill-defined ailments. Though her body is bulky, and she thinks constantly of losing weight, she is in fact starving and may be just as desperately in need of vital nutrients as the emaciated inmate of a concentration camp.

It takes only a moment's thought to realize that putting such a person on a total fast is tantamount to courting disaster. If she takes nothing but water, she may very well begin to burn up the reserves of fat which have been accumulated. Unfortunately, however, fat stores, especially in such people as this, do not contain the necessary quotas of other important nutrients that are needed for the metabolic activities that will be fueled by the fat. If, in defiance of common sense, such a person insists on doing a water fast, nutrients for vital metabolic processes must be pulled from other tissues. The result will be that strategic organs such as the heart, brain and liver, which were already suffering from a short supply of crucial nutrients, will become even further depleted. Whether the outcome is a mental and emotional breakdown or the development of a grave physical illness will depend on the constitution of the person in question and which organ systems are most susceptible.

This is not to say, of course, that fasting cannot be very beneficial. It is important to realize, however, that when the person fasting has been on an "average American diet" or its equivalent for some time, that he should be supplied with a whole spectrum of nutrients during the time he is on the fast. While vitamin and mineral supplements have been used in some cases for this purpose, the calculation of the appropriate dosage for individual persons is, as we have seen in earlier chapters, difficult to say the least. Besides, we are never sure that the supplements that we provide include all of the many components or carry all of the properties of fresh, live food. What's more, fat cannot be converted into the glucose necessary to keep blood sugar up to fuel the nervous system. If a small amount of carbohydrate is not present in the diet, then protein will be broken down for conversion into the needed sugar. The result is not fasting—it is starvation.

THE JUICE FAST

In the ancient Asian traditions, fasting is termed a process of "making one lighter" *(langhana)*. When properly done, rather than starvation, it is a process of revitalization. This means that one should be offered all the most nutritious aspects of the best quality of food with the exception of most of its carbohydrate content. At least this is true when fasting is done primarily to reduce weight. If the purpose of fasting is simply to let the digestive tract rest, one need not cut carbohydrates so drastically though he should be careful to eliminate fiber, taking his nutrients in a form that can be easily and quickly absorbed and will leave little residue.

The ideal technique for successful fasting is the use of fresh, raw fruit and vegetable juices. On such a diet, the full spectrum of nutrients is supplied in an easily assimilated form, so the digestive tract is able to remain essentially at rest. With the wide variety of juices that can be prepared, it is possible to select those which contain the right amount of carbohydrate and especially large quantities of certain nutrients which may be particularly needed. For instance, one who is fasting for weight loss should use sparingly such juices as carrot, apple and even orange. Grapefruit and cucumber juice, by contrast, can be used liberally and are especially beneficial when they are combined with the juice of a dark green leafy vegetable such as romaine lettuce.

If one is not fasting for weight loss, combinations of carrot, apple and lettuce juice or simply fresh squeezed orange juice or the extracted juices of other fruits and vegetables can be used in generous quantities. It is necessary, however, as we shall see in the next chapter, to be careful in using the stronger tasting vegetables for juice since they may contain significant quantities of medicinal substances that could have undesirable effects and might disrupt or undermine the beneficial effects of the fast.

In general, it is unwise to continue a fast for more than

Fresh Juices

Fresh juiced fruits and vegetables supply abundant amounts of vital minerals and vitamins. They are a natural counterpart of multiple vitamin pills. Each juice has its own special flavor and pharmacologic properties.

Juicing removes the nutritionally rich liquid from the "boxes" of fiber surrounding it, so they should be taken as soon after extraction as possible since they are no longer protected from oxidation and tend to lose many of their beneficial properties fairly quickly. There are many juice extractors currently on the market, but for all except citrus fruits, electric grinders with mechanical presses are probably best, especially for the seriously ill, since the juice made with them is thought to retain more nutrients. Their use is, however, a two-step process and too time-consuming for most people. Centrifugal and rotary juicers are simpler and less expensive. Liquifiers and blenders are not really juicers as they do not remove the pulp.

Produce should be thoroughly washed before juicing. Apples and cucumbers should be peeled, as should root vegetables. The peels tend to be strong, bitter, gritty or coated with wax. All tough portions (husks, stems, seeds) should also be removed. One half inch should be cut off of either end of the carrot, for example. If the soil in which they were grown is questionable, root vegetables should be washed again after peeling or even dropped briefly in boiling water to sterilize. For those who have difficulty digesting raw juices, they may be cooked a little in ghee in which onions and spices are sauteed and then served as soup.

The juice of some vegetables is strong-tasting and should be used sparingly, diluting it with milder juices such as carrot or cucumber. Juices are easily combined to make tasty drinks. Carrot and celery juice are staple ingredients, with other juices such as lettuce, spinach, cucumber and sometimes cabbage being supplemental. Apples, pineapples and pears are popular fruit juices. Though fruit and vegetable juices sometimes don't mix, certain combinations such as carrot, apple and leaf lettuce (in proportions of 5, 3 to 1) are both delicious and healthful.

three days without the guidance of a physician, even when one is using properly prepared and selected juices. Long fasts are, in any case, disruptive and interfere with the harmonious rhythmical functioning that might have been established by the body.

While many people find it beneficial to carry out a three-day fast monthly, weekly fasts of one day's duration are probably less disruptive and have a gentler and more consistent effect. Of course, the most ideal frequency for fasting is daily.

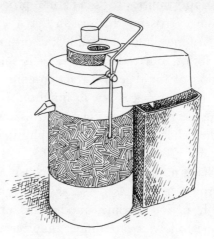

THE DAILY FAST

The primary function of fasting, as we have seen, is to allow the gastrointestinal tract to rest and permit the system to turn its energies away from the processing of a continuous incoming stream of food, concentrating instead on the process of cleansing. Just as a conscientious *hausfrau* would never consider cleaning while in the process of receiving guests, so does the body await that opportunity which comes between feedings to carry out its processes of cleansing. Receiving food, like receiving guests, requires a different set of activities. Once the guests have gone and time is available, the curtains come down for washing, and all the dirt that had been hastily swept under the corner of a rug is uncovered and hauled away.

In a metaphorical way, we might think of many degenerative conditions of the human body as resulting from too much dirt that had been too often swept under too many rugs, so that the time for spring housecleaning had been postponed indefinitely. While fasting may be of some value as a therapeutic measure in such cases, prevention of the problem lies in providing regular and consistent opportunities for the natural processes of elimination and cleansing. It is for this reason that the most ideal fast is that which is done daily. Probably the optimal duration for such a fast is about fourteen hours. This is sufficient time for the major portion of the digestive tract to empty itself, rest and undergo the restoration necessary to function well the following day. The natural time for carrying out this fast is, of course, during the night, when outward-directed physiological processes tend to slow down.

It is perhaps no accident that in English the first meal of the day is termed "breakfast," suggesting that, for at least some respectable period of time, one has abstained from taking food. When one follows a late dinner, however, with a train of TV snacks that extends far into the late movie, stepping out of bed the next morning to a cup of coffee and toast, he violates this time-honored and common-sensical tradition. The result is a digestive tract that is forced to start a new day's work after having labored through the night shift. A gradually cumulative state of internal pollution is the usual result, dulling one's sense of vitality and alertness and setting the stage for the development of a wide variety of illnesses. Breakfast, in any case, need not be heavy since the digestive system and metabolism are not geared to the assimilation of food very early in the morning. The body is still undergoing the process of cleansing, and overburdening it with food at this point is not healthful. Though there has been much talk in recent years about the necessity of "a good breakfast," this seems to be a matter of fashion in nutritional thought. Quite the opposite idea was current thirty or forty years ago. At that time there was a "no breakfast plan" which emphasized the healthfulness of omitting breakfast entirely. But this fast, like any other, is likely to be especially unpleasant for just those people who need it most, since they will feel the effects of more wastes being "dragged out" for excretion. Cleansing is most unpleasant when it is overdue.

Actually, people's needs are different. It is probably best for those who have no appetite in the morning not to eat. A large glass of juice or a cup of hot milk is usually adequate for such a person. In any case, a light breakfast is usually sufficient. If the heavy meal is to be had in the evening, then a light lunch can also be taken. If the larger meal is taken at midday, then the arrangement can be reversed and the lightest meal—supper—can come in the evening.

When meals are planned with an understanding of the basic mechanics of the digestive system in mind, and with an awareness of one's own capacity and limitations, then one can provide for his nutritional needs and still allow sufficient opportunity for the processes of elimination. This ensures not only strength, stamina and health, but also a sense of clarity and alertness. Of course, there is one further factor which has an important bearing on how food is handled by the digestive system, how much is useful and how much is waste. That is how it is prepared. Cooking and other techniques of food preparation can change the availability of most nutrients. These processes can also alter other substances in food, such as those which have no nutritive value, are not even classified as fiber and are present in very small amounts, but have the power to affect the body as well as the mind. These are the pharmacologically active substances in foods.

IV

The Pharmacology of Nutrition

The events that transpire in the intestinal tract are, as we have just seen, at least as important in determining whether one will get what is needed as the nutritive value of the food itself. We have introduced another whole set of variables into the study of nutrition: the unique physiological characteristics of the person who is eating. Yet the nutritive value of the food and the characteristics of the person eating it, complex as they may be, still do not complete the picture of human nutrition. There is a very important intervening area between the two: how the nutrients are prepared and processed and what other substances accompany them into the body. This we will call the "pharmacology of nutrition." This area of study covers the intricacies of food preparation, including the complex traditions that govern the use of seasonings and spices. It also encompasses the role of those compounds present in foods, either added or naturally present, which have no nutritive value but which have the power to affect the body and even the mind in obvious or in subtle ways.

An exploration of the ways in which food can be altered has led at worst to its overprocessing and its adulteration and contamination with harmful substances. But at best it has led to an appreciation of how man's intelligence and ingenuity can be turned to transforming available foods so that they become more healthful or more ideally suited to a particular person whose physiology may be unbalanced or whose digestion may be poor. Such knowledge is the basis of what we call the art of cooking. It is also the foundation of many traditional systems of medicine and healing around the world, who as we shall see, regard the proper preparation of food as the most important of the tools a physician uses, as well as one of the most important factors in maintaining good health.

Beyond Nutrients

13

In addition to carbohydrates, fats, protein, vitamins and minerals, there are other substances in the food that we eat. Besides the additives contained in most processed foods, a variety of compounds that are not nutritional in the usual sense are found even in whole, natural foods.

Some of these we have mentioned before, such as phytic acid, which is found in the bran of grains and the outer coating of legumes and which can tie up minerals like calcium, iron or zinc and prevent their absorption. Oxalic acid, a compound found in spinach and other fruits and vegetables, has been accused of the same thing, though that this is really a practical problem is doubtful.[1] Other substances in food may have a pharmacologic effect on the intestinal tract, speeding it up so that the absorption of nutrients is hindered. Prunes, for example, contain a substance which is thought to have a medicinal effect on the bowels, promoting their action. Some foods contain frankly toxic material, such as the cyanide-like compound that is found in the cassava root from which tapioca is made. As it is prepared for consumption in the West, the poisonous substance is removed chiefly by grating the cassava root and drying it in the sun. In Africa, however, where natives sometimes eat inadequately treated cassava, poisoning can occur.[2]

Honey can also be toxic if the nectar from which it is made is gathered from poisonous flowers. In America those which most commonly cause trouble are members of the rhododendron family which includes such flowers as mountain laurel and azalea. Yellow jasmine has also yielded a honey which has been fatal to humans.[3] Usually, of course, nectar which is poisonous is avoided by the bees, but in these cases for some reason the bees are not susceptible to the toxin, while man is. From a practical point of view, honey is not a danger since beekeepers are careful that honey from known toxic flowers doesn't reach the market.

A toxic substance is also found in certain beans (*khesari dhal* or *Lathyrus sativus*) that are grown in India and North Africa. Generally, of course, if there is something toxic in a plant, seed or fruit, it is not considered a "food" and will not be consumed. In this case, however, the bean is very drought resistant and in dry years will produce a crop when everything else fails. For this reason it is still sown in India, usually along with wheat. If the weather is good, the wheat takes over, but when the rains don't come, the beans grow. When eaten in small quantities they are harmless, but in dry years when they come to make up more than half the diet and nutrition is otherwise poor anyway, a debilitating neurological disease that paralyzes the legs[4, 5] can result. Raw kidney beans and the black beans which are favored by many Latin Americans contain toxic substances which interfere with digestion. If the beans are incompletely cooked, one can become quite ill with vomiting and diarrhea.[6] Thoroughly cooked in water,* they are a wholesome food and

---

* Dry heat may fail to destroy the toxic compounds. Thus the advisability of adding the flour of such beans to bread dough has been questioned.[7] Of course, the flour of beans which do not contain these properties (such as Indian besan, the flour of a sort of chick pea) may be added with benefit as has been done for many generations in India.

serve as a major source of protein for many millions of people. Another bean grown since Roman times in Italy and the Mediterranean area, the broad bean or "fava" bean, can cause anemia, jaundice, fever and even death in certain people if it is eaten in sufficient quantities and improperly cooked.[8] We would expect that if some plants have significant amounts of toxic materials, then other plants, which might also be used for food, would contain smaller amounts of such compounds. In fact, it turns out that they do. Many foods contain tiny amounts of substances which, if taken in larger quantities, would be toxic. A little bit of caffeine, for example, may produce alertness, while in extremely high concentrations, it can cause nervousness and even psychosis. In general, a substance that is active pharmacologically at a low concentration will be toxic at a higher concentration.

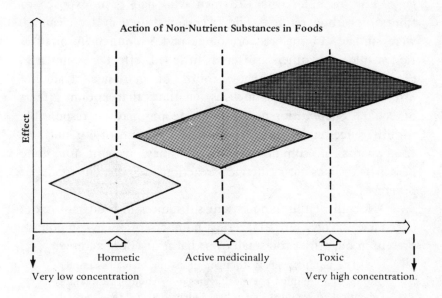

But caffeine is only one of the many active compounds found in commonly used foods and beverages. Tea, for example, contains nearly 30% by weight of a family of substances known as phenols, examples of which sport such impressive names as epicatechin, quercetin, kaempferol, leucoanthocyanins, gallic acid, chlorogenic acid, theogallin and ellagic acid.[9] The nature of the action of these compounds on the body is little understood. Being more of a drug-like plant than a food plant, tea would, of course, contain more pharmacologically active substances than most foods. Yet many of the compounds in tea are found in other plants, many of which play an important role in the diet. Buckwheat, mango and rhubarb contain large quantities of phenols as do most bananas. Nearly all fruits and vegetables contain 250 to 500 mg of such active compounds per pound.[10] Small amounts of such mildly toxic compounds in commonly used foods might produce a noticeable reaction only in those people who are susceptible since people, too, vary in their biochemical makeup.

For example, when 78 men who had been exposed to fumes of carbon tetrachloride, a chemical used in dry cleaning, were studied, 15 suffered poisoning and 6 required hospitalization while the others suffered little ill effect.[11] Similarly, researchers have found that a fourth of an ounce of alcohol affects some people, as much as ten times that amount affects others.[12] Such differences among people may be responsible for differences in sensitivity to the small amounts of non-nutrient components of common foods and may account for some personal dislikes or "allergic" reactions to certain foods or beverages.

Not all of the non-nutrient substances in foods are toxic, of course. There are staggering numbers of such compounds present in quantities too small to be harmful. For example:

> The potato, usually thought of as one of man's simpler foods, is a complex chemical aggregate. About 150 distinct chemical substances have been identified in this natural product, among which are the solanine alkaloids, oxalic acid, arsenic, tannins, nitrate and over a hundred other items of no recognized nutritional significance to man. Forty-two chemical entities have been found in orange oil, including 12 alcohols, 9 aldehydes, 2 esters, 14 hydrocarbons and 4

ketones.   The orange as a whole includes a host of other chemical substances.   All vegetables and fruits and other natural food products are similarly complex.[13]

In some cases, these compounds have been studied enough to know that they may be beneficial.   Garlic and onions, for example, not only contain medicinal substances which decrease blood fats and help decrease the "stickiness" of blood, but garlic also has an active substance in it which has antibiotic activity.[14]   In other cases, little research has been done, yet tradition has it that a food has medicinal value.   For example, in the East, cucumbers, especially the seeds, are prized for their diuretic effect, that is, their ability to rid the body of accumulated water, and many melons are said to have this same property.

Sometimes the pharmacologic effects of a substance are sought out not for medicinal reasons, but because they produce a pleasurable effect.   Coffee and tea are common examples and chocolate is similar.   Chocolate contains considerable amounts of theobromine,[15] an alkaloid which is somewhat similar to caffeine but has less powerful effects on the nervous system.   However, it tends to have more effect on the muscles, kidneys and heart. It has been used in medicine to stimulate the kidneys to rid the body of excessive accumulations of fluid and to relax smooth muscles in the treatment of asthma.[16]   Yet the chocolate contains 40 to 60 percent fat which is of nutritional value and therefore it must be considered a food.   This contrasts it, of course, with coffee, tea and the various herbal teas that are often used which do not contain any nutritional value to speak of but are used primarily for their medicinal effects.   They are, in fact, more drugs than foods.

In our Western scientific way of thinking, "drugs" and "foods" are quite distinct, yet it is obvious that there is a great deal of overlap between the two, and in fact, there may be times when it is difficult to know in which of the two categories a substance should be put.   For example, onions and chili peppers both have obvious pharmacologic effects, causing flushing, burning and nasal discharge when taken in generous amounts as well as their less obvious medicinal effects. Yet they are also foods. Chili peppers are rich in vitamin C while onions are high in carbohydrate as well as various vitamins and minerals. In the traditional medicine of the East where drugs were always natural substances and were found widely dispersed in nature, they were often intimately bound up in this way with what was used as food. For this reason, foods and drugs were not considered to be separate and distinct.

IS YOUR FOOD MEDICINAL?

In the ancient medical writings of India, the general term *dravya* is most often used since it includes both foods and medicines. Nearly all foods were acknowledged to have, in addition to their nutritional value, some medicinal effects, while it was also appreciated that many of the natural medicinal plants and substances contained some food value. Even today in traditional schools of medicine in India, pharmacology and nutrition are treated as the same subject. Perhaps this will be clearer if we think of a food as a substance which contains primarily nutrients and relatively little pharmacologically active compounds while a medicine is a substance which is primarily made up of pharmacologically active compounds but contains very little food value.

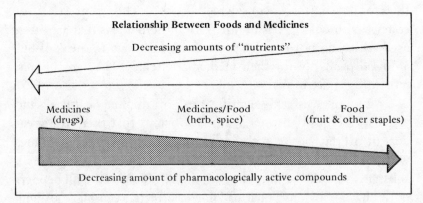

Relationship Between Foods and Medicines

Decreasing amounts of "nutrients"

Medicines (drugs)   Medicines/Food (herb, spice)   Food (fruit & other staples)

Decreasing amount of pharmacologically active compounds

These are in fact two extremes on a spectrum, and it seems likely that the majority of what we eat lies somewhere between these two extremes.

Though most of our food contains at least tiny quantities of a variety of complex and little understood compounds, this is less true of foods that have been highly processed. White sugar is a good example. It is refined to the point that it is more than 99% pure.   Other foods, however, even whole grains, contain small quantities of other compounds besides vitamins, minerals, fats, carbohydrate and protein. Oats, for example, contain an alkaloid which makes oatmeal mildly stimulating and anti-spasmodic.   In times past, when strong chemicals were less common and there was a greater sensitivity to subtler compounds, an infusion of oats was used as a "nerve tonic."[17] Fruits and vegetables are even more likely to contain a variety of trace amounts of complex, naturally occurring biochemicals which lend the distinctive flavor and character to the food. Old-fashioned fruits with strong tastes were often reputed to have medicinal value. Quince syrup, for example, was used to stop vomiting and to "strengthen the stomach"[18] while wild huckle-berries were said to rid one of worms.[19]   In most cases, such claims have been ignored by modern researchers. When a closer look has been taken, however, the results have sometimes been intriguing. In New England, for example, cranberry juice was a time-honored folk remedy for urinary infections. Upon careful study it was found to contain large amounts of a compound that is converted into another substance, hippuric acid, which acts as an antibiotic when it is excreted in the urine.[20] For hippuric acid to kill bacteria, it must be highly concentrated and the urine must be acid. The researchers found cranberry juice to be in-adequate as an acidifier and hippuric acid concentrations "only occasionally" to reach high enough levels to kill bacteria after one had taken an equivalent of one to two pints of pure juice a day. Many other foods also elevate urine hippuric acid levels, however. Unfortunately, the authors did not explore possible diets that would potentiate the effects of the cranberry juice, nor did they consider that cranberries might contain other active compounds that could work in conjunction with hippuric acid. Meanwhile, many persons have found cranberry juice helpful for urinary problems. More than eight ounces a day of the pure juice could be excessive, however, since the berries probably contain other medicinal substances too. By and large, it has been assumed that if the substances present in a food do not cause any toxic effects then they are inconsequential. In those cases where the amounts of non-nutritional compounds in foods seem too small even to have a medicinal effect, they have been largely ignored. The subtler effects that very small doses might possess have been studied only sketchily or not at all. It may turn out, however, that they are more important than has been thought.

HORMESIS

In 1929, Alexander Fleming noticed something strange about a specimen of bacteria which he was growing on a little dish of culture medium in his laboratory. The plate had become contaminated by a spore of mold which had apparently floated in through the open window where the dish sat on the window sill. Where the mold had grown, something interesting had happened. There was a surrounding area of destroyed bacteria. Fleming showed it to one of his co-workers, remarking that, "It might be important." The mold was a strain of penicillium which had the power to kill bacteria. From it was extracted penicillin, and the era of "miracle drugs" was born. In recent years, the nature of antibiotics and their interaction with bacteria has been studied in more detail. When concentrations of the antibiotic are lowered enough, there comes a point, as one would expect, when the tiny amounts no longer have a toxic effect on the bacteria. Much to the surprise of researchers, however, if the concentration of antibiotic is lowered even further, it actually begins to stimulate growth. A substance toxic to bacteria, when given in extremely low concentrations, reversed its effect. Instead of being toxic, it actually promoted growth.[21]

This was not an isolated instance. Further research has demonstrated that the same principle applies in many biological systems: where an agent is harmful or toxic in moderate quantities, at very low concentrations it can become instead a stimulant, having exactly opposite results. As we have seen before, antibiotics in the feed of chickens are used to increase growth. This was thought to be effective because the antibiotic was able to alter the bacteria of the intestinal tract since when the antibiotics were given in special laboratory chicks kept free of intestinal bacteria, there was no effect. If, however, the concentrations of antibiotic given to the germ-free chicks was extremely low, then there was again a stimulation of growth. This demonstrated that besides the ability of regular doses of antibiotics to alter the microbes growing in the intestinal tract, much smaller doses exert a completely different effect. This second effect by very tiny doses has been called *hormesis.*[22]

The term *hormesis* was coined to indicate the effect of tiny sub-pharmacologic doses of substances which can affect the organism in subtle but important ways. Such substances are acting not in the usual pharmacological or nutritional way, but rather as stimulants of certain biochemical processes much in the way that hormones act. Hormones, of course, are internally generated, manufactured by one's own body for the purpose of tuning metabolism and turning off or turning on certain metabolic processes. Only recently has research begun to suggest that compounds from outside the body could similarly affect metabolic processes in extremely low concentrations. While these compounds may be stimulants at very low concentrations, when the amount of substance is increased, the body's reaction reverts to the expected or usual one.*

* In the case of penicillin and its interaction with bacteria, this may make more sense than meets the eye. Most fungi live in the soil which they "share" with those bacteria that break down organic matter into humus. While the fungi "need" the bacteria, they

Actually this is the rediscovery of a well-known principle. It is a basic law of pharmacology that while large doses of a substance may be toxic, and moderate doses pharmacologically active, smaller, homeopathic[†] doses are stimulating. This is true in the above experiments with penicillin but has been documented for a wide variety of compounds such as insecticides and other toxins. Insects exposed to tiny doses of insecticides have shown a paradoxical effect such as that seen with bacteria and penicillin. They not only thrived, they turned out to grow much larger than usual.[24] Agricultural experts have even begun to expect that some such principle underlies the current tendency among farmers to use larger and larger amounts of insecticides. If the field is sprayed only once, the insects are initially killed, but as the poison is washed away by rain and weather, concentrations reach a critical low point at which time the insects suddenly begin to multiply and grow rapidly. One dose of spray can eventually produce a race of "super bugs," so more and more is needed.[25]

It seems likely then, that food contains a wide variety of non-nutritional substances, some mildly toxic, some with little effect and others that stimulate various metabolic processes, depending on the compound and the amount present. This makes an assessment of the "effects of food" quite complex. Moreover, compounds that act in this way are not limited to

don't need them *too* close or they impinge on the territory of the fungus. We have known for some time that most fungi produce antibiotics to protect themselves from being overwhelmed by bacteria. in view of their cohabitation in the soil, however, it would not be surprising to find that their antibiotic substances not only prevented bacterial growth in the immediate area around them, but stimulated it beyond that. This might be one of the factors operating to keep the microbes of the soil in proper balance. There is evidence that certain fungi that grow where the soil touches the root are constantly manufacturing small amounts of antibiotics which are absorbed through the rootlets of the plant into the stems and leaves.[23] These minute quantities of antibiotics if present in tiny concentrations in many fruits and vegetables could have some hormetic stimulating effect, and one may wonder if they might account for some of the subtle and "energizing" effects of fresh, organically grown vegetables and fruits.

†   Actually, over the last two centuries those who have worked extensively with the use of very small doses of active compounds have found that at this level they are most likely to be active only for certain persons to whom they are particularly suited. This matching of the active substance to the patient is what makes a treatment "homeopathic."

those naturally present in food. Traces of insecticides could affect the human consumer as well as the bugs in the field. There are in addition many other chemicals that find their way into our food supply today.

HOW DO YOU KNOW YOUR FOOD IS SAFE?

Other substances in foods which may play a similar role are those which are added intentionally to prevent spoilage, or to enhance the flavor or appearance or texture of the food. There are presently about 2,000 such chemicals which are used in commercially available foods.[26] The exact effects which these have on human subjects is poorly understood in many cases. A century ago, additives were used with no control at all. Whatever would preserve the food or enhance its color was added surreptitiously by unscrupulous food manufacturers. Formaldehyde was added to milk so it would keep until marketed, copper compounds were put in canned peas to make them bright green, and flour was added to expensive ground spices.[27] Fortunately, most foodstuffs were purchased directly by the consumer from the grower or from the butcher or baker and since they were held personally accountable, good quality was the rule.

By the turn of the century, however, shipping, cold storage and mass marketing had begun to spread and matters became more impersonal and subject to abuse. Spoilage was an economic disaster much more real to packer, shipper and retailer than was the possible danger of preservatives which were, after all, it was reasoned, used in small quantities anyway. Meanwhile, more and more chemical preservatives were being patented, and other additives and adulterants were used with a free hand.

By 1904 the public was beginning to take notice. The State Food Commissioner of North Dakota, for example, reported that 90% of the butchers in his state were using preservatives for their meat, 70% of the chocolates examined were adulterated, and that although "potted chicken" and "potted turkey" were sold widely in the state, none of the cans he had found so labeled contained either! There were other reports of plaster of Paris in candy, nutmegs made of wood and sawdust in black pepper.[28] About this time, Harvey Wiley, M.D., a federal official who had been crusading for regulation of food purity for decades began to attract more attention. One of his targets was sodium nitrate which was used at the time to retard spoilage of sausages, bacon, etc.* Wiley's rousing speeches stimulated the spirit of reform in many, and he soon had a wide following. Public indignation was further excited by popular books and articles such as Upton Sinclair's 1906 novel, *The Jungle*, which described the filthy conditions in Chicago's meat packing houses and how diseased animals, such as those with tuberculosis, after being rejected by inspectors, found their way back into the packing line.

> There was never the least attention paid to what was cut up for sausage; there would come all the way back from Europe old sausage that had been rejected, and that was mouldy and white—it would be dosed with borax and glycerine, and dumped into the hoppers, and made over again for home consumption . . . . There would be meat stored in great piles in rooms; and the water from leaky roofs would drip over it, and thousands of rats would race about on it . . . . These rats were nuisances, and the packers would put poisoned bread out for them; they would die, and then rats, bread and meat would go into the hoppers together. This is no fairy story and no joke; the meat would be shovelled into carts, and the man who did the shovelling would not trouble to lift out a rat even when he saw one—there were things that went into the sausage in comparison with which a poisoned rat was a tidbit.[29]

The book and the growing furor came to the attention of the President, Theodore Roosevelt, who sent investigators to Chicago's meat packing plants to see if Sinclair's descriptions were

---

* Interestingly enough, though its use continued despite Wiley's efforts, research in recent years has shown it to play a role in the causation of cancer.

accurate.   After surreptitiously infiltrating the plants and observing conditions, they reported back to Roosevelt. The novel,
they said, was not true to life. The situation was even worse than
described. The President responded by backing a Pure Food Law
that became effective in 1907. Though this legislation was not
stringent, it was helped along by the development of brand
names.   Once a brand became well known, the publicity associated with seizure of a contaminated or illegally labeled shipment
stuck in the shopper's mind and the loss of a good reputation
meant the loss of business.

Though obviously spoiled and adulterated food and the
use of known toxic additives decreased, the chemical and food
industries were using increasingly complicated processing techniques and more clever labeling and advertising. The industry
had also developed a whole host of new chemical additives, such
as coal tar dyes used to color foods. 1938 saw a new law passed
which was called the Food, Drug and Cosmetic Act. This set
standards for the identity and method of preparation of some of
the more common processed foods and set forth regulations
aimed at preventing misleading labeling and packaging. Additives
found to be harmful in any amount were prohibited, but the
burden of proof lay in the Food and Drug Administration
(FDA). After World War II, the use of new chemicals increased
dramatically and the FDA was swamped. It could not test them
all.

THREE POUNDS OF ADDITIVES A YEAR

Public concern again grew and President Eisenhower
appointed a committee to study the matter. It reported in 1960
that chemicals causing cancer in experimental animals could
cause cancer in man too. A careful study of food additives was
recommended. The climate was right, so an amendment to the
Food, Drug and Cosmetic Act passed. This threw responsibility
for testing back in the lap of the Food Industry. If they couldn't

prove an additive was safe, then they couldn't use it. Of course, one can never prove that a substance is harmless in *every* situation and at *any* dose—there would be too many possibilities to test. So in order to be practical, the amendment softened the definition of "safety" somewhat: an additive would be permitted if "it was safe in the amount and under the conditions in which it appears in the food." At the insistence of Representative Delaney of New York, a clause was included which specified that no agent which had been shown to cause cancer could be used in *any* amount. Since many chemicals can cause cancer if given in doses much larger than those normally used in food, this "Delaney Clause" has remained a thorn in the flesh of the food industry and there are periodically efforts made to repeal it.

The tests suggested for the food industry to prove the safety of a new additive included:
1) tests feeding animals a high dose to see if they become acutely ill or died,
2) long-term toxicity tests feeding the chemical extending over two years,
3) long-term feeding tests with rats for two years,
4) long-term tests injecting rats for two years,
5) further tests if the first four leave any doubt of safety,
6) if the chemical is suspected of causing cancer, much more elaborate tests are required.

The cost of testing a single chemical in this way would run between one and 200,000 dollars and would easily require five years.[30]

Hundreds of additives were already in use by this time. Some of them were time-honored and naturally-occurring like turmeric or black pepper. To test all of these would cost a fortune and take years. Meanwhile, the food industry would be crippled. The compromise was to draw up a list of additives that were already in general use before 1958 and were "generally recognized as safe" (GRAS). There are 768 of these and they include preservatives, sweeteners, stabilizers and artificial flavors.

Their continued use was, and is, permitted without testing, though new ones have to be thoroughly tested and proved safe[31] before they can be included in foods. Thus, the use of many additives of which we know relatively little continues, and research continues to turn up incriminating evidence. BHT, for example, which is used to prevent rancidity in oils and many other foods is listed as GRAS. It has even been suggested that because of its antioxidant effects it might be beneficial.[32] Recent research, however, has implicated it as contributing to the tendency to develop cancer.[33] If this is true, at any dose, under the Delaney Clause, its use must stop.

Since 1960, however, the use of convenience and ready-prepared foods has skyrocketed, and so the consumption of additives has continued to increase. What the results of the regular use of such substances in the diet will be we cannot say. Their consumption by the public at large amounts to a large-scale experiment, and their pharmacologic effects may be responsible for many problems while their action along the principle of hormesis might stimulate growth. It has even been suggested that this may account for the general increase in height among today's youth.

ADDITIVES AND HYPERACTIVITY

Though tiny quantities of additives may have a hormetic effect, larger amounts can produce definite though sometimes mild states of intoxication. Monosodium glutamate is famous for this, and although it is available in supermarkets for home use, it is in Chinese restaurants where large amounts of this compound are often used to enhance the flavor of foods. Its use can result in a state of uneasiness with a flushed face and a clouded mind, and a "Chinese restaurant syndrome" has been described in medical literature.

Recent research has suggested that additives may cause the restlessness, difficulty in learning and "hyperactivity" which is becoming increasingly common among American children. Though this has not been proved conclusively nor is it clear which additives are most dangerous in this respect, there is a growing feeling among pediatricians and psychiatrists that such chemicals can contribute to behavior disorders in children. The author of this theory, Ben Feingold, M.D., claims that if such children are put on an additive-free diet [34] before school age, they very quickly calm down and their disposition improves. Other researchers have not found this to be so.[35, 36] It's possible that the elimination of additive-containing snack and junk foods in Dr. Feingold's diet results in children eating more fresh, wholesome, natural foods and that behavior improves because of a general improvement in diet rather than simply the elimination of the chemical additives.

It is possible that the medicinal effects from food additives may be in part responsible for their appeal. The question of whether a sort of mild addiction to certain food additives might be important in stimulating sales of snack foods and sweets has not really been explored. When we stop to realize that the average American eats two to three pounds of chemical additives a year, then it becomes obvious that their effects, whatever they may be, deserve close scrutiny. Until more is learned about food additivies of recent origin, a wise shopper reads labels and avoids technical-sounding names which are obviously not natural foods. This may eliminate a whole Pandora's box of unidentified horrors, but it doesn't eliminate all questions about naturally occurring non-nutrient substances.

There are many "additives" which are not synthetic but which occur in nature and have been used for hundreds or even thousands of years. These we generally call herbs or spices, though in fact some of them have been used for the same range of effects as modern synthetic additives. Spices were particularly prized in the Middle Ages, both for their ability to prevent the spoilage of meat as well as their tendency to cover up the odors and tastes that resulted when the meat was not fresh. Tumeric is often used in Indian dishes to lend a yellow color and is added to ground mustard seed in the West to make the familiar yellow "prepared mustard" that is commonly marketed as a sandwich spread. Saffron, an herb which is more expensive because it is the tiny pistils of a flower, is also used to give foods a yellow color, but it has more pronounced pharmacologic effects. In substantial doses it produces a pleasant mania with sudden changes from hilarity to melancholia. In very large doses, it can create headaches, cough and even hemorrhaging. In the small amounts usually used in cooking, however, it is both harmless and pleasant, and according to ancient tradition, has a rebalancing and calming effect.

A NEW DIRECTION FOR NUTRITIONAL RESEARCH?

When we recall how many non-nutrient substances are naturally present in plants and that each of them has a possible range of activity extending from its toxicity, through its pharmacologic properties down to its potential as a stimulating agent at very tiny doses, we begin to understand the complexity of the effects of even whole natural foods. It becomes increasingly obvious that we cannot rely on a simple assay of traditional "nutrients." The amount of fat, carbohydrate, protein, vitamins and minerals may be only the crudest and most obvious of a food's properties. The smaller amounts of "non-nutrient" substances present may account in complex ways for the many distinctive and sometimes important properties that the food may have. Many common items of diet such as the carrot, which is usually not considered to contain any active pharmacologic ingredients, are considered by traditional physicians in many cultures to have important effects on the functioning of the human being—effects that go far beyond the simple supplying of nutrients. Chronic diarrhea is treated in some cultures with a diet of pureed carrots. Clinical studies in America have shown that this is quite effective,[37] and yet there is no indication that

other similar yellow vegetables which are primarily carbohydrate
are effective for the same purpose.

Whether such properties as the anti-diarrhea effect of
carrots are due to the action of tiny amounts of as yet unidentified antibiotics from the soil, to small amounts of other constituents of the root, or to properties that we have not yet even
suspected, remains to be seen. It is clear, however, that beyond
the matter of nutrients which are conventionally recognized,
there are many other qualities and substances in a plant that may
have a bearing on its ability to influence the body and mind. As
many well-known nutritionists have admitted, there may be a
number of "unknowns" in nutrition yet to be explored. Though
some of these "unknowns" may be vitamins and trace minerals
in the classic sense, it seems likely that others may involve the
"non-nutritional" substances whose effects are so subtle and
which are present in such numbers. Though we know of 150
in the simple potato, there are countless others:

> . . . . many chemical components of natural food products
> have been identified. It is likely, however, that even more
> have not. The greater number of chemical substances dis-
> covered in any single food studied . . . reflects an almost
> endless variety of specific chemical compounds that remain
> to be discovered in all the foods that make up the diet of
> man. At each step in the continuous increase in the sensi-
> tivity of our analytical methods, more and more discrete
> chemical entities will undoubtedly be found.[38]

An understanding of the subtle effects of these substances
may open up a whole new area of understanding of how foods
affect man. They may, in fact, be the "vitamins" of an exciting
future era in nutrition research. Such an understanding may
require us to examine with new respect complex and widespread
traditions regarding the unique properties of individual foods
which have been dismissed as unscientific or superstitious from
the point of view of our current limited understanding of the
known nutrients. Moreover, the fate of such compounds may
vary with different methods of food preparation.

THE PHARMACOLOGY OF COOKING

Cooking alters active substances in many ways, though this does not mean that cooked food is completely devoid of properties that are non-nutritional. Cooking does, however, have the tendency to break down or alter many of the substances present in moderate quantities which may be pharmacologically active. While little research has been done on this subject, too many patients comment, "I can eat cabbage cooked but not raw" or vice versa, for such reactions to be attributed to imagination. Similarly, some people find themselves unable to eat cooked carrots while they are able to eat them raw. On the other hand, raw onions upset some people's digestion while cooked ones do not.

In a much more obvious way, cooking is sometimes used to remove medicinal properties from foods by boiling them in water and pouring off the liquid. This is especially true for some leafy green vegetables where a strong, bitter taste suggests that there are high concentrations of harsh, medicinal substances present in the leaf. While long cooking is successful in rupturing the cellulose cell wall and allowing the nutrients to be freed and the strong taste can be covered up with other substances, traditional wisdom has it that this is not sufficient preparation for such a vegetable. It should, according to the ancient scriptures of Ayurveda, be boiled for some time in water which is then poured off. The leafy greens should then be squeezed after which they are cooked with an appropriate amount of fat and certain mildly pungent seasonings which promote their digestion. Otherwise, the dish will be heavy and difficult to manage. Unfortunately, such cooking is too often regarded with naive disdain. The discovery that throwing away cooking water resulted in the loss of certain vitamins led to the idea that no vegetable should be boiled in water that is discarded. Though with some vegetables the loss of vitamins could be crucial, most greens contain such huge quantities of vitamins, minerals and protein, that this is not a cause for concern. Besides, cooking them properly allows so much more of the vegetable to be eaten and assimilated that this easily compensates for what is lost in the process. Removing the irritating or possibly harmful medicinal substances by boiling and pouring off the water and rendering the contents of cells available by breaking down the cellulose through long cooking are probably much more important than vitamin and mineral loss. Many green leafy vegetables such as mustard, collards and turnip tops which were formerly the stand-bys of sturdy peasant people, have been abandoned because the modern cook, who feels he must quickly boil the vegetable in a small amount of water and eat it while it is still nearly crunchy, finds them strong-tasting, unpalatable and heavy to digest. For this reason they have largely disappeared from supermarkets and home gardens. Yet such green leafy vegetables are one of the best sources of calcium, protein, vitamin A and other vitamins and minerals. When properly cooked, they can be an extremely valuable part of the diet.

Cooked versus Raw

14

Perhaps as long as man has been a village dweller, or even a farmer for that matter, he has looked back wistfully toward his wilderness origins. It must have been a time of innocence, a time when one moved in harmony with nature and did not split himself off with his walls and villages. This nostalgia for the pre-historic past finds its highest expression in the writings of Jean Jacques Rousseau who idealized the "noble savage" during the Romantic era of European literature. Such a notion has its counterpart in the field of health and diet: if much of man's misery can be attributed to his intake of unnatural food, then perhaps he can be restored to a pristine state of innocence and perfect health by reversing this process and returning to a diet that is thoroughly natural and unaltered. If man evolved in the jungle eating wild plants and game, then surely his digestive tract and his physiological and metabolic apparatus is ideally suited to just such food. Would it not follow that, plant cell and animal cell having been evolved together, man's physiology is designed to digest raw, natural food, as his ancestors must have eaten it plucked from the tree as they stomped through the jungle, and not to digest food after it has been altered by cooking? Is it not then possible that by reverting to natural, unaltered, uncooked food, the tendency to disease might be removed?

THE RATIONALE FOR RAW FOOD

Such reasoning has led to the rise of a popular school of nutritional philosophy which, though it remains outside the mainstream of modern academic medicine, nevertheless commands the loyalties of many. In the last century, John Tilden attracted quite a following with his book entitled *Toxemia, the Cause of All Illness.* In this little treatise, Tilden decried the use of denatured and processed food and claimed that a return to a more natural diet could remove the tendency toward most diseases. Fasting and raw foods have been advocated by Dr. Tilden's followers since that time, and one currently popular lay writer claims, for example, that arthritis can be cured by taking nothing but raw foods.[1] Recently, articles have appeared in some of the more conservative medical journals indicating that there is also a growing interest among physicians in the value of raw foods as a treatment for certain diseases. There is a report of one diabetic, for example, who was found to be able to reduce his insulin requirements dramatically on a diet of raw foods while another discontinued the medication entirely.[2] An even more extreme version of the raw food regimen is the "fruitarian" diet, composed only of those foods which naturally fall from trees and require no cultivation or harvesting. Such a diet of fruits and nuts is said by its advocates to be the purest replica of the diet of early man.

The simplicity of this way of thinking is appealing. At this point in time, when we're suffering from an over-processed and unprecedentedly chemically contaminated diet, it is indeed refreshing to think that we might totally reverse the whole picture by recapturing a completely natural, uncooked diet that would divest us of all the ill effects of generations of poor eating.

Making Green Salads

By cutting those which are strong-flavored into smaller pieces, almost any fresh, tender vegetable can be included in a salad. There should be a balance with something green and leafy, something crunchy, something red or yellow, and usually, something slightly sour.

Iceberg lettuce adds little taste or nutrition to a salad and is useful primarily for "diluting" it. Leaf lettuces like romaine are preferable. Spinach is also good when it is young, tender and mild. Alfalfa sprouts are one of the most delightful additions to, or replacements of, green leafy ingredients in salads. (See box p. 203). Most other sprouts are too fibrous or strong-tasting to be used in any quantity in raw salads.

The "crunchies" in a salad give it texture and make it fun. Celery is the most commonly used, but small amounts of the more tender stems of spinach, broccoli and romaine lettuce (unless they are bitter) are good if cut thin. Cucumbers are also crisp and green peppers are sometimes suitable but should be used with caution since their taste is strong. Raw onions are crunchy, but have no place in most salads since they overpower other flavors. Leeks and chives, which are milder, can be used in small quantities, but are actually seasonings.

Yellow vegetables add color and a special sunshiny energy. Carrots are most often used and may also replace other crunchy ingredients. Fresh baby yellow squash have a subtle taste and can be added in small pieces. Fresh tomatoes, when they are in season, are a favorite. If they are not available, a bit of lemon juice will supply tanginess.

More substantial ingredients are especially appreciated when the salad is the major part of the meal. Pumpkin and sunflower seeds, crumbled cheese (paneer) and tofu (beancurd) boost the protein of the salad tremendously as do cooked garbanzos, especially if one includes a sprinkling of toasted bread squares (croutons).

Dressings

A yogurt-based dressing is good. Oil should be minimized or avoided. In many cases a sprinkling of fresh herbs and lemon juice will be found to be all that is necessary to make a salad delicious. A low (or non-) fat dressing with body and "richness" can be made with paneer (see box p. 277). Put enough of the fresh cheese into the blender to cover the blades well. Add onion salt (or powder) to taste and enough dried parsley flakes to give a light green color. With blender running, add liquid (water, whey or milk) until dressing reaches a fluffy, whipped consistency. Similar dressings can be made from tofu and occasionally, for variety, from avocado.

The enthusiasm for raw foods has not been without its impact. Whereas in the 1800's raw foods and even freshly cooked vegetables were seen as carriers of disease and during one epidemic banned entirely from the city of Washington,* one is more likely these days to think of uncooked fruits and vegetables as being, at least in moderation, "healthful." Salads, for instance, have become a popular part of the diet, whereas a century ago they were virtually unheard of. In the last century the term "salad green" meant a pot herb, i.e., a green leafy vegetable that was cooked. Among Appalachian folk even today, a dish of cooked leaves of the pokeberry plant is called "poke salad." In general, however, the word is nowadays understood to mean something raw. So go the fashions in nutritional thinking.

Actually, there is no good evidence that our jungle ancestors were free of health problems, despite their uncooked diet. Though those of the primitive ape-men who survived life in the jungle must have been robust, at least through the age of reproduction, we have no reason to think that many who were less fit to survive did not die from various diseases. In fact, in recent digs by anthropologists in East Africa, the most complete skeleton of one of the earliest man-like creatures, dating back three and one-half million years (dubbed "Lucy") was discovered to have evidences of arthritis, with the same spurs on the spine which are so common today. How could this be if arthritis is a disease of civilized diet? Actually, the fact that it occurred among man's ancestors does not rule out the possibility that it is due in part to a poor diet. Their diet was often based on expedience—what was there, they ate. If, due to shifting climatic patterns and loss of vegetation, their diet was primarily meat, this may have been a contributing factor in arthritis. A meat-free

* Such actions were probably based on more than superstition. A century ago hygienic measures in most cities were abysmally poor and fresh produce probably was responsible for transmitting infections. In many areas of the world this is still true, and raw foods are best avoided by the traveler.

diet has relieved many arthritics, and traditional wisdom in many parts of the world associate the two. In any case, the problem could not have been due to cooking, a practice which was not to be adopted for another few million years.

Technically, cooking is the heating of foods to a high temperature, most often and originally by exposing them to fire. The heat accomplishes several things. When plant foods are cooked, the heat causes the starch inside the cell to swell. This ruptures the tough cellulose wall of the plant cell which "locks in" the nutrients, liberating the cell's contents so that they become accessible to the digestive process. In the case of meats, the heat converts to gelatin the connective tissue which otherwise makes it difficult to chew and may interfere with digestion. Inevitably, of course, some nutrients are destroyed by the heat. Some of the vitamins, like vitamin C for instance, are more sensitive to high temperatures and a large percentage of them may be lost, while other vitamins remain relatively unaffected.[3] The cell is, of course, killed by the heat, and breaking down the cell's protective wall exposes its contents to oxidation by the air. For this reason, after food is cooked it should not be kept for long periods of time before it is eaten.

However, some breaking down of the cell's contents can be helpful. Research has shown that protein molecules of the large, intricate variety are sometimes more easily digested after they have been exposed to heat. The denaturation that results breaks certain cross linkages that hold the long chain in its folded and coiled position. This exposes the chain more completely to those digestive enzymes which break it down into amino acid units. This is usually true of vegetable proteins where protein and starch are mixed, especially when the heat is moderate. Heating also destroys a factor in beans that otherwise inactivates one of the protein-digesting enzymes.[4] If the heat is extreme, however, then protein molecules are damaged, so that the amino acids may be destroyed or cannot be easily released by enzymatic action.[5] Meat proteins can also be made less digestible when overcooked since the muscle proteins coagulate, making them tough and less accessible to the digestive enzymes. For breaking down the tough connective tissue that would otherwise keep one from chewing meat, fine grinding might be more ideal, as is done with "steak tartar" (a Central Asian dish made with raw ground beef). But dangerous microbes are sometimes present in raw meat, so cooking remains a practical expedient. In fact, a major advantage to the application of heat is that it kills microbes. This sterilization process helps prevent the entry of harmful bacteria, fungi and viruses to the digestive system.

The active non-nutrient compounds contained in vegetable foods include not only the strong irritants in green leafy vegetables which are broken down or removed through cooking, but others such as some of those in raw onions which can cause the face and eyes to burn and leave consciousness cloudy. Yet it is felt that the diet of man's ancestors consisted of huge quantities of leafy greens which he apparently plucked from the tree. If man evolved around the use of such quantities of raw green leaves, how is it that the traditional writings of an ancient culture caution against taking such food without careful cooking? The answer probably lies in the marked differences between these early predecessors of man who lived in the wild and man himself as he lives in the civilized world today.

Digestion must be vigorous to handle large quantities of raw food. According to the ancient teachings of Ayurveda, the vigor of the digestive "fire" is dependent on many things, one of which is the amount of exercise and activity. When the body is constantly engaged in vigorous physical activity, then the digestive fire is fanned. Primitive man, running through the jungle chasing his food and fleeing his enemies, had no doubt a more vigorous digestion to match his more robust physical health. Civilized man, who sits for long hours using his mind rather than his body, often suffers accordingly. The digestive system is less invigorated and the digestive fire "weaker." According to the ancient tradition, the fire which cannot be supplied by the digestive system to burn the food is partially replaced by the fire that is added during the cooking process.

Eating raw food in the quantities that were necessary to sustain his high degree of physical activity, primitive man was probably required to eat very frequently. In fact, according to some writers, he ate almost constantly. What he ate was what he happened upon, and feedings were apparently both longer and more frequent. As a result, his consciousness was more continually focused on the intake of food and its digestion. As man became more civilized, he invested more of his consciousness on higher pursuits. He came to understand that the cooking fire helped him with his digestion and also permitted the concentration of food into a few discrete feedings through the day so that the rest of his time need not be occupied with matters of food.

It has also been suggested that cooking, which softens food, permitted structural changes in the jaws and skull. The prominent brow ridges and heavy jaw of the Neanderthal man could be reduced in size. Reducing the need for chewing allowed the face to be refashioned for the more subtle nuances of speech.[6] Some anthropologists have gone so far as to maintain that cooking food is one of the prime causative factors in human evolution.[7] Just as the habit of erect posture and walking on two legs alone freed the hands for all of their delicate skills, so the use of fire for cookery freed the face for its intricate task of communication. Basing survival on the development of skills and cleverness along these lines, the brain grew.[8]

ADVANTAGES OF COOKING

In terms of sheer quantity, one can take more of a food when it's cooked than he can of the same food raw. When vegetables, for example, are cooked according to the traditions of Himalayan people,[9] they are condensed without losing much of their integrity or vitality. Once the skill of cooking in this

Stir-Fried Vegetables
(Indian Subzi)

By roasting vegetables in a flat, cast iron skillet, they are seared and sealed so that they retain their integrity and flavor even when "cooked down." The result is referred to simply as *subzi* "vegetable" in North India. Given the basic procedure, one can create delightful variations each of which is unique. The way a vegetable is cut has much to do with how it cooks. Tough, fibrous and indigestible parts should be removed. Firm vegetables should be cut smaller and cooked longer. Tender ones can be left in larger pieces, added later, or allowed to cook apart, forming a sauce or gravy.

Cooking is begun by adding 1 teaspoon of turmeric, 2 of ground cumin and 3 of ground coriander to 2-3 tablespoons of ghee. Other seasonings may also be used on occasion. When these are well browned, 2 medium onions which have been cut into ¼ inch rings, are added and browned. The degree to which this mixture is cooked will vary the taste greatly, and experience will become one's best guide. As the vegetables cook it is important to repeatedly scrape up the darkened portion that sticks to the pan. This adds a rich flavor to the dish. Next, 1½ cups mushrooms, a green pepper, and 1½ cups green beans, broccoli or asparagus are added, all cut into bite-sized pieces. These are spread out in the ghee and spices so they fry well and salt is added. A bit of water can be poured on when the vegetables dry out or they can be covered with water and allowed to cook submerged until it boils away. Another approach is to bring out the natural moisture of the vegetables by keeping a lid on part of the time. In any case none of the juices of the vegetables are ever discarded or lost. Covering the skillet will soften tough vegetables but not all the vegetables should be mushy. Cooking time depends on the vegetables used and the effect desired. One may allow the *subzi* to end up either quite soupy or dry enough to be served on a plate. When the fat begins to ooze out forming a film on top of the liquid, the vegetables are ready.

Milk, yogurt or soy powder dissolved in water can be added toward the end of cooking to make a creamy sauce and boost the protein content of the dish. Other ingredients such as tofu, paneer, green peas, spinach, tomatoes, chopped celery or parboiled mustard greens can be used with or in place of the vegetables already mentioned to add variety. The result is concentrated, delicious and easily digested.

Condensed from:*Himalayan Mountain Cookery* by Mrs. R.Ballentine, Sr. which contains dozens of recipes that are variations on this theme.

way has been mastered, one can easily see a difference in the food. The vegetables "cook down," yet maintain their shape and their distinctive flavor, so that a large quantity of vegetables can be reduced to a small serving without their becoming mushy. This cooking technique involves proper use of selected fat and spices and herein lies the genius of much of Indian cooking. The Indian method of cooking vegetables tends to reduce their bulk and make them more tender, thus giving one access to a larger quantity of nutrients. In the Zen tradition this process is called "yang-izing" which means the food is pulled in, concentrated, made more strong and meaty. Such food will have a more centering effect—tending to bring one down to earth. Raw or lightly cooked foods, by contrast, are more "yin," and their watery substance and medicinal effects tend to leave one feeling "spacier." In Ayurvedic terms, it would be said that they are likely to be more *vatic*, "vat" (literally "the wind") being that which tends toward restless activity, jumpiness and rapid motion. That, of course, is alright if you're running around in the jungle, but not so great if you have to sit still in an office or classroom.

Vegetables and fruits which are weak, anemic and chemicalized are also more "yin." If vegetables are deficient in vitamins and minerals, cooking them down according to the method mentioned above is very effective in helping to bring to a manageable bulk of food the necessary amounts of the nutrients that are needed. Of course the Zen cook would say that one who is too tight, too assertive, too "yang" can benefit from a little food which is less cooked and more "yin." Nevertheless, in the Zen tradition, as is the custom in India, it is rare to eat a large quantity of raw food. Vegetables are usually prepared by the "cooking down" method.

The issue of whether foods should be taken cooked or raw is not a matter of black and white. The problem is obviously much more complex. The appropriate degree of cooking will depend on the particular food, its medicinal properties, its toughness or amount of fiber, its digestibility, etc. Moreover, the degree of cooking will also be partly dependent upon the person who is to eat the food. Important here is his way of life, his amount of physical activity, his constitution, etc.

ADVANTAGES OF RAW FOOD

Regardless of the degree of cooking that is found to be optimal, it remains true that food which is cooked is different in nature from that which is raw. There are certain important properties of the live plant cell which are delicate and subtle and which are probably very valuable, and perhaps even necessary in some quantity, for good nutrition. Though vegetables are taken cooked in most cases in the East, fruits are usually taken raw and serve to provide that little bit of fresh vitality which should be included in the diet. In some communities a bit of freshly plucked mint leaves are chopped into a dish of yogurt, while the Punjabis have a custom of taking a handful of raw bean sprouts each day. Even most Americans feel something is not quite right if they miss their salad, grapefruit or glass of fresh juice for several days. There seems to be a universal recognition that a little bit of some unidentified something in raw foods is needed each day. While the vitamin C complex is probably one aspect of this, it is unlikely that we have identified all the aspects of this "freshness" which are of value.

A SECOND LOOK AT THE CELL

When we explored the cell in Chapter One, we saw it as an extremely complex and intricate lattice-work of huge inter-connected protein molecules. Within this "jungle-gym-like" framework of protein, we saw a fluid and a mobile mixture of smaller molecules which moved from position to position, under-going various biochemical reactions and changes. Despite the apparent complexity of the picture we painted, we have in fact overlooked a great deal and simplified to a remarkable extent.

Fruit Salad

Each fruit has its own special personality, and they should each be treated differently when preparing them. Citrus fruits, for example, are most appealing in a salad if cut in half and the sections removed, leaving the tough membrane to be discarded after the juice is squeezed out. In this way, their light, juicy and delicate quality is not ruined by a chewy, tasteless skin. Grapes, cherries and berries should be carefully washed under running water, pitted or hulled and peeled if the skin is tough. Apples, peaches, pears and even ripe figs are usually best peeled. Blanching peaches slightly may help in removing their skins. The skin may contain some nutrients, but pesticides and other contaminants accumulate there as well and skins of such fruits as apples are not very digestible anyway. This is especially true when they have been coated with wax to protect them and make them shine. Organic, tree or vine-ripened fruit is always preferable when available.

Generally a combination of two or three fruits is optimal to make a fruit salad. Some favorite combinations include bananas, pears and grapes; orange, grapefruit and pineapple; and peaches, plums and cherries. It is said that melons are best taken alone, while citrus and acid fruits such as cranberries do not mix very well with sweet fruits like bananas and dates. However, when individual ingredients are combined, the mixing forms a new entity with unique properties of its own. Eating a banana and then a wedge of melon, for example, may produce a different reaction in the digestive system from eating the two when they have been cut up, stirred together with a sauce, allowed to stand a few minutes and served as a single dish. Rather than following certain rules, one is best advised to follow his own taste and intuition. Many fruits such as ripe figs or fresh berries taste best when taken alone with fresh cream or a whipped curd and honey topping. Fruits should, of course, be served as soon after preparation as possible as they quickly lose their vibrancy. Tofu (soy bean curd) beaten in the blender with honey until fluffy makes a tasty dressing for fruit salads. Paneer can be used the same way and has an even more subtle flavor, yet is substantial enough to turn a fruit salad from a dessert into a meal. Toppings made of pureed fruits such as bananas and honey are lighter. Yogurt and honey make an intermediate topping, while raw honey thinned with fruit juice is quite delicate. Experimenting with such condiments as ground coriander, cardamon or chopped fresh mint is occasionally refreshing. Nuts and seeds like roasted sunflower seeds make a salad more substantial and occasionally provide a nice contrast in texture and taste.

In fact, the complexity of the arrangement is even more staggering. We did not even bother to ask, for example, what produced the motion of the small molecules through the intercellular fluid. Our tendency is to regard the protein, fat, vitamin and mineral molecules floating through the space within the cell much as we would visualize so many automobiles being piloted down the street. Yet there is no "little man" inside each molecule steering it from place to place. In fact, there is an incredibly complicated interaction between each molecule and those surrounding it. There is a field of forces and energetic interrelationships that determine which molecule is held in place against adjacent molecules and which one is repulsed and propelled away.

Sometimes we tend to think of the components of the inside of the cell as so many little tinker toys. In fact, our models of molecular biology are made up of ping pong balls connected by toothpicks to show the "chemical bonds" holding atoms together to form that complex we call a molecule.

But each molecule is a study in itself: it is surrounded by a huge variety of other biochemical structures which "touch" it in different points. The result is a variety of interactions involving the force fields of each. One molecule is never simply "lying beside" another. Positive and negative fields of one must always have some effect on the positive and negative fields of each of those nearby. This determines whether that molecule will remain stationary, whether it will move, in which direction it will move and what changes it will undergo as a result of the movement. There is, in other words, an extremely complicated "ecological" balance that exists inside the cell so that each component influences all the others.

It is this complex entity, which we call the cell, that is the basic foodstuff around which animal life has evolved. This cell is, in fact, the "nutritional standard." It is this which our bodies are really designed to use. It is on the breakdown and assimilation of these energetic complexes that we base our metabolism, our physiology and our existence.

BEYOND ANALYSIS

What happens to the intricate energy relationships between molecules within the cell during the processes of cooking, chewing and digesting, and how their reorganization, their disentanglement, their breaking down and their reunion within the body occurs remains yet to be fully understood. We have identified certain complexes, certain molecular structures, certain atoms that we know our bodies are unable to do without. These we have labeled vitamins, minerals, proteins and so forth. We have begun to realize that there are other "non-essential," non-nutritional compounds which may effect us in significant ways. Yet we must increasingly come to see that even after our painstaking analysis, our decades of laboratory research, there may still be many essential qualities of food, many aspects of the intricate interrelationships between molecules and even within molecules, which have so far eluded our grasp.

In view of the complexity of the cell and its constituents, it is clear that an analytic approach to assessing the nutritional value of foods is not only inadequate but cumbersome. Besides the constituents and properties of foods, we must deal with the variation among people. Not only is the food complex and variable, but so is the person who is to eat it. It would require, in fact, a battery of computers to plan a single meal if, indeed, all the information necessary could be identified, collected and put into the computer! Moreover, both the program and the information would have to be changed from day to day and even from hour to hour. In search of proper food, we would starve to death, pushing buttons and waiting for another printout.

For such reasons, the traditional approaches to nutrition from ancient civilizations come as a refreshing relief. The intricacies and exasperations of nutritional analysis are shortcut in ingenious and practical ways. The obvious resolution of the dilemma is as simple as placing a morsel of food in the mouth and tasting it. As one modern physiologist observed: "Our senses of taste and smell constitute a most astonishing chemical laboratory. In a fraction of a second they can identify the chemical structure of compounds it would take a chemist days to analyze by the usual laboratory methods."[10] What's more, our senses are not limited to the identification of simple compounds. They are expressly designed for the identification of whole foods. Not only do our senses of taste and smell grasp the gestalt of a slice of home-baked bread or the complexity of a piece of fresh fruit, but they simultaneously match them to our own needs of the moment.

While our senses are designed to lead us to what is the most suitable nutrition, this process is subject to disruption and confusion. For this reason, in some traditions such as that of Ayurveda, certain rules or guidelines for the evaluation of foods and their appropriateness through the senses of taste were laid down. This permits an objective and systematic assessment of foods that remains nevertheless grounded in personal experience and sensitivity to one's requirements.

Ayurvedic Nutrition

15

In the ancient medical system of India, we find what is one of the oldest and most time-tested approaches to nutrition. Its science of food and diet is an integral part of a philosophy of man, his consciousness and his relation to the universe. The result is an approach to diet that is unsurpassed both in its profundity and sophistication as well as in its practicality and simplicity. Here the selection and preparation of food is seen as inseparable from the treatment of disease and the cultivation of vibrant health. Both these goals are part of traditional Indian medicine.

The traditional system of Indian medicine is called *Ayurveda*. *Ayur* means "life" and *veda* means "science," so *Ayurveda* means "the Science of Life." It comprises a body of medical tradition that extends back at least several thousands of years. Moreover, it has continued to be practiced without interruption during this period of time, its present form having been shaped primarily by the writers Charaka, Shushruta and Vag Bhata prior to 500 B.C. It is thought that this codification represents a transfer of oral tradition into written, and it is considered likely by historians that the spoken tradition dates back much further.   The form and organization given to the Ayurvedic system of medicine by Charaka and Shushruta has persisted, and these textbooks [1,2] are still taught and used by medical students in the schools of traditional medicine throughout India today.

Through its long history, it would appear that Ayurveda witnessed the rise and fall of many schools of therapy ranging from herbal medicine to physical therapy and massage, surgery, psychiatry, the use of meditation, mantra and many other treatment modalities.   Each of these apparently was integrated into the physician's practice, and the conceptual scheme expanded to accommodate them.   As a result, the school of Ayurveda has a breadth and depth that could be unparalleled in the history of medical science.   This also made it possible for Ayurvedic physicians, or *vaidyas*, to develop, over thousands of years, an extremely complex and complete science of herbology and pharmacology.   Long before we discovered their use in the West, traditional Indian physicians were using such preparations as reserpine to lower blood pressure and calm nerves, cardiac glycosides similar to digitalis to regulate the rhythm of the heart, and fungal preparations similar to penicillin as antibiotics.   Their practice of surgery was astonishingly advanced for the time, and as early as 1,200 years ago, there are accounts of successful plastic surgery such as the replacement of ears and noses that had been severed in battle.   Moreover, even in ancient times, the treatment of mental illness was advanced, and the treatment of physical disorders often involved definite mental, psychotherapeutic and meditative techniques.   In fact, perhaps the one thing that can be said most clearly about Ayurveda is that it admits no distinction between mind and body, and that it provides one of the most comprehensive schemata for understanding psychosomatic interaction.

The science of nutrition in Ayurveda is vast and comprehensive and is not separated from pharmacology.   Since no distinction is admitted between foods and drugs, herbal and mineral substances that are used in the preparation of food are thought to be equally important medicinally as those that are given separately.

TRIDOSHA

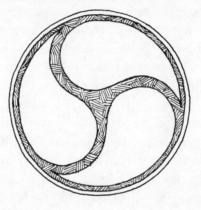

Those few people who are familiar with the name of Ayurveda know that it is often taken to be synonymous with the concept of tridosha. Tridosha is that conceptual framework which forms the heart of Ayurvedic medicinal science. It is also the great-grandfather of most of European medicine, and a proper understanding of its meaning has been greatly hindered by this fact since most Western students tend to assume that the meanings of the terms used in tridosha are equivalent to the "humors" of Greek and medieval European medical thought. Though the "bile," "wind" and "phlegm" of the Europeans are apparently descendants of the ancient Indian concepts, they were (and are) too often corrupted by overly literal interpretation.

Tridosha is essentially a system of conceptualizing mind, body and their interaction in dynamic terms that cut across the usual categories of Western thought. Tridosha means the system of "three doshas." The *doshas* are dynamic factors of vectors whose interaction produces that complex known as the psychosomatic entity, or person. The *doshas* are called *Vata, Pitta* and *Kapha*.* In Sanskrit, *Kapha* signifies all that about the psychosomatic complex which is heavy, dense, gross, sluggish, coarse and tending toward the material. *Pitta* indicates that aspect of the total system which is hot, energetic, assertive, capable of doing work and having the property of fire. *Vata*, the last aspect of the psycho-physiological system, represents that which is least tangible, least perceptible, most subtle, most active, erratic and unpredictable. For this reason, it is often translated "wind." It is the wind which we cannot see, which moves in such subtle and erratic ways, yet which has the power to generate electricity, move ships or destroy cities.

Pitta is most often translated as fire, since in the natural world it is the flame which most closely corresponds to this aspect of the psychosomatic system. The flame is hot, quick, angry, aggressive, yet full of warmth, energy and the ability to act in the world. The normal "home" of this fire in the Ayurvedic system is the "solar plexus" whose name reflects the ancient recognition that the organs of digestion were the primary site where fuel is broken down and the whole process of energy production begins and is to a great extent regulated. Modern physiologists acknowledge that a significant amount of energy may be produced during the digestion and assimilation of foods.†

Kapha is difficult to translate. It designates that aspect of the system which is most material. Sometimes it is connected with the earth or water since these are the material, tangible, grosser aspects of the universe. In the context of medicine, *Kapha* is often translated as "mucus," and as we noted earlier, there seems to be some etymological relationship between the

---

* Or *Vat, Pit* and *Kaph*. In Sanskrit the final consonant is usually lightly vocalized with a neural (a) but this is difficult to render in Roman characters and so neither of the two transliterations is precisely accurate and authors vary in their usage.

† This is called the Specific Dynamic Action of a food, and though current physiological theory has not been able to explain it very well, it follows easily from Ayurvedic notions.

English *cough* and the Sanskrit *Kaph*, both of which are connected with the accumulation of mucus in the respiratory system. In a similar way, *Pitta* is often translated (though perhaps regrettably so) as "bile" since it is bile which is the identifiable fluid most closely connected to the digestive and heat-producing catabolic and digestive processes of the body. *Vata*'s translation as "wind" is taken in the context of physiology to mean gas in the intestinal tract or elsewhere in the body. This is, of course, a limited aspect of its meaning, and the literal translation of the *doshas* as mucus or phlegm, bile and wind is clearly a misinterpretation of their intended significance.

Tridosha can perhaps be most aptly understood in the context of Western science if its derivation is likened to a process of factor analysis: if we can imagine the ancient physicians working primarily on the basis of empirical evidence gathered through self-scrutiny, careful clinical experience and keen observation, if we can imagine their trying to analyze the multiplicity of psychological, emotional, mental, spiritual and physical phenomena into manageable terms, then we might see that their efforts amounted to something quite similar to what a computer does to a pile of data when it carries out a factor analysis. The reduction of the multiple variables into functionally-grouped categories not only brings order out of the chaos, but brings an order which is most meaningful and revealing of the basic nature of the system being studied. This "factor analysis" carried out by the traditional physicians of India apparently revealed three major functional "forces" or groupings involved in the psychosomatic system, and these were designated as the *doshas* (that is, three main categories as far as understanding and dealing with disease).

It is through examining and evaluating in each patient the predominant activity, quality and imbalances in these three functional entities that the physician arrives at a conceptualization of the disease process. For instance, in some diseases *Pitta* might be greatly accentuated while *Kapha* is normal and

Vata is deficient. Diagnosis is more complex than this, of course, since any one, any two, or all three of the *doshas* may be either accentuated, vitiated (i.e. irregularly or unevenly active), or decreased. The various combinations are many.

Of course, the use of the conceptual scheme is not limited to dealing with "disease." It is not necessary that one be disabled, nor that he apply to a physician for help to avail himself of the insights that tridosha can provide. In fact, the Ayurvedic writings not only clarify diseases and functional disorders through use of tridosha, they also conceptualize the "normal" person in these terms. Though the ideal situation is one where the three doshas are in perfect harmony, such an ideal state rarely exists. Each person's makeup or constitution determines that he will tend to slip out of balance in certain characteristic ways, e.g., one may tend toward anger, volatileness and have a reputation as being "hot-headed." The red face, quick assertive manner and aggressive actions all suggest the *"pittic"* constitution. If there is, in addition, an erratic nature, an inconsistency and spaciness, then there is also an element of *Vata* involved. The person who is heavy, staid, unshakable, with perhaps a tendency toward lethargy and indifference, would be called *kaphic*.*

TRIDOSHA AND TASTE

Ayurvedic science is, as we have seen, experiential and practical. It is first and foremost a way of organizing one's experience. Therefore, it is not surprising that its methods for judging the properties of foods and naturally occurring medicines (herbs, spices, mineral substances, etc.) is simple and part of one's everyday experience. In fact, as mentioned before, the

---

* The correspondence to modern typologies such as Sheldon's ectomorph, mesomorph and endomorph is striking but not complete. There are differences. The *kaphic* person may be well-formed (mesomorphic), for example, and the *pittic* type is often slight of build (ectomorphic).

properties of food and medicines as conceptualized in Ayurveda can be deduced by their tastes in most cases. There we find the sense of taste put in a different perspective: it has evolved to help us apprehend the dynamic qualities of foods so that we can judge their effect on us. Whether it's the *vaidya* in his pharmacy or the cook in his kitchen, one of the most important guides to the properties of food or drug is its taste.*

Effects of Different Tastes on the Doshas

	KAPHA (substance-like)	PITTA (fire-like)	VATA (wind-like)
Bitter	⇩ (open, down)	⇩ (open, down)	⬆ (dark, up)
Pungent	⇩ (open, down)	⬆ (dark, up)	⇧ (open, up)
Astringent	⬇ (dark, down) watery	⇩ (open, down)	⇧ (open, up)
Salty	⬆ (dark, up) i.e. watery kaph	⬆ (dark, up)	⇩ (open, down)
Sour	⬆ (dark, up) i.e. solid kaph	⬆ (dark, up)	⇩ (open, down)
Sweet	⬆ (dark, up)	⬇ (dark, down)	⇩ (open, down)

Each taste has definite effects in terms of the 3 doshas. The darkest arrows are the most prominent effects. Direction of the arrows indicates increasing or diminishing effects of the particular dosha. For reasons that will become apparent in the last chapter, this is a rather crude approximation.

Taste reflects certain qualities in the food—its ability to modify certain principles *(doshas)*—therefore one can know from

---

* This does not mean that a good Indian cook is constantly tasting the food as he cooks. In fact, a good cook in the best tradition never tastes the food until it is fully prepared and those for whom it was made are served.

the taste of the substance how it will affect the dynamic equilibrium of the body-mind complex. By looking at the chart, we can see how it is that one can, by assessing the taste of a food or herb, immediately know how it is likely to affect the *doshas.* He can then know, if he is aware of the dynamic balance of the three *doshas* within himself at the moment, whether this is the food that he should eat. The Ayurvedic pharmacology of taste is essentially a way of putting into formal terms the intuitive and experiential sense of what is right and proper to eat at any moment.

A person who is overweight, for example, and who is dull and heavy and lethargic, will find that he feels livelier, more active, and has less tendency to gain weight if his foods are predominantly pungent and bitter. His tendency, however, is likely to be the opposite of that since it is often this which has led him to over indulge in sweet foods in the first place. By contrast, a person who is very nervous, shaky, "spaced out," flighty and unable to "keep his feet on the ground," should not take a preponderance of bitter substances. If he does, he will tend to become even "spacier," and may even lose contact with reality. Such a person, the typical ectomorphic, intellectual, dreamy, paranoid recluse can usually benefit from some starchy, fattening food. This is the secret, perhaps, of much of the success of the macrobiotic diet which emphasizes whole grains, especially rice. Among the wandering youth of the mid and late 1960's, the "macrobiotic" diet gained quite a reputation. A steady diet of predominantly brown rice is often very settling, bringing the "spaced out" veteran of "mind-expanding" drugs down-to-earth and helping him feel more in touch with the world around him. Centers offering assistance based on such dietary practices have sometimes been dramatically helpful. Foods which are hot and spicy stimulate digestive fire, and it is thus that traditional cooks the world over add chilis and pungent spices to their bean recipes so that the difficult-to-digest legume can be handled better and will not cause so much gas. The *kashaya* or astringent substances are a special case. Astringency is almost more of a sensation than a taste, strictly speaking. It is a drawing or pulling together, and according to Ayurvedic thought, this means that a cool, dry contraction is produced.* Such a dynamic effect is useful where there is a preponderance of watery *Kapha*. Any discharge or flow from the body will be reduced by this, thus the universal use of astringent compounds in such cases from the American Indians' blackberry root or oak bark tea for diarrhea to the current use of alum compounds in underarm anti-perspirants.

The appreciation of the taste-related properties allows one to be less crude in his understanding of the effects of foods. For example, before ripening, the banana has a subtle but distinct astringency. When properly cooked, it is therefore useful in such disorders as diarrhea and runny, drippy colds. When the banana ripens, however, it loses its astringent taste and becomes quite sweet. At that point, the drying and "drawing closed" effect is lost and increasingly replaced by its opposite, so that banana (which to most people means ripe banana) is notoriously "mucus forming."

There are other *gunas* or properties that food contains besides simply that of taste or *rasa*. Another is, for example, *virya,* which means the effect that the food has on the temperature of the body—does it create heat or does it make one cold? For instance, sesame seeds tend to generate heat in the body while mung beans tend to do the opposite. This is despite the fact, it should be noted, that both contain roughly similar quantities of protein, carbohydrate and fat. Here we are dealing with a subtler system of analysis than the laboratory method of simply determining the quantities of known nutrients. There is something about the non-nutritional compounds or properties of the sesame seed that has a specifically warming effect on the body and something about the mung bean that is the opposite.

* See Chapter 20, The Philosophy of Nutrition.

Meats were classified in that way too by the ancients, and whereas most kinds of fish will tend to produce warmth, other meats do not seem to. Of course most spices, with the exception of cloves, are heat-producing, while fruits are generally cooling, though here, too, there are exceptions. In both the tropical plains of India and the icy Himalayan slopes, heating or air-conditioning are still used very little. The traditional wisdom about *virya* is therefore adhered to carefully. A heating *(ushna)* food taken in the hot season can produce considerable discomfort. Sesame confections, for example, cannot be found in Indian sweet shops during the warm months, whereas in the winter they are especially favored by those who suffer from the cold.

Altogether, there are twenty-two pairs of *gunas*, like heat-producing *(ushna)* versus cold-producing *(shita)*. The more important of these are lightness versus heaviness and oiliness versus dryness. Among beans, for example, *mung* beans are considered light *(laghu)* and easy to digest, whereas kidney beans are heavy *(guru)*. Both, however, have the quality of dryness *(rooksh)*. *Urad dahl*, on the other hand, another kind of legume, is considered oily or unctuous *(snigdha)*, the opposite of dry.

Whether a food is drying *(rooksh)* or oily (unctuous or *snigdha)* is of some practical importance. Those who have problems with dry, hard bowel movements may find they have been eating foods that were predominantly *rooksh*. An increase of foods that are *snigdha* such as fats, ripe bananas, coconut, sugar and salt, can correct this. Similarly, one who is having a runny nose and eyes can often greatly relieve his discomfort by temporarily limiting his diet to more drying foods, herbs and seasonings like chick peas, honey or black pepper. The *bajra chappati*, made from the flour of a dark millet, is remarkable in its ability to dry up a drippy nose—especially in cool, damp weather.

Many of these properties are in line with common sense and do not come as a surprise because they are consonant with our experience.   Most of the others follow logically from the principles of taste pharmacology. However, there is another set of properties which are not so apparent or logical. This is the "taste" *(rasa)* of the food after it has undergone some process of digestion.   This is called *vipaka*. For instance, most starchy foods, after chewing, become sweet, and the post-digestion "taste" is sweet *(madhura)*. But starchy foods tend to be classified as sweet *(madhura)* anyway, so the taste *(rasa)* is the same as the *vipaka*. Sometimes, however, this is not true, so that a predominantly starchy substance like mung beans, becomes pungent or *katu* after digestion. Thus the value of mung beans, for while they may be agreeable in taste to those who prefer mild, sweetish foods, they will not be unduly fattening and actually help to stimulate the digestive fire.

THE PHARMACOLOGIC USE OF SPICES AND FOODS

An understanding of the *doshas* and their relationship to the taste and other properties of food are part and parcel of common knowledge and folk culture in India. Everyone educated in the traditional way understands, at least to some extent, these basic concepts. Classically, the selection of foods from the table and the choice of things to cook are based on seasonal and other considerations with an understanding of how they affect the doshas and what sorts of foods would be appropriate.

An appreciation of tridosha and the science of taste pharmacology also explains much of the use of spices in Indian cooking. When the seasonings and spices are added to a food, they change its taste. Therefore they change its properties and the effect that it has on the body. For instance, rice with salt and pepper will have quite a different effect on the physiology than rice alone. Though in Western scientific terms it is said that the spice has little nutritional value, in Ayurvedic terms it has a very specific pharmacologic action, such that the whole processing of the food and the net effect on the body is changed.

EFFECTS OF ANIMAL FOODS ACCORDING TO AYURVEDA

	TASTE						VIRYA		DOSHA			POST DIGESTION EFFECT			PROPERTIES				
	SWEET	SOUR	SALTY	PUNGENT	ASTRINGENT	BITTER	HEATING	COOLING	KAPH, substance	PIT, fire-like	VAT, wind-like	SWEET	SOUR	PUNGENT	HEAVY	LIGHT	OILY/SMOOTH	DRY/ROUGH	
FISH (general)	X						X				C				X		X		Strengthening
BEEF			X				X				C						X	X	Useful for excess gastric fire
PORK	X				X			X			C				X		X		Appetizing, promotes perspiration
RABBIT					X			X	C	C	C			X				X	
MUTTON	X							X		C				X	X				Strengthening
CHICKEN	X				X			X	C	C	C					X			
COW'S MILK	X							X		C					X		X		
BUFFALO MILK	X							X							X		X		
CAMEL'S MILK			X		X		X		C							X		X	Relieves & prevents constipation, worms, hemorrhoids
GOAT'S MILK	X							X			C					X			Relieves diarrhea, cough, fever
YOGURT (mature)		X					X						X				X		Good for digestion, diarrhea and painful urination
BUTTER					X														Reduces hemorrhoids, promotes intestinal absorption

X property of the food
C indicates that the food "cures" (restores to balance) the dosha in question

It is perhaps for this reason that the average Indian can eat a predominantly starchy diet made up of rice, *chapatti*, potatoes and *dahl* with a *madhura rasa* (sweet taste) as long as he adds his spices—cumin, coriander, pepper, ginger, and so forth, which are predominantly *katu* or pungent with some bitter and astringent taste. They serve to balance the food and prevent it from having a fattening or *kaphic* effect. Of course, it is common sense, even to the Westerner, that seasoning a food so that it becomes hot and pungent decreases its mucus-forming properties and "cleans out the sinuses."

During ancient times when the Ayurvedic scriptures were written, it seems that a more varied diet of fruit, vegetables, grains and wild and leafy greens was much more easily available. The population was less dense and there was more vegetation per person. At that time, it seems likely that the need for spices was less, and they seemed to have been used predominantly as medicine. But as the diet became increasingly domesticated and agricultural, and the population density greater, food became less varied and more starchy with a predominantly sweet taste *(madhura rasa)*. It was then that the spices moved from the pharmacy into the kitchen, and their use became a daily necessity. Unfortunately, a very starchy diet sometimes leads to the heavy-handed use of the least expensive and most potent spices such as chili peppers. The result can be caustic, irritating and inflaming to the intestinal tract. In fact, the use of chilis, brought only a few hundred years ago from Mexico, might be regarded as a corruption of classical Indian cuisine. Many people have had tearful and burning experiences with so-called Indian food as a result of eating in East Indian restaurants. Actually, restaurants are not used by most people in India, and the preparation of food is carefully done at home. A mastery of subtle seasoning is the mark of a cultured and well-educated cook, and the judicious use of spices is considered a crucial part of turning out a meal that is not only nutritious but that can promote a gentle rebalancing of the system.

EFFECTS OF FATS, OILS and SWEETNERS ACCORDING TO AYURVEDA

	TASTE						VIRYA		DOSHA			POST DIGESTION EFFECT			PROPERTIES				
	SWEET	SOUR	SALTY	PUNGENT	ASTRINGENT	BITTER	HEATING	COOLING	KAPH, substance	PIT, fire-like	VAT, wind-like	SWEET	SOUR	PUNGENT	HEAVY	LIGHT	OILY/SMOOTH	DRY/ROUGH	
CASTOR OIL	X						X		←	↯	↯				X				Helpful in chronic fever, some heart disease
WHITE MUSTARD OIL	X	X		X			X		↯	↯	C								Helps itching skin (topically)
LINSEED OIL	X	X					X		↯	↯	C			X					
SAFFLOWER OIL							X		↯	↯	↯			X	X				Excessively irritating
SESAME OIL	X				X		X		—	←	→			X					Strengthening, good for skin, increases gastric fire
OIL (in general)								X	←	⇒	⇒				X		X		
GHEE	X							X	←	⇒	C						X		
HONEY	X				X		X		←	↯	←			X	X			X	"Cuts" mucus
CHEWED SUGAR CANE	X							X	←		←								Laxative, strengthening
GUR; SUGAR	X							X	←		←			X	X		X		Increases fat and tendency to worms

*Solid raw sugar (sugar cane juice cooked down – no refinement.)

X property of the food
C indicates that the food "cures" (restores to balance) the dosha in question
↯ the food vitiates (arouses and irritates) the dosha
≀ weakens the dosha
← strengthens
⇒ diminishes

Because so little distinction is made between the pharmacy and the kitchen in traditional Indian culture, we find in Ayurvedic medical schools that pharmacology and cooking are taught as the same course. The culinary spices like cardamom, cumin, coriander, turmeric, etc. have always been an important part of the armamentarium of traditional physicians. Cardamom, for example, is an important cough remedy, and even today can be found in Western over-the-counter cough syrups. Moreover, many of the items which we regard as strictly foodstuffs are considered by the traditional physician to have important pharmacologic action. For instance, onions, honey, clarified butter, sesame seed oil, milk, many meats, etc., are ascribed very specific and important medicinal effects.

Milk is a laxative, as is honey. *Ghee* (clarified butter) promotes digestion as do most fats, which is in accord with research which has shown that full-fat soy flour is digested with less gas than the defatted preparation.[3] One can easily compile a list of over a hundred plants which are used in India both as food and as medication. This is another reason why both foods and medicinal substances are subsumed under the term *dravya*, and why in the discussions of taste and of the properties of foods and medicines, so little distinction is made between the two. The same methods of preparation, processing, handling, and selection are applicable to the major part of this spectrum of substances. It is for such reasons, too, that cooking and the preparation of medicine can be taught at the same time. In fact, the Ayurvedic physician who would attempt to prescribe medication without seeing to the preparation of the meals taken during the course of the day by a patient would be considered a fool.

Even among the Ayurvedic physicians, the matter is regarded as extremely complex, and even the most extensively tested rules, evolved over thousands of years, like that of the taste pharmacology, are not always completely accurate. The properties of perhaps 80% of foods and medicinal-like herbs can be deduced according to their taste *(rasa)*. Another 10% or

EFFECTS OF LEGUMES (BEANS AND PEAS) AND SESAME SEEDS

PREP'S OF LEGUMES	TASTE						VIRYA		DOSHA			POST DIGESTION EFFECT			PROPERTIES				
	BITTER	ASTRINGENT	PUNGENT	SALTY	SOUR	SWEET	COOLING	HEATING	VAT, wind-like	PIT, fire-like	KAPH, substance	PUNGENT	SOUR	SWEET	DRY/ROUGH	OILY/SMOOTH	LIGHT	HEAVY	
PREP'S OF LEGUMES (in general)						X	X		↩						X			X	Dehydrating. "Take in small quantities with pungent, fat and salty things."
GARBANZOS		X				X	X			C	C						X		Very dehydrating
RED LENTIL (massur)		X				X	X										X		Dehydrating
MUNG BEANS		X				X	X			C	C	X			X		X		
URAD*						X		X	C	C	C					X		X	Strengthening
ARAHAR* (tuar)							X		←	←	←								
KIDNEY BEAN		X				X		X	C		C				X			X	Laxative
SESAME	X	X				X		X		←	←					X			Strengthening

*Though not commonly used in the West, these beans and peas are easily available at Indian food stores. Therefore they are included here.

15% must be explained by what happens after digestion occurs *(vipakha)* and a few others by the *virya* or other *gunas*. For example, honey, which is sweet in taste, is converted upon digestion to a pungent *(katu)* substance. This means that after it is processed by the body, it is transformed so that it does not have the effect that most sweet substances do. It does not aggravate the tendency toward obesity, nor does it increase the formation of mucus. Thus, instead of being a *kaphic* food, it is one which stimulates *pitta* and has exactly the opposite effect of most sweet foods. Because it is transformed by the body into a pungent or "hot" substance, it helps one lose weight, stimulates body heat and tends to dry up mucus. For this reason, it is sometimes used along with milk or yogurt to reduce their mucus-forming tendencies. The Ayurvedic scriptures say that yogurt is an excellent food if it is taken with honey. On this basis it is also said that the diabetic can take honey without harm, whereas he should avoid sugar assiduously. Conventional modern medicine, by contrast, has tended to forbid honey to the diabetic on the rationale that it is a carbohydrate. Interestingly enough, however, honey contains primarily fructose which, as we have seen, is different from most sugars in that it does not require insulin for its metabolism. If taken in excess, however, honey can overstimulate and unbalance or disturb *pitta*, causing digestive problems that may be difficult to correct. For this reason, though it is an excellent food, one is counseled to take honey in proper measure (for most people more than two tablespoons a day is unwise).

All in all, there may be one food, herb, or spice in a thousand which falls into a special category which is called *prabhava*, meaning "it can't be explained!" This means that neither the taste, the *virya*, nor the *vipaka* can account for the effect that the food has on the body. In fact, these classifications are for convenience, simply a way of organizing the information that has been accumulated. Though they usually can be reasoned out and followed through, the designations were, and still are, derived

EFFECTS OF SPICES AND HERBS ACCORDING TO AYURVEDA

	TASTE						VIRYA		DOSHA			POST DIGESTION EFFECT			PROPERTIES				
	SWEET	SOUR	SALTY	PUNGENT	ASTRINGENT	BITTER	HEATING	COOLING	KAPH, substance	PIT, fire-like	VAT, wind-like	SWEET	SOUR	PUNGENT	HEAVY	LIGHT	OILY/SMOOTH	DRY/ROUGH	
FRESH GINGER ROOT				X			X		C		C								Promotes digestion, aphrodisiac
HOLY BASIL*						X	X		C	←	C								Relieves cough
DRY CORIANDER				X	X	X		X	C	C	C	X					X		Appetizer, promotes digestion, good for asthma, worms
DRIED GINGER				X			X		C		C	X					X		Improves digestion
BLACK PEPPER				X			X		C		C					X			Dehydrating
CUMIN				X			X		C		C					X			Promotes digestion, decreases diarrhea
TURMERIC				X	X	X	X												Helpful for peptic ulcer, diabetes
GARLIC				X			X								X		X		Reduces intestinal worms
SALT			X				X								X		X		Laxative, improves digestion; appetizer

* This is different from Western basil.

empirically. That is, different foods were tried and their results *(gunas)* were catalogued, and thus they were designated a certain *rasa*, a certain *virya* or a certain *vipaka*. It is for this reason that the *rasa* (taste) sometimes cannot accurately predict the *vipaka* or the *gunas* (properties). Moreover, foods and plants not described in the ancient writings must be tested out today, as well as new varieties of the ancient plants or even those grown under vastly different conditions or on markedly different soils.

AYURVEDA AND THE PATTERNS OF NATURE

The properties of the substance may be evident from the source of the food itself. For instance, the goat has the quality of being "dried up" and small. It also has a quickness, a lightness and a jumpiness that goes along with this.* The ability of goat's milk to reduce diarrhea and tighten the bowel movements is not surprising if one looks at the goat itself, whose feces are small and hard. The milk or meat of the water buffalo, however, stands in contrast. The water buffalo is an animal which is heavy, large, calm, quiet and slow to anger or movement. Its feces are copious, loose and mushy. Its products are considered to be very good for people who are underweight, undernourished and nervous. It tends to calm them down, to make them heavier, to strengthen and nourish them. In a similar way, the meat of certain birds is said, according to the traditional teachings, to be very good for heavy people. This is not as true, on the other hand, of those birds which are water dwellers.

The world of nature and the predominance of wild fruits, vegetables, herbs and game provided the Ayurvedic physicians with a rich store of foods having a wide variety of very specific effects. By prescribing food alone, along with a few herbal seasonings, they were able to have a great impact on a person's

---

* How the dry, constricting qualities of the goat's milk relate to the *vatic* aspects of his nature is reflected partly by the astringency of the milk. This can be better understood in relation to the *bhutas*, as demonstrated in Supplement I.

EFFECTS OF SPICES AND HERBS (CONTINUED)

	TASTE						VIRYA		DOSHA			POST DIGESTION EFFECT			PROPERTIES				
	SWEET	SOUR	SALTY	PUNGENT	ASTRINGENT	BITTER	HEATING	COOLING	KAPH, substance	PIT, fire-like	VAT, wind-like	SWEET	SOUR	PUNGENT	HEAVY	LIGHT	OILY/SMOOTH	DRY/ROUGH	
CELERY SEEDS	X			X					↓	↑	↓					X			Helpful in urinary disorders and nausea
ANISE SEED				X			X		↓	↑	↓					X			Promotes digestion, helpful in fever
DILL SEED				X			X		↓	↑	↓					X			Used in menstrual disorders, uterine pain
AJWAIN*				X		X	X			↑									Helps get rid of worms
CINNAMON	X			X		X				↓	↓								Decreases thirst, prevents dryness of mouth
CLOVES				X				X											Promotes digestion, helpful even with hyperacidity
SAFFRON						X			↓	↓	↓						X		Helps some headaches, reduces vomiting
FENUGREEK						X			↓		↓								Helpful in fever, some arthritis

*Also called "king's cumin," not commonly seen in the West.

health and often reversed serious chronic diseases.* Moreover, their theoretical framework, their conceptual scheme, based on *tridosha* and a holistic approach to observing the world of nature around them, permitted them to benefit from the complexity of natural substances.

This is why in Ayurvedic nutrition, one can deal with milk in dimensions that are quite impossible from the point of view of Western nutrition. Though goat's milk can be said, through the laboratory analysis of Western nutritionalists, to contain a bit less butterfat and perhaps more protein than cow's milk, according to Ayurveda, its unique properties can be deduced from its taste, which is somewhat astringent *(kashaya)*. Thus its tendency is to draw together, pull tight and cure diarrhea. This would lead one to think that it would be very effective in reducing weight which it has been found from experience to do, while the milk of the water buffalo has the opposite effect which the difference in its taste as well as the nature of the two animals would lead one to expect.

Ayurvedic nutrition is based on the concept that for each food, whether it is meat, fish, vegetable, fruit or milk, there is an essence or energy state or quality that can be identified and formulated. It can be partially identified through its taste and partially through the other properties which it is observed to manifest. Partly it can be identified by the observation of the personality or role of the plant or animal as it participates in the overall ecological system. Finally the essence of the food's effects can be formulated by using tridosha, a conceptual system that allows the physician enough breadth and depth to express such a holistic understanding. It is tridosha which has given the

---

* In India today, that capability has been greatly reduced. Not only are most of the foods domesticated, but their supply is short. In the Ayurvedic hospitals, where there is a basis for understanding which foods to prepare and prescribe, often it is not possible to provide them. In a land where there is overpopulation, specialized foods are an impossible luxury. In fact, to simply provide rice with a few beans and a little wheat is often sufficient strain on the hospital budget. For this reason, the best in Ayurvedic dietary treatment will seldom be found being practiced in India today, even though the knowledge is there.

	TASTE						VIRYA		DOSHA			POST DIGESTION EFFECT			PROPERTIES				
	SWEET	SOUR	SALTY	PUNGENT	ASTRINGENT	BITTER	HEATING	COOLING	KAPH, substance	PIT, fire-like	VAT, wind-like	SWEET	SOUR	PUNGENT	HEAVY	LIGHT	OILY/SMOOTH	DRY/ROUGH	
CARROT	X				X				C		C								Reduces hemorrhoids; avoid if pitta is disordered
ONION									↓	−	C				X				Appetizing, strengthening
MUSTARD GREENS*									↓	↓	↓								
CUCUMBER								X							X				
LAUKI (Indian summer squash)								X							X				Laxative
DILL GREENS									C	C	C								
TENDER RADISH									C	C	C								
LAMB'S QUARTERS	X				X		X		C	C	C					X			Stimulates digestion, helps hemorrhoids
OXALIS		X			X		X		C	C	C					X			
COOKED GREENS* (in general)	X														X				Loosens feces, slows digestion

* Should be boiled, drained and mixed with oil or fat. This removes strong medicinal principles.

EFFECTS OF VEGETABLES ACCORDING TO AYURVEDA

Ayurvedic physician the capacity to express his understanding of food in a way that is usable and practical since it can relate the uniqueness of the food to the present state of the person who is to eat it. Modern nutritional science in the West stands in dramatic contrast to this, of course. Here we have succeeded in attaining greater accuracy, dependability and predictability by studying much more limited and isolated components of food. By separating out the carbohydrates, the protein, or certain vitamins or minerals, we can make accurate predictions about how each will effect the body. Unfortunately, this is often difficult to relate to natural foods since each vegetable contains many nutrients and one may vary dramatically from the next in terms of its exact content of vitamins or minerals, and may include besides many other complex substances and properties which our analysis has overlooked. Thus, we might say that our Western analytic science of nutrition has attained greater precision at the expense of a sort of impoverishment: an apprediation of the richness and individuality of natural phenomena, both in the world of foods and in the world of human physiology, is lost.

Moreover, as we have seen before, a study of vitamins, minerals, and the other isolated components of food leaves us ill-equipped to deal with the practical situation of selecting this apple rather than that or one seasoning instead of another or one method of preparation of food instead of a second. The practical, everyday, experiential situation of eating or preparing food seems far divorced from Western laboratory research on nutrition. By contrast, the Oriental science of nutrition is organized around and based on personal experience. It is through the inner experience of taste and one's reaction to the food that he formulates its properties. It is one's individuality and experience of himself that allows a conceptualization of how his system is functioning, i.e., a "diagnosis" in terms of tridosha. The focus of Ayurvedic nutrition is on the interaction between the person and the food and the directly observed and experienced reactions that occur.

FRUIT	TASTE: SWEET	SOUR	SALTY	PUNGENT	ASTRINGENT	BITTER	VIRYA: HEATING	COOLING	DOSHA: KAPH, substance	PIT, fire-like	VAT, wind-like	POST DIGESTION EFFECT: SWEET	SOUR	PUNGENT	PROPERTIES: HEAVY	LIGHT	OILY/SMOOTH	DRY/ROUGH	
PEAR	X				X			X			←				X				
GRAPE	X							X	⟿	⟿	C						X		Strengthening, helps reduce alcoholism
RIPE PEACH	X						X								X				Strengthening, easily digested
COCONUT	X							X									X		Strengthening
FIG	X							X							X				Nourishing, delays digestion
APPLE	X				X			X											
GREEN BANANA					X				—										Constipating
BANANA (ripe)	X							X	←		C				X		X		Laxative
ORANGE	X	X					X				C				X				Increases appetite; difficult to digest
POMEGRANATE	X	X			X		X		— C	C	C						X		Stimulates digestion, reduces mucus

EFFECTS OF FRUITS ACCORDING TO AYURVEDA

Though Ayurveda is a medical science, its application is not limited to the physician. An understanding of the rudiments of Ayurveda is an important part of traditional education, and the physician's role is merely to be an expert or consultant in this area. The patient's role is to learn from the physician what he can about his own inner state, how it has become imbalanced, and how he can correct and prevent this through the proper selection of foods, herbs and condiments. The Ayurvedic physician is a teacher, and the patient takes over from him as treatment is terminated, the role of studying his own system, taking the management and maintenance of balance into his own hands.

Cooking

16

Perhaps it was the light of fire that pulled man into social contact, drawing him in groups around the mouth of his cave at night to savor the warmth of glowing coals and to recount the daily adventure of searching for food. It was perhaps his desire to show his find to his friends or to share it with them that led to his accumulating food and making a common meal. Some think that it was the wish to infuse the food with added energy that led to exposing it to the fire, roasting and cooking it. Whatever the precise origins, the complexities of food preparation seem to have begun with the birth of social gathering and to have increased with the development of agriculture and with the growth and expansion of villages, towns and cities, keeping pace with the freeing up of consciousness for the creativity and exploration that has characterized civilization at its best. At the present time, however, during this era of huge metropolises, things done in food preparation have become so numerous and lengthy as to fill shelves with cookbooks and in some cases to leave the food itself barely recognizable.

As we have seen, however, there are many pharmacologic

properties of common foodstuffs, such as compounds which are not nutrients in the usual sense of the word. Though this is especially true of seasonings, it is also true of the blandest fruits and vegetables. Heat can alter their properties, as can other techniques of food preparation, whether it be fermentation, marinating, or simply chopping and mixing together. When we stop a moment to remember the innumerable constituents and properties of the food and consider the almost endless ways that they can interact, we can only be awed by the complexity of what is too often dismissed as a menial job. Obviously, food preparation cannot be a science alone. Too many variables are involved for a logical analytical approach to be practical. An element of art is required, and our understanding of the chemistry and physics of cooking must be integrated with an humble study of the culinary traditions of those cultures where there is the most continuity and the best health.

If digestion is to be good, it is also important that food please the eye and that it appeal to the palate. Creative and constructive food preparation must be consistent with this principle. Properly performed, this task is an adventure. By contrast, when recipe books are slavishly followed without understanding why various ingredients are used, how they affect the body, or what purpose they serve in the dish, then cooking can degenerate into a chore which is boring and tiresome. But recipes need rarely to be followed exactly. There is actually little need to ever prepare the same dish twice. When one understands the basic principles of food preparation, he needs no recipes and he can combine the fresh and seasonal ingredients at hand into delicious and healthful meals. Though much of the art of cooking is best learned through personal experience of working in the kitchen with a truly accomplished cook, the following pages will at least give the aspiring student some grasp of the fundamental principles that underlie it.

COOKING WITH ACIDS

There are many processes through which food can be changed, altering its properties and its effects on the body. Exposure to heat is the most obvious and universally used, but "cooking" with acid is also a frequently used technique. In Central America, coastal peoples make a dish called *ceviche*, consisting of raw fish and minced onion "cooked" overnight by steeping it in lemon juice. A more commonly used dish which can be prepared by the use of acidic substances is curds (paneer), the homemade cottage cheese described earlier. This fresh cheese is highly valued for its ability to supply easily assimilated protein. In Ayurvedic terms, it increases solid *kapha*, that is, it promotes the production of tissue, lending substance to the body. The whey, by contrast, tends to pull water from the body and has a cleansing action. It is prized in the East for its ability to wash out the kidneys. Having had its solids removed, it is in a sense "empty" and thus capable of taking up and removing unwanted wastes from the body.

Through the simple process of adding lemon juice to milk, two distinct substances are created—cheese and whey. Their properties are vastly different from those of milk or lemon juice, and yet an analysis of the milk and lemon juice before and after the transformation would certainly show the same total quantities of carbohydrate, fat, protein, vitamins and minerals. What has occurred is, in fact, a pharmacologic process creating from one food a new one which will have different effects. Besides lemon juice, other acidic substances such as vinegar are also used for this purpose in the preparation of marinated meats, beans, and so forth. In this process, the acid begins the hydrolysis of the protein in much the same way as hydrochloric acid in the stomach does, and both reactions aid digestion by beginning the breakdown of protein chains. Even foods cooked in tomato sauce probably take advantage of this principle to some extent. Sometimes "cooking" by acids results from fermentation. In part, this is what happens during the making of cheese though the initial curdling is accomplished by the addition of rennet, an enzyme extracted from the stomachs of calves.

COOKING BY MICRO-ORGANISMS

After curdling, aged cheeses are stored for some time during which a variety of microbes begin to grow. The protein is broken down somewhat by the acids produced during this "ripening" process. The exact bacteria, fungi and yeasts which grow in the cheese determine the flavor and consistency that it develops. The longer such cheese is aged, the more the protein is "pre-digested," but at the same time, the compounds produced by the growth of microbes increase in quantity so the taste is "stronger" and the likelihood of significant amounts of medicinal substances being present is increased. Some cheeses, for example, tend to elevate the blood pressure.[1]

The art of making such cheeses is a delicate one, and the techniques which evolved over hundreds of years have been handed down from generation to generation. The development of the necessary microbes is easily disrupted when the cheesemaking process is shifted from one locale to another or when milk from cows pastured on different land is used or when the cheese is made in a different season. For these reasons, many of the modern commercial cheeses that are made in an attempt to reproduce the flavors of traditional ones are of inferior quality.

Unless one can be sure that aged cheeses were produced with skill, care and understanding, it is best to avoid them. Fresh cheeses, such as those made with lemon juice, provide a convenient alternative. Soft curds which are not aged are marketed in the West as "cottage cheese," but most of them contain a number of added conditioners, flavorings and other superfluous ingredients which may detract from their nutritional value and which certainly ruin their taste.

"Processed cheese" is made by heating aged cheese which has been ground and mixed with certain chemical compounds that help it to melt and maintain its consistency. After it is poured into containers it hardens and keeps well, probably because most of the microbes are killed.[2]

The growth of micro-organisms is used in many dishes throughout the world to initiate the digestion of protein. This is part of the reason for making miso, a soybean paste produced by the growth of microbes which break down the soy protein into smaller chains that are more easily absorbed. In much of the South Pacific, where soy beans are a staple, over 70% of them are eaten in the form of *tempeh*. This is produced by mixing the pre-cooked beans with a culture of a local fungus which soon converts them into a tight, fuzzy, mold-covered lump that can be sliced and fried. As unappealing as it may sound, the finished product is often quite delicious, resembling fish or chicken in taste, and its protein is much more easily assimilated than that of the unprocessed beans.

During the Second World War, Americans in a Japanese prisoner of war camp tell of having great difficulty digesting the soy beans they were allotted when they were simply boiled for as long as their scanty supply of fuel permitted. One of the prisoners, who was Dutch, recalling his experiences in the Dutch East Indies, threw a gunny sack over the soy beans, and allowed them to mold. The improvised *tempeh* was easy to digest and became a popular dish thereafter for those in the prison camp. Moreover, during the preparation of *tempeh*, there is an increase in some B vitamins, riboflavin, niacin, and especially B_{12}[3] which may be a crucial matter for vegetarians who eat no milk products or eggs. Some nutrients such as thiamin (vitamin B_1), lysine and methionine are reduced, however.[4] The latter are essential amino acids which already tend to be low in the vegetarian diet.

Unfortunately, the action of molds can be unpredictable

so that flavor and properties vary. This probably means the production by the mold of potentially active pharmacological substances. Even when the culture which is used is pure, there is no insurance against the growth of contaminating spores. Related molds, *Aspergillus flavus,* produce aflatoxins which are highly toxic.[5] In the South Pacific, however, one day's *tempeh* is used as a starter for the next day's batch, and the appropriate molds predominate in the air and dust. The culture is incubated by wrapping it in a banana leaf and leaving it in the warm, tropical air, and so results are probably wholesome. Nevertheless, no research has yet been done on the possible untoward effects of substances produced by undesirable molds growing during *tempeh* production.

These forms of "cooking" deserve that term because they initiate, in some way, the process of digestion. The application of heat also does this, and therein lies its primary value. The exact degree and manner in which this predigestion is carried out will determine to a great extent the properties and effects of the food.

IRON SKILLETS AND COPPER KETTLES

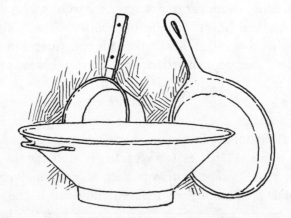

Cooking with heat is, of course, the most common method of predigestion used, but it is by no means the least complicated.

It also breaks down the complex molecules to some extent, but it may change them into new compounds as well. These effects are balanced by the positive aspects of cooking such as the rupture of cellulose cell walls which, as we have noted, makes the nutrients more available. Exactly how the constituents of food are altered chemically during the process of cooking probably depends on a multitude of factors. Not only is the degree of heat important, but it is likely that there is also a role played by the kind of cooking oil and seasonings which are used, and by the type of utensil involved. The metal with which the food comes in contact during the chemical reactions of cooking is very important since metals may serve as catalysts during some of these reactions.[6] If in fact the organic compounds in foods can act as chelating agents, taking up metals from the surfaces of such cooking utensils, quite valuable trace elements may be produced. This could be the reason that certain cooking utensils have been traditionally preferred.

Cast iron utensils such as skillets are among the most ideal for cooking since they are usually thick and heavy and thus distribute the heat more evenly, maintaining the cooking food at a more uniform temperature. This prevents having one part of the food underheated while another part is being scorched. The heavy-bottomed skillet permits a sort of roasting of vegetables so that, held at a constant temperature in the absence of water, they can be tenderized, dehydrated to some extent, and yet maintain their shape and flavor.

Cast iron utensils should be manufactured in such a way that the inner surface is smooth and not of a rough-grained texture. In order for them to perform satisfactorily, one must care for them properly. Abrasive cleaners should be used sparingly, though any accumulation of food or burnt material should be removed until the inner surface is smooth and clean. After each use the skillet should be well dried by setting it back on the fire for a moment and then it should be oiled. When cared for properly in this way for some time, the surface of the cast iron develops a smooth, tough coating of carbon, and the tendency of food to stick to it is diminished. Cast iron pots and pans should never be left with water or acid foods standing in them since they will then begin to rust and/or discolor the food. It is said that some of the vitamin C in foods may be destroyed during this reaction. Though the iron which is taken up by the food during its reaction with the utensil is probably not harmful and may even be useful, the inner coating of the utensil is broken down by this and its interaction with the food is further accentuated. If it is maintained properly, however, cast iron is essentially care-free. In addition, it is time-tested and almost universally considered to be healthful and safe.

Pottery cookware has been used even longer than iron, and grains or beans baked in an earthenware pot have a remark-able flavor. In India, specially made crockery pots are used over the fire. Modern pottery, however, is often glazed with com-pounds which contain lead, or, if the glaze is red or yellow, cadmium. Cooking foods in such pots for a long period of time, or allowing foods, especially those which are acidic, to stand in contact with glazed surfaces may leach out some of the lead or cadmium and contaminate the food. This is much less true of glass or white porcelain.

Stainless steel, though a relatively modern innovation, seems safe and is quite serviceable. There has been some sug-gestion that the chromium in the stainless steel might combine with the foods that have been cooked in such utensils though there is no indication that this is harmful. Copper and brass are, however, according to tradition in India where they have been used since antiquity, not suitable for cooking. Again, this may be because of their tendency to release copper into the food, thereby elevating copper levels in the body, a situation which, as we have seen, can cause significant problems. On the other hand, copper and brass kettles are considered excellent for boiling water and are thought in some way to purify it.

Aluminum utensils are relative new-comers to the kitchen,

and the safety of their use is controversial. Foods cooked in aluminum pots and pans take up small amounts of aluminum from the utensils.[7, 8] More, however, is taken up when the food is alkaline.[9] It was shown many years ago that when such aluminum was ingested, it was absorbed into the blood,[10] but it was thought that the small quantities entering with food in this way from cooking utensils were harmless. Aluminum compounds occur in generous quantities in the earth's crust and it was reasoned that if such quantities of aluminum were harmful, surely man and many animals would have shown signs of toxicity long before aluminum pots and pans came along.[11] Moreover, the quantities present in natural foods are greater than those obtained from pots and pans. However, the naturally occurring forms are not necessarily identical to those resulting from an interaction of the food and the utensil and could even have opposite effects in the body. Although aluminum is absorbed only in small quantities, the majority of it combines with phosphorus in the intestine, creating insoluble compounds which pass out with the feces.[12] Some thought that this could lead to calcium deficiencies, since phosphates were thought to be necessary for combination with calcium if it is to be absorbed, and some writers even suggested that aluminum, by indirectly depriving the body of calcium, was responsible for many allergic symptoms.   There have been reports of improvements when allergic patients who had been exposed to aluminum were given calcium supplements.[13]

Based on this principle, very large doses of aluminum have been recently used to intentionally tie-up and remove phosphorus in patients who are on an artificial kidney and unable to get rid of phosphates. This was considered a safe treatment since the aluminum compounds were thought to be harmless, but it has been found that the dose must be carefully regulated or one can pull too much phosphorus from the body.[14] It seems possible that the use of large amounts of antacids (which are usually aluminum gels) could do the same thing.[15]   Though letters

continued to appear in reputable medical journals deprecating
the "myth of aluminum toxicity,"[16] more serious problems
began to emerge. In one study, a number of patients on kidney
machines fell ill with a mysterious brain condition, causing
mental disturbance, inability to speak clearly, recurrent epileptic seizures and finally death. On autopsy it was found that
the involved areas of the brain contained four times the usual
levels of aluminum.[17] A similar brain disease has been produced
in experimental animals by injecting aluminum compounds.[18]
The idea that aluminum is responsible for such brain damage has
not been universally accepted, and controversy continues, but
the evidence that it is seems to be accumulating. Of course
patients such as those on a kidney machine or ulcer patients on
antacids are taking aluminum in much larger quantities than one
gets through contamination from pots and pans. Nevertheless,
recent articles in respected medical journals have begun to raise
the question of whether small amounts of aluminum ingested
regularly might not produce a slight but significant degree of
damage to the brain.

Besides contamination of food from pots and pans, aluminum also enters the body in baking powders, most of which
contain high percentages of it. Though some cities even add
aluminum compounds to the water supply to eliminate murki-
ness, there are so far no standards set for the amount of aluminum permissable.[19] Case reports from physicians have trickled
in steadily over the years, suggesting that aluminum in the diet
could cause a whole spectrum of ills, ranging from colitis to
stomach ulcers and asthma.[20, 21] It is well known that aluminum
compounds such as those in popular antacids can cause constipation, though again the dosage may be important.

While it may be true that the small doses of aluminum
may have relatively little effect in some people, in others, who
happen to be more sensitive to even tiny amounts, small quantities may be important. Meanwhile in the East, aluminum utensils
are universally regarded as "the poor man's " pots, and their use

is considered to be unhealthy. No one who can afford better will use them.

An even more recent addition to the available selection of kitchen utensils is plastic coated metal such as teflon. These surfaces have become popular because they prevent food from sticking to them, but the effects on food cooked in contact with such materials has not been carefully explored. It is well known that chemical reactions can occur between food and plastic containers.[22]   On the one hand, cooking on a utensil with a plastic surface might be expected to accelerate reactions between the plastic and the food since temperatures are higher than those used for storage, while on the other hand, one might argue that any active compounds in the teflon coating would be taken up by the food during the first few times it is used, thereby rendering it safe for subsequent usage. In any case, the use of such synthetic materials on a large scale is another experiment of sorts, and with time we should have a better understanding of what it does.

POTS AND PANS: DEEP OR SHALLOW?

The metal of which a utensil is made is not the only important variable. The shape of a pot or pan is also a consideration and has a great deal to do with the way the food cooks. Deeper pots tend to hold moisture inside and keep much of the cooking food submerged. This is especially true, of course, when a deep pot is filled. This is one reason why it is usually found that when large quantities of a dish are prepared the results are different from those produced when a small amount is made. Sauteed or stir-fried vegetables made for twenty-five people often turn out limp and sad even though the proportions of ingredients are carefully controlled. Stews, porridges and bean dishes, however, are favored for cooking on a large scale and give good results. Foods cooking in the center of a huge vessel apparently undergo a more constant temperature and a somewhat increased pressure.

This effect can be magnified by cooking in a pressure cooker. Here the expanding gases resulting from the heat are trapped, and the pressure is forced to increase in the pot.

The use of pressure cookers has been somewhat controversial, some people claiming that they reduce cooking time and thereby minimize the destruction of nutrients, whereas others have discouraged their use, claiming that they destroy the food through the increased pressure. Probably both are true and the two effects usually cancel each other out,[23] as long as cooking time is carefully regulated. It is certainly true, however, that pressure cookers should be used cautiously since food can be very quickly overcooked and turned into mush.

It has been said that pressure cookers are a "new" device and that, since we have had insufficient experience with foods cooked in them, we therefore know too little of their effects to justify their use. Actually, however, the use of pressure cooking is not as new as one might think. In many cultures, heavy iron lids have been used for centuries, and during the preparation of certain foods, further pressure was often created by placing huge stones on top of the lid. It is clear that pressure cooking provides great savings in time and fuel, especially in the preparation of certain dried beans and peas, such as soybeans, that are hard to cook. It is also very helpful in cooking some vegetables such as collards or other leafy greens which would otherwise be too tough or fibrous to be properly digested or enjoyed.

Even when an unpressurized, lidless pot contains only a small amount of food, if it is deep it will give a different effect than one which is shallow. If sauteing is attempted in a deep pot, the high sides prevent moisture from escaping and the pieces of food tend to cook "wet." This is the principle of the "waterless cooker" which, while not necessarily deep, is covered to give the same effect. Though vegetables break down and lose liquid as a result, this is served along with them. A steaming rack which unfolds in the bottom of a pot allows cooking of a similar nature, but it is the rising steam from boiling water underneath the rack that does the cooking. This is often said to cook the food at a lower temperature, but in fact not enough research has been done to know its exact effects.[24] It is obvious that the vegetables lose some liquid into the steaming water, which is colored and strong in taste, and this probably represents a significant loss of nutrients. Nevertheless, steamed vegetables are light and refreshing and may have other valuable properties not yet identified.

In a shallow skillet, since the food is more exposed to air and evaporation, moisture is lost more easily than in deeper pots, and foods cook "drier." A wok (or, as it is called in India, "karhai") creates a more complicated situation. Because of its conical structure, it allows a fairly high degree of drying, but this at the option of the cook. The food can be spread up the slanted sides of the wok so that it functions much as a skillet, or it can be scraped down into the center where it cooks as though it were in a pot. This means that a certain degree of skill is required on the part of the cook. Actually, the situation is even more complex than that, for a temperature gradient is also created along the sides of the wok. At one level the temperature will be quite high, much as that required for quick frying, whereas above or below that, the surface will be somewhat cooler so that the food cooks in a more gradual way. The result is such that when one sautes or stir-fries in a wok, he must be constantly tuned in to the pieces of food, rearranging them and turning them as necessary to assure the effect desired.

Where the hottest level along the side of the wok is located depends to a great extent on the intensity and shape of the heat source beneath it. When a fire is used, the shape of the flame is important. Using a wok over a ring-shaped gas flame is quite different from using one on a wood fire. A wide ring of flames will leave the center cool while overheating the sides whereas a small circle of flame overheats the center while leaving the sides cool.

There may be other differences between foods cooked

over various kinds of heat sources, but our laboratory techniques have not been sensitive enough to detect them. Despite this lack of scientific verification, the people of many cultures maintain that food cooked over an open wood fire tastes better, and in some traditions it is believed that the value of the food is highest when so cooked and that it decreases as one moves from wood to coal to gas to electric heat.

Modern microwave cooking involves a totally different principle, however. Heat is not applied to the food—it is generated in it. Exactly what this does to the delicate molecules of the foodstuffs or to what extent the human body is equipped to handle food cooked in this way remains to be seen. In any case, it is clear that the food is affected differently by microwave radiation than it is by fire. Microwaves cook the food from the inside out so that the central part of a baking potato for example, gets hot first. It is this which allows the delighted owners of a microwave oven to boil a cup of water in a plastic cup without melting the cup. Cooking with heat, by contrast, cooks food from the outside inward and is more successful in shrinking, contracting or "yang-izing" vegetables. When heat is used, foods can be roasted with their surface in contact with the utensil, a cooking oil, or water, and selected spices, seasonings, salt, and so forth can be added. The result is a complex interaction which can be varied in a multitude of ways, each combination giving a subtle but characteristic twist to the cooking process.

This is especially true on the surface of food where temperatures are more extreme. Here there is something called a "browning reaction," one example of which involves an interaction between amino acids and sugars in the food.* As a result of this, the amino acids may be converted into compounds which cannot be used by the body. Most often the amino acid involved is lysine, one of the essential eight.[25]   Since lysine is

---

* The sugar must be present either as a natural constituent of the food, or as an added ingredient. Thus a loaf of bread which contains natural sugars browns well, but a ham must be glazed with added sugar to develop a rich color.

the limiting amino acid in most grains, browning may significantly decrease the usable protein in a diet which is mainly grains.   Legumes are relatively more rich in lysine, however, and if they are taken with grains, one need not worry so much about the losses incurred during browning.   When the browning is primarily of carbohydrate, the process is called "caramelization."   Though the flavor and color produced is familiar, the way in which the nutritional value of the caramelized sugars and starches is altered is not well understood.   Such reactions are an important part of other cooking techniques that develop the flavors we rely on to make our food more appetizing.   They may even alter it in beneficial ways which we don't yet understand.   Certainly it is true that despite the losses incurred through browning reactions the roasting of wheat cakes and breads is common throughout the world and the sale of electric toasters continues unabated.   As we have seen before, these processes may be important in disrupting the chelation of important minerals by partially or completely destroying the large molecules which hold them.   Thus, while a moderate degree of browning may enhance certain properties of a food such as flavor and aroma, if it is overdone, minerals may be reduced to an unusable form or a significant amount of vitamins may be destroyed by the heat.

Browning reactions also affect taste.   The way in which an onion is roasted, for example, will change its flavor entirely. Different methods of cutting (in rings, chopping, etc.) and different rates of stirring while cooking at different heats produce different results as well.   Slow roasting produces a sweeter flavor, while roasting the onion a long time at medium heat will produce a rich meaty taste that is very much favored by those who have not yet become accustomed to a vegetarian diet or who like hearty meals.

Adding water early in the cooking will ruin the roasted flavor of the onion, but even after having cooked in water, onions can dry out, brown around the edges and produce interesting and unique flavors. A few well roasted onions can become a seasoning which stimulate the appetite, perhaps even adding something unknown but valuable to the food.

Fats are also altered by high temperatures, and this may, as we saw earlier, convert them into toxic compounds. This is especially true when foods and oils are kept at a high temperature for a long period of time or are used repeatedly. Vegetable oils especially tend to become rancid as a result of this, picking up highly reactive oxygen that tends to damage the cellular components. They may also polymerize, forming new harmful compounds such as benzene. When oils and fats are used in small quantities to fry or "saute" foods, the oil is then incorporated into the dish and the moisture of the vegetables, for example, keeps temperatures down, reducing the possibility of their being overcooked or damaged. Besides this, an important dietary goal is a low percentage of fats in the total caloric intake.

FATS AND OILS IN COOKING

In the Far East, where dairying is not common, vegetable oils are usually used for cooking purposes. Peanut oil is particularly prized because it deteriorates less than other oils upon heating and will not "gum up" utensils like corn oil will, for example. However, the safety of vegetable oils in general is questionable, as we have previously seen. Nevertheless, in South India, because of their availability, vegetable oils are used as a cooking medium in much the same way as they are used in China and Japan. Here, however, more tropical vegetable oils and fats, such as coconut oil and palm oil, are used. Sesame oil is occasionally used and is said to be the slowest of all vegetable oil to deteriorate on storage. Safflower oil *(kusumms)* is considered the most dangerous and harmful of all the vegetable oils.[26] Mustard seed oil is sometimes used for special effects or by those who cannot afford clarified butter, but is not considered ideal.

In Northern India, by contrast, where the use of dairy products is traditional, clarified butter or ghee is the most highly regarded of all cooking media. Clarified butter is preferred as a cooking fat because it is considered to have unique properties. It is said that this ghee has the power to retard deterioration of food and to magnify the nutritional value of its constituents. There is no laboratory research to support the notion that vitamins or minerals become more active or effective or are better absorbed when they're taken with butterfat except in the case of calcium where there is some evidence that this is so.[27] It is known, however, that the clarification of butter by heating it until the water-soluble part can be removed does eliminate most of the perishable constituents of the butter and that the clear liquid or ghee which can be poured off will keep for long periods without refrigeration, undergoing little or no deterioration. If it is properly prepared, ghee seems to retain almost all the nutritional value of the butter.[28] Unfortunately in much of India, the use of hydrogenated vegetable oil has, because of its lower price, largely displaced clarified butter much as it has displaced the use of lard in other parts of the world. Sold under the name of "vegetable ghee," it has become so common that genuine ghee is virtually unknown to many Indians.

Ghee is certainly more convenient for cooking than unprocessed butter since it will not scorch or turn black when heated to the temperatures that are needed for frying or sauteing. The water soluble milk solids that turn black when butter is used for frying are removed during the ghee making process. This principle is also familiar to the French who often use clarified butter in their *haute cuisine.* According to Indian tradition, ghee, when fried with spices, takes on the properties of those spices, diffusing them through the food. The combination of ghee and spice may be used as a seasoning agent *(tarka)* for food or as a medicinal preparation. Because of the properties ascribed to it, ghee is often used in traditional medicines, and there is, in fact, a whole category of Ayurvedic medicines called *ghritas* which are prepared from a base of ghee.

COOKING WITH SPICES

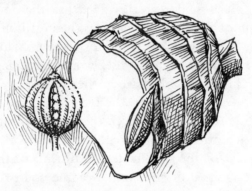

Although Indian dishes have a reputation for being hotly spiced, this is not true of all regions of India. In the non-urban areas of the North and in the Himalayas, seasonings are simple though tasty and are especially designed to enhance the health. In fact, most Indian dishes, whether they are primarily of vegetables or of beans, rely on mild spices fried in ghee to give them flavor, preserve their quality and increase their digestibility. The good cook uses these seeds and herbs in moderation to subtly complement the natural flavors of the food. A wide variety of such seasonings may be used, depending on the region, on what is available locally, and on the tastes and customs of the people.

In other areas the spices used are quite strong and medicinal, and while they may be of particular value in one season, in one food, or for one particular person, they may well be undesirable under other circumstances. Asafoetida, for example, (or *hing* as it is known in the East) an aromatic resin with an overpowering (and to most people, offensive) odor which comes from a Middle Eastern tree, was a highly regarded medicine in Europe and America in earlier days. It was worn around the neck in the wintertime to scare away colds, which it most likely did, along with anyone who might have one. In India and Pakistan it is used in tiny quantities for the unique savor that it lends spicy dishes, but those who are not accustomed to it may develop a puzzling diarrhea after having inadvertently eaten it. Asafoetida is also reputed to be a powerful antidote to homeopathic remedies.

The exact blend of spices and herbs and how they are cooked and combined with the food is a fine and extremely delicate art. A few seconds more of frying a spice may totally distort or destroy its properties, changing it from a beneficial addition to a harmful one. Practice soon brings a satisfying skill, however, and varying the technique of frying can produce an endless variety of taste experiences. Of all the herbs and spices used in Eastern cooking, there are a few whose use is most universal because they are most often appropriate, mild and are practically never harmful. Probably the most common of these in India are cumin, turmeric and coriander, and there are few dishes which do not contain these three basic spices. Actually, "spice" is not really the correct term in this case because these three seasonings do not have the harshness nor the pungent aroma one usually associates with a "spice." They are much milder and less obtrusive and are used primarily for their ability to promote digestion rather than merely for their flavor. It is consonant with Ayurvedic theory, however, to find that they do improve the taste appeal of the food. Using them with different degrees of cooking or roasting can produce a wide spectrum of effects, lending foods a hearty, meaty kind of savor which vegetarian dishes often otherwise lack. These seasonings, called collectively *masala* in Hindi serve much the same purpose in Indian cooking as does miso in the cuisine of Japan. Both give a rich body to the dish, although because of the problems with miso mentioned earlier, a *masala* of turmeric, cumin and coriander will usually constitute a seasoning of more dependable quality.

Such a combination of spices can be added to the water in

which vegetables and beans are cooking to cook along with them, but it is more common to fry them in fat before they are added to the food. Not only do they aid digestion in a general way, but each of these three seasonings has its own unique properties. Turmeric is considered to have beneficial effects on the skin, and it is said that Indian women owe their velvety complexions to the daily intake of turmeric in their foods. Researchers in India are presently looking into the traditional belief that turmeric prevents cancer and that it has a beneficial effect on diabetics. Turmeric is a tropical plant, and South Indians eat its bright yellow root raw like horseradish, the taste of which it somewhat resembles. The turmeric powder familiar to most Americans is made by boiling the roots and then drying them, after which they are ground.

Cumin is mentioned several times in the Bible, and the Romans took the ground seed medicinally, regarding it highly as a condiment. Even before that, it was used in Egypt, India and China, and today its addition to bean dishes is traditional around the world. A true Texan would not consider cooking his pinto beans without the cumin (or "comino") which also serves as the major ingredient in his "chili powder." The Indian or Pakistani also regards cumin as an essential ingredient in *dahl*, the staple dish made from dried beans or peas which is taken with nearly every meal. This is not surprising since cumin has long been used medicinally to correct intestinal gas, to stimulate digestion, and as a remedy for colic or for the headache that comes from an upset stomach.[29] In India, cumin water (*jira jala*) is still taken after meals by those who have digestion problems. Cumin is usually used in somewhat larger quantities than turmeric, but probably the seasoning used most generously in Indian cooking is coriander.

Coriander has been used since antiquity in India, Europe and Africa. Even the indigenous peoples of Peru and much of Latin America consider it an essential part of their traditional cooking. It was also a favorite of American settlers who used it to season their sausages and meats. Ground coriander seed was also used as a flavoring in confections, and it is still sometimes preferred to cinnamon for spicing an apple pie. The part of the plant which is used is the "seed" (which is actually a fruit). These are gathered after they have been dried and then are ground for cooking. Because of its pleasant flavor, an extract of coriander seeds is often used in medicines to disguise their unpleasant taste. In the case of laxatives, for example, it also reduces their cramping tendency. The medicinal oils in the coriander powder have long been known for their ability to reduce gas in the intestinal tract. In many areas of the world, the leaves are also used and are called "celantro" in Spanish America, where they lend a characteristic flavor to soups and rice dishes. Known as "Chinese parsley" in areas where Far Eastern cooking is familiar, they are chopped into many Oriental dishes. In India, the green leaves are considered the most healthful of all vegetables and are universally used whenever available.

Other spices and herbs are also used in Indian cooking. Black pepper, ginger, black mustard seeds and fenugreek are among the most commonly used of the milder and more healthful seasonings. Though black pepper is a native of South India, it very early became popular in Europe. It is said that Attila the Hun demanded, among other items, 3,000 pounds of black pepper in ransom for the city of Rome. Even today it is the one Indian spice which has worked its way onto the table of every American home. Its medicinal properties depend on a pungent resin which is a carminative, that is, it decreases gas in the intestinal tract. Pepper corns are prepared as an Ayurvedic remedy which is used in treating sinus and digestive problems. The pepper stimulates the mucus membranes of the rectum and so is good for constipation. Its stimulating action also aids upper intestinal digestion as well. It is said to be helpful when the stomach is sluggish, or in Ayurvedic terms, it is said to stimulate the digestive fire. Black pepper is usually not fried as much as other spices like cumin, turmeric and coriander and may be added toward the end of cooking. White pepper is really black pepper with the black outer cover of the pepper corn, which is the most pungent part, removed before grinding.

Ginger is the tuberous root of a tropical plant that apparently originated in India. It is sliced as a vegetable into some pungent Chinese dishes, but in India it is generally grated or browned and may occasionally be fried along with the *masala* (spices) to lend variety to the seasoning of vegetable and bean dishes. It is also an important ingredient of some sweet Indian relishes or chutneys, where it may be used along with other ingredients such as apples, raisins, cloves and cinnamon. The flavor and texture of the ginger root varies according to the season when it was gathered and the length of time it has been stored. The older roots tend to be tough, fibrous and strong tasting whereas the younger roots are more tender and mild. Ginger roots are seen in every market place in India as well as in the West Indies and are now often available in Western supermarkets. When the root is dried, it can be ground into the ginger powder which is familiar to those living in non-tropical areas. Ginger tea, made by simply steeping ground ginger in boiled water, is sometimes helpful for those who have excessive mucus.

Black mustard seeds have similar properties to ginger and black pepper and are fried along with other seasonings until they begin to pop. Ground fenugreek is used and has a calming effect despite its bitter taste. It has a maple-like flavor and aroma and is an important ingredient in many commercial "curry powders." Actually, a good cook will not use pre-mixed *masala* but will make his own "curry powder" as he cooks, adding the various seasonings in their proper proportions as they are needed. Using a base such as turmeric, cumin and coriander fried in a bit of ghee, and occasionally adding other spices such as fenugreek, mustard seed, ginger or a dash of red pepper for variety, one can create a wide variety of tastes and effects. These spices, cooked in ghee with onions, form the basis for many Indian dishes such as *dahl* which is made from legumes.

Preparing Legumes
(Dahl)

Beans and peas are the key to a healthful vegetarian diet. In fact, it is difficult to plan a healthy meatless diet without using legumes in some form or other. The preparation of the legume, however, is one of the greatest challenges to the skill of a good cook. If they are improperly prepared, they taste coarse, bland and are an unpleasant cause of troublesome intestinal gas. If they are properly prepared they can be delicious, flavorful and easily digested. The key, of course, is combining them correctly with oil, spices and heat.

In preparing legumes, the first step is to carefully sort them to eliminate any pebbles, debris or defective beans. Next, they should be washed with lukewarm water. Soaking the legume overnight (especially soy beans or chick peas) increases their vitality and digestability. The following basic recipe for dahl can be adapted for any bean or pea:

Place two cups of washed and sorted mung beans in a pressure cooker and add three or four inches of hot water. Cover, bring to pressure and let cook for ten to fifteen minutes. The more delicate legumes such as split mung require little cooking time while the heavier ones such as whole soybeans need more. After it has been pressured for a while, turn off the heat and let the dahl cool without opening the pot.

Meanwhile, as the legume is cooking in the pressure cooker, place three tablespoons of ghee in a cast iron skillet and heat it on a medium flame. When it is hot, fry one teaspoon of turmeric, then two teaspoons of cumin and finally three teaspoons of ground coriander until brown, being careful not to burn the spices. Mustard seed or grated ginger root is sometimes added. Next, fry one large sliced onion until browned and then one cup of sliced mushrooms until they are also browned. Green pepper and tomato are also used on occasion. The fried vegetables and seasonings should be well-browned, or, if a heartier taste is desired, quite dark.

Now, open the cooled pressure cooker and pour the mixture into the beans, adding one and a half teaspoons of salt and hot, boiled water if necessary to thin it. Turn up the heat under the pot and cook the mixture uncovered for another five to ten minutes, or long enough so that the beans are soft and the mixture soupy.

Only a small amount of dahl is necessary to balance a meal, usually less than a ½ cup, and in India it is dished up in tiny bowls, serving as a gravy to be spooned over rice, a dip for bread, or a sauce to be stirred into the other ingredients of the meal.

* See *Himalayan Mountain Cookery* by Mrs. R. Ballentine, Sr., p. 89-109 for various dahl recipes.

Beans and peas are the key to a healthful vegetarian diet. In fact, it is difficult to plan a healthy meatless diet without using legumes in some form or other. Research has also shown that they are important in combating arteriosclerosis and heart disease[30, 31] so that they are also a healthful addition to the diet of meat-eaters. Of course, one of their major functions is complementing the protein contained in grains and increasing its value. As we saw earlier, by adding ten to twenty per cent as much legume as grain to a meal, its nutritional value is greatly enhanced.

But the preparation of the legume is one of the greatest challenges to the skill of a good cook. If they are improperly prepared, they taste coarse, bland and unpleasant and are, as mentioned earlier, notorious for their tendency to cause troublesome intestinal gas. If they are properly prepared, however, they can be delicious, flavorful and easily digested. The key, of course, is how they are combined with fat, spices and heat.

European cooking traditions include the use of leafy herbs such as rosemary, thyme, marjoram, sage and oregano. In most cases these also have digestion-promoting qualities, but each of them has other medicinal qualities as well and should be used advisedly. They are generally added near the end of cooking, since the leaves are more delicate and the aromas are destroyed by too much heat.

REFINING AND PRESERVING

Flavorings and seasonings are usually added to pre-packaged convenience and snack foods by the food industry, not on the basis of their ability to promote digestion or add healthful qualities to the food, but to increase taste appeal and to cover up the unpleasant effects of other additives or to restore flavor to an over-refined food. Food refining is another important way of processing food, and in some ways its purpose is similar to that of cooking or fermenting. It is often carried out to remove the less digestible part of the food, making it easier to break down and absorb. Beyond a certain point, of course, this becomes more harmful than helpful, since one eventually begins to remove valuable nutrients from the food. For example, we have seen that a 93% extraction rate flour may be more easily handled and more healthful than whole wheat. But in most of the commercial flours in America, more and more of the wheat is removed until, when one reaches a 60% extraction rate, 40% of the grain has been lost and its nutritional value is seriously compromised.*

More often than not, refining is carried out to remove the more perishable parts of the food so that it can be stored better. This is the case with refined flour, from which the perishable germ has been removed. Preservation is also sometimes given as a rationale for refining sugar. In other cases, storage time of foods is increased not by removing the perishable components but by sterilizing it and enclosing it in an air-tight, germ-free container. Though it may be done in glass jars, this process is generally called "canning" since, when it was first done in Europe, hand-made metal containers were used. In order that they might not rust, the inner surfaces were coated with tin. This practice persisted, and even today Englishmen speak of "tinned" food, though many cans are made of other metals now. More recently it has become practical to freeze food, storing it at a low enough temperature that the bacteria and other microbes which would return it to the soil cannot take hold. In each case, however, the rationale remains the same: nutritional value is sacrificed to gain prolonged storage.

Before the technological capacity for canning and freezing was available, whatever food preserving occurred was primarily done through salting and drying the food. Salting creates such a chemically impossible situation for microbes that they cannot grow. Drying accomplishes much the same purpose by removing

* See Chapter 4, Carbohydrates

all the moisture that would be necessary for the growth of micro-organisms. Drying is of particular interest here since in many cases it appears that the tissue of the fruit or vegetable continues to function to some extent during at least part of the drying process. In any case, there is a transformation that occurs so that after drying, fruits high in manganese, for example, are found to contain less manganese but more iron.[32] Formerly, most drying was done through exposure to the sun, but nowadays, special drying ovens are used. Apparently no research has been done to explore the difference in these two processes.

Some fruits and vegetables can be stored alive. This is particularly true of root vegetables such as onions, potatoes and carrots which, in the days before refrigeration, freezing and canning, were the mainstays of a winter diet for most people living in temperate climates. Many such vegetables can be stored in a root cellar, though onions need a drier environment. In fact, in most areas, root crops can be wintered over if they are covered with a heavy mulch. They can then be pulled fresh as needed. Sprouts are invaluable in winter. Dried beans, peas and grains which are also in a natural storage form are always available and can be transformed with a few days exposure to moisture into a live fresh vegetable. They are often soaked for a few hours or overnight even when cooked in the ordinary way, to begin to "bring them to life," but the longer this process continues, the less the bean or grain is a "seed" and the more it is becoming a fresh, leafy "vegetable."

When combined with occasional sprouts, the use of such root crops, along with grains and beans which are also in a natural storage form, can largely eliminate the need for canned, frozen and refined foods. While in some situations, the occasional use of artificially preserved foods is unavoidable, on the whole it is best not to remove foods from the flow of nature. To do so encourages the growth not only of bacteria, but insects, rats and all of the other vermin by means of which nature tries to recycle that which is stagnant and to which the hoarders of civilization usually fall prey.   Besides, if the food is processed so as to be unsuitable nourishment for scavengers, then it is not likely to be particularly healthful for the human body either, and a diet made up primarily of refined and preserved foods has been universally associated with deterioration in health.

OTHER PROCESSING

Even the chopping, peeling, slicing and mixing of raw food is a processing of sorts, and there is evidence that the food is altered significantly thereby.   Shredding, for example, exposes raw foods more thoroughly to oxygen, and browning reactions with the destruction of vitamin C can result.[33]   Such preparation, however, does improve the appeal of the food, and it is said in the East that the blending of such foods intermingles their essence or energy so that even without cooking they are made into one dish rather than many, so that their digestion is simplified and their properties are altered.

CONCLUSION

The preparation of food is a complex matter and cannot be reduced to any simplistic rule.   Cooking is a great art, and equipped with sensitivity and knowledge, one can gradually cultivate a capacity in this area.   Extremes should be avoided, and we must be wary of those who wish to tell us that our diet should be the same as that of our jungle ancestors.   Our consciousness is now different from that of those early man-like creatures, and as a result, the total body-mind complex functions differently.

We should also beware of those who wish to persuade us that our diet can be adequate and satisfying when it consists of processed, preserved, dead, embalmed and otherwise devitalized foods, despite the fact that their preparation or consumption might be more convenient at times.   We must instead become serious students of the delicate and crucial art of cooking, cultivating in ourselves a sensitivity to the subtle life and lifegiving properties of food, learning how to preserve and cultivate them.

The person in the household who selects the food, prepares and serves it bears a heavy responsibility. He or she can, in subtle and gentle ways, nourish health and consciousness in the family or gradually, through carelessness and ignorance, weaken them. When cooking is thought of as a matter of indifferently opening cans or laboriously preparing complicated conglomerations, it becomes either boring on the one hand, or exhausting on the other. When, however, it is appreciated as the delicate art of choosing and preparing natural foods in such a way that their life-giving qualities are unharmed and so that they are pleasing to the eye and refreshing and delightful to the palate, then cooking becomes a joy.

Because processed, preserved and chemicalized foods are usually easier to prepare, more convenient to store and often cheaper, it has been easy to develop unhealthy eating habits. Modern advertising, attractive packaging and other social pressures tend to perpetuate these practices, and tastes acquired over many years, even for synthetic and obviously harmful foods, have a strong effect. In the face of all these influences, the cook's challenge is an enormous one. Yet it can be met. Where economic necessity, cultural prejudices, taste and nutritional considerations are carefully balanced and brought together to create meals that are both healthful and appealing, the food that results will encourage those who eat it to develop a more subtle sensitivity toward what they eat and their body's reaction to it.

In the Zen Buddhist tradition, the kitchen is regarded as the altar of the house. It is said that plant life is sacrificed there in order that human consciousness might be created and sustained. The fullest human consciousness cannot be created by food which is unhealthful, misused, or carelessly prepared. Among the strictest Brahmins, a hired cook is unknown. The wife carefully prepares the food after having bathed, put on clean clothes and readied herself to approach the kitchen with serenity and devotion.   Only she can perform the ritual of preparing food.   Her motions are carried out with a studied grace, and her mind is kept focused and calm through the repetition of special mantras. Though she never tastes the food until it is blessed, dedicated to ennobling the spirit and until she has fed those for whom she has prepared it, she remains closely attuned to its changing properties and seldom fails to add the right seasonings or the proper amount heat at the precisely correct moment necessary to create a delicious and healthful dish.

In many such traditions, there is a profound appreciation for the importance of how food is prepared. The preparation of food is the key, the crucial step, between all the events that occur with the sun, the water, the soil and the air which result in the creation of the plant and all the events that occur in the digestive system, the bloodstream, the nervous system and the mind which result in the creation of consciousness.   It is the preparation of the food that lies at this strategic juncture between the two worlds of plant and man.   It is at this point that man's intelligence and intuitiveness can play such an important role if he understands the subtleties of cooking.

For this reason, it might be said that food preparation is perhaps the greatest art and the greatest science.   It is a great science because it is the primary activity which can be performed in an external, observable and objective way to influence and effect the whole human being: his body and its physiological workings, his health, his mental and emotional outlook, his energy, and even his consciousness.   It is a great art because it involves a creative involvement with the intersection of so many variables: the selection of the food, the conditions under which it was grown, the mixtures of ingredients, the temperature of cooking and the suitability of the preparation to the temperament, digestive system and state of health of the person who eats it. If one were to deliberately and logically ponder each of these variables before he added another ingredient or cut another vegetable, he might well go mad before he prepared his first meal. Man's mental computer bogs down in the face of such complexity. Consequently, he must rely instead on his intuition and look for guidance to the traditions of those who preceded him in the painstaking evolution of cooking.

The art of preparing food is both extremely difficult and at the same time potentially very rewarding. It can also be a matter of utmost importance. There is a story of the Chinese nobleman who, lying ill, was heard to say, "I don't need a doctor. I need a good cook."

V

Food and Consciousness

We have examined the science of nutrition in a very systematic fashion: looking at the soil, how it relates to the quality of foodstuffs, analyzing the biochemical nutrients, where they are found and how to get enough of each. We have examined the intricacies of the digestive system and even surveyed the pharmacological complexity of the non-nutritional compounds in foods and the effects of cooking techniques. Yet there is one issue we have repeatedly skirted. That is the relationship between nutrition and the mind.

We have mentioned that thiamin deficiency is often seen in persons who are weak and nervous or that B_{12}, folic acid and vitamin C levels are often low in those who have psychiatric problems. Niacin deficiency, we have seen, classically produces pellagra, a disease which may fit the picture of schizophrenia. Too little zinc and manganese or too much copper may also aggravate such a situation.

Non-nutritive substances in food also play an important part, not only because of toxic and/or pharmacologic effects on the body, but because of similar effects on the nervous system which can precipitate mental and emotional disturbance. Strong spices, for instance, in those who are not accustomed to them, can cause giddiness, intoxication, or more simply, a headache. Nutmeg is a case in point, and even coriander, a mild seasoning, when used in extremely large quantities, can have a sort of narcotic effect.

Though dietary intake affects the mind, this is more than a one-way interaction. The mind also affects what we eat. One's thoughts and feelings influence his choices as he walks down a cafeteria line. Moreover, the mind also plays a big part in determining what is absorbed after it is eaten. We mentioned in our discussion of the digestive system, that emotional and psychological factors can affect the physiology of the intestinal tract in profound ways, determining the microbes that grow therein, affecting the mobility of the intestinal tract, and playing a major role in determining how much of which digestive juices are secreted.

If the mind is so closely tied to issues of nutrition, we must make some attempt to unravel their complex interrelationship in order to understand more clearly its implications. This is no small challenge, but what awaits us are some surprising insights today—such as the debate about megavitamins—and a realization that a reexamination of the philosophical premises that underlie our methods of studying diet is long overdue.

Interaction between Diet and Mind

The mind and diet relate to each other in a sort of double feedback fashion. What goes in psychologically affects the diet in many ways. And then, the resulting change in nutritional status has important effects in psychological functioning. This means that a continuous interplay exists, and that this can, if allowed to run amok, carry one to great heights (or depths) of mental and physical disorder. Of course, with the proper understanding this interaction becomes a means of promoting the health of the whole person.

CARBOHYDRATE AND HYPOGLYCEMIA

Not only the presence of non-nutritive substances or deficiencies in vitamins and minerals but also irregularities in the intake and assimilation of such nutrients as protein, carbohydrate and fat, can also affect the mental state. The most dramatic of these is of course carbohydrate, and an uneven and irregular alteration of the blood sugar can be most disrupting to psychological functioning. When the blood sugar climbs abruptly, one will usually feel a surge of energy, but when it drops, equally abruptly, there is a feeling of weakness, irritability and often anxiety. The sensation might be described as "I feel as though I'm falling apart." In those persons whose ability to control blood sugar levels is poor, such a drop occurs especially after eating refined carbohydrates like soft drinks, candy, pastries, etc. The episode of low blood sugar is called "hypoglycemia." (*Hypo* means low, *glyc* indicates glucose, the major sugar transported to the cells and *emia* refers to the blood.) It has become recognized in recent years that this situation is not uncommon.[1] In fact the feeling is familiar to many people. It seems likely that the increased consumption of sugar has played an important role in the development of this tendency. Because of the fact that sugar is "naked calories" it, of course, increases one's nutrient debts. This will weaken one's functioning in many areas including carbohydrate metabolism. Yet it is unfortunately true that one can temporarily escape from the tremulous, weak, hypoglycemic state by simply having another dose of sugar! This immediately relieves all the symptoms or, at least, decreases their severity. But relief is short lived. Besides, the next time around, the feeling is worse, and the amount of sugar required to stop it is more. This picture has led some to term heavy sugar use an "addiction." If so, it is a hidden addiction, since many people are unaware of the connection between their periodic feelings of restlessness, irritability and tiredness and their habitual use of sugar. A closer look reveals, however, that contemporary lifestyles are usually structured to provide frequent doses of sugar, an observation borne out by many findings, from the sugar listed on canned vegetables and meats, to the sweetened beverages provided every few hours by airlines to the passenger who is confined and unable to be out foraging for his own favorite sugared "fix."

Though large amounts of sugar in the diet will inevitably run up nutrient debts and eventually result in the breakdown of some system of the body, it need not be carbohydrate metabolism that fails.   Not everyone suffers hypoglycemic attacks from eating sugar.

Several factors normally prevent the blood sugar from bouncing up and down and help hold it at a steady level so that one's energy supply is even and consistent.   The first of these factors is insulin, which regulates the movement of glucose from the blood into the cells.   If insulin is supplied by the pancreas in appropriate amounts at appropriate times the blood glucose is controlled by removing any excess from the blood into the cells where it is either used for energy or converted to fat.   A person whose insulin is well-regulated may therefore eat sweets without suffering a hypoglycemic episode, though he is likely to gain weight if he does so often. Glucagon, another hormone, has an effect which opposes that of insulin; it raises blood sugar by releasing sugar that is stored.

Some of the people who are subject to precipitous drops in blood sugar, or hypoglycemic spells, have this problem because they are unable to regulate insulin secretion properly.   After eating a meal heavy in sweets, insulin is slow to appear, so glucose cannot move from the blood into the cells and blood sugar begins to soar.   Finally, when insulin secretion does come, it comes in full force, and so much glucose is removed from the blood that blood sugar drops drastically and one begins to experience the characteristic weakness and shakiness.   The glucose tolerance test demonstrates this.

The whole sad picture, however, cannot always be blamed entirely on the pancreas and the insulin-secreting cells.   Actually such large quantities of sugar should never reach the bloodstream in the first place.   Food absorbed from the intestines is taken up by the portal vein and goes directly to the liver.   Here all blood is filtered and nutrients are sorted out, some put in storage and others released for immediate use, according to what is appropriate.   If the liver is healthy and is able to "triage" nutrients and to store glucose, then excessive amounts of this sugar are not dumped wholesale into the blood.

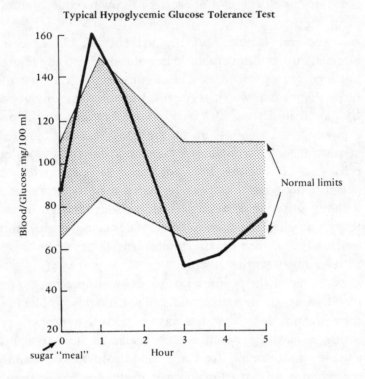

Typical Hypoglycemic Glucose Tolerance Test

Hypoglycemic attacks, then, may be due not only to an inappropriate insulin response but to a weak or sluggish liver which is unable to perform its duties properly. This is especially well illustrated by alcoholics where the liver is damaged from habitual drinking. They are often hypoglycemic. This may even be true before the liver is damaged, since alcohol, like sugar, relieves the unpleasantness of low blood sugar and this may be one inducement to drink.

When it is poor liver function that is the primary cause of hypoglycemic attacks, the high protein diet that is often used for the condition is unsuitable. Large amounts of protein put a further burden on the liver, and though the absence of carbohydrate may afford some immediate relief from the hypoglycemic episodes, over the long haul the situation will become worse.

Even earlier in this chain of events, the disaster can be averted. There is no real reason why a flood of sugar has to be delivered to the bloodstream or to the liver. Whether it is or not depends, as we saw earlier, on what kind of carbohydrate was eaten. White sugar, which is a simple carbohydrate, is ready to be absorbed rapidly from the intestine; starch chains, a complex carbohydrate made up of many sugar links must be broken down gradually. The breaking off of sugar units from the starch results in a piecemeal release of sugar into the blood, so that having a meal of a grain, like rice, in the digestive tract produces quite a different effect from a piece of candy or a sweetened drink.[2] If the grain is a whole grain, and taken along with a protein source, such as a legume for example, and combined with a fat such as butter or ghee, absorption is further slowed and sugar uptake is even more gradual.

The blood sugar is generally controlled then, by these three lines of defense: the use of complex carbohydrate, a well-functioning liver and proper insulin regulation. If it is not, the jolts of high and low blood sugar can be quite trying.

If the blood sugar drops too low the nervous system is endangered. The brain relies on blood sugar for its functioning, and if it is deprived of it, it cannot continue. This is what happens when a diabetic gets an overdose of insulin, for example, and all the sugar enters the cells. There is none readily available for the brain, so the person lapses into a coma. Though such a drastic drop in blood sugar is not usually experienced by the hypoglycemic, the decrease is still interpreted as a danger signal, and the adrenal glands usually respond by secreting adrenalin. This helps mobilize stored glucose from the liver, but it also sets off a general alarm, alerting the whole body as for emergency action. One may feel apprehensive, tremulous, and find that his heart is beating rapidly, his hands are becoming cold and clammy and he is breathing in a rapid and shallow way. Of course the reaction is not always so dramatic. How severe it is depends on how low the blood sugar drops and how drastically the adrenal glands respond.

It has been demonstrated that those who experience drastic dips in their blood sugar levels excrete more of the breakdown products of adrenalin in their urine. They are repeatedly responding as though to danger. The result can be an overall feeling tone similar to what we call "anxiety."[3] It has been proposed that drops in blood sugar constitute a sort of "internal stress" and may create a great deal of wear and tear on the individual, both provoking mental problems, aggravating emotional crises, and increasing irritability and difficulty in working with others.   Such chronic stress and the resulting chronic anxiety could be a primary factor in the development of ulcers, headache, or simply general nervousness and exhaustion.

Though hypoglycemia may be one aspect of the development of any of a variety of disorders, it cannot itself be called the "cause" of anything. Nor is it proper to call it a disease. It is rather one link in a chain of events which begins with the improper selection of food (usually too much refined carbohydrate), continues with an overworked and disabled liver,* worsens with a disrupted insulin response and ends almost anywhere, depending on the other characteristics of a person, his weaknesses, his habits, etc.

Here we must distinguish between two rather distinct uses of the term "hypoglycemia." In some cases it is used to describe a state of moderately low blood sugar which can occur in almost anyone who eats a great excess of purified sugar, sending the blood sugar very high so that it subsequently drops below normal. Sometimes, however, the term hypoglycemia is used to indicate a clinical diagnosis, which means that the person in question has an unusual tendency for his blood sugar to respond by dropping rapidly to an extremely low point[4] even with little provocation. In other words, although some people are particularly prone to experience low blood sugar, others are

---

* See Chapter 10, Digestion.

relatively resistant.

Normally the body responds relatively well to the sugar load. Even if blood sugar begins to drop, there are mechanisms for meeting the challenge. Glucagon, for example, another hormone secreted by the pancreas and the walls of the intestinal tract, releases stored sugar from the liver without setting off the alarm reactions caused by adrenalin. In some people, however, glucagon secretion may be sluggish or inadequate, just as insulin response can be excessive, or poorly tuned. Why some people "use" the pancreas in one fashion while others use it differently is not known. However, a particular tendency for the blood sugar to drop is correlated with certain psychological and personality traits. In one study of patients with mental and emotional problems, 70% of those who had been diagnosed as schizophrenic exhibited some form of hypoglycemia[5] as did many neurotics.

The fact that the endocrine system is so intimately involved in sugar metabolism suggests that the glucose tolerance curve is testing more than a single physiological function. Rather it reflects the way that the whole person, as a psychosomatic unit, reacts to fuel. In other words, it tells us something about the characteristics of a personality and how it handles its source of energy. An oversecretion of insulin, for example, floods the cells with a rush of sugar, a sort of physiological "greediness" that parallels the overconsumption of sugary food that preceded it.

The way insulin is regulated depends to a great extent on the autonomic nervous system whose functioning is closely related to the mind and emotions. Why one secretes insulin too rapidly causing the blood sugar to plunge may be due partly to some momentary emotional disturbance, but we might wonder whether it may also be due to a sort of "physiological habit." If one eats a concentrated dose of sugar, driving the blood sugar up and stimulating the pancreas to pour out insulin, he may gradually "train" his pancreas to function in this fashion. At first it may be the kind of food eaten which creates the unfortunate course of events: physiologically, a rapid rise and subsequent fall in blood sugar, and psychologically, a rapid high followed by a sinking to a state of low spirits. Eventually, however, this may happen without the stimulus of poorly chosen food. Such a mental/emotional/physiological pattern of response might come to be ingrained and easily triggered by almost any

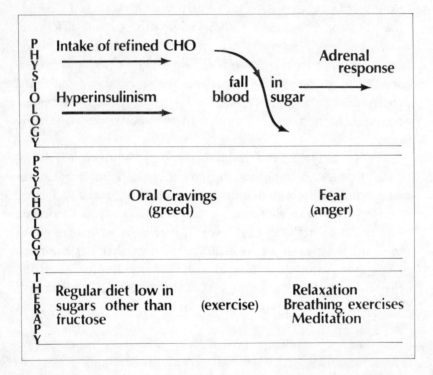

Physiological, Psychological and Therapeutic Aspects of Hypoglycemia

stress. The result would explain the frequently observed tendency to be quick to anger, seen in such persons who often "fly off the handle for no good reason" or tend to become sarcastic or overly sensitive to criticism. Gradually, however, new habits can be formed by being careful to supply the nutrients needed for the metabolism of carbohydrate such as the B vita-mins* and chromium, by not using concentrated sugar in the diet, by changing one's emotional stance in relation to disturbing situations, and by helping the autonomic nervous system to function differently through the use of such techniques as relaxation and breathing practices.

THE LIVER AND DEPRESSION

What emerges from our discussion of hypoglycemia is that the liver plays an important intermediary role in maintaining an internal homeostasis and balance. All the nutrients coming from the intestinal tract (with the exception of a large propor-tion of the fats) go to the liver, where they are processed before they are released in the bloodstream. If it is functioning well, it can "smooth out the bumps" in absorption and make sure that the blood is supplied with an even flow of sugar and other nutrients. This in turn insures that the adrenals and the nervous system do not have to cope with "internal emergencies" which are created by having too much or too little of this or that. The liver, then, serves to provide a constant internal milieu in which the nervous system can function, and if it does its job properly it contributes greatly to one's ability to maintain a sense of equanimity, calm and peace of mind.

Of course, as we have seen earlier, the liver does more than this. It is also responsible for filtering the blood and removing any wastes, contaminants, or toxins which might damage the cells throughout the body or interfere with their function. For example, it removes pesticides, insecticides and other toxic materials which might be absorbed along with food, as well as many metabolites which are created within the body itself. If, however, the liver is not functioning properly and

---

* Thiamin is often a problem here. It is needed in large quantities to handle heavy loads of carbohydrate, yet it is absent from sugar and many sweets such as candies, and soft drinks are not "enriched" with thiamin..

fails to do this job as completely as it should, then many of these toxic materials remain in the blood and are circulated throughout the body. This can cause an overall heaviness, achiness and soreness, as well as an unmodulated supply of nutrients. But it is particularly important to us here because of the effect that it can have on the nervous system. These circulating wastes, metabolites and contaminants are in some cases able to enter the nervous system and may directly interfere with the functioning of the brain and central nervous system. This can create a feeling of apathy, lethargy and often depression.

In fact, it has been suggested by some authors that the primary cause of most "depression" is liver dysfunction.[6] If due attention is given to removing stresses from the liver and to not overburdening it, allowing it to recover its normal capacity, the symptoms of depression will often clear. First and foremost, of course, is the proper regulation of the diet since the liver is forced to cope with whatever is absorbed by the intestinal tract and brought to it by the portal vein. If there are huge quantities of nutrients, such as those resulting from overeating or those resulting from eating overly-refined food which is absorbed too rapidly or damaged in such a way that much of it is not useful and must be removed; or if there are large amounts of chemicals resulting from eating food which is contaminated with insecticides, herbicides, or other incidental pollutants; then the liver's job becomes doubled, tripled, or even quadrupled. In such a case it cannot recover but must inevitably weaken further.

Overeating overworks the liver. As the liver becomes overburdened it begins to function poorly and its modulating influence on nutrition is lost. One's ability then to provide himself with an even flow of energy from food is compromised. He may be sometimes flooded with nutrients which the liver cannot handle and which enter the bloodstream while between meals he is deficient, since the liver stores are not adequate to fill in the gap between feedings. It's either feast or famine. Moreover he is constantly toxic from internal pollutants which the liver is not removing. He begins to feel a sense of uncertainty, not being able to "trust his liver." The irritability and suspiciousness that results is projected onto the world and comes to characterize his personality. The liver patient may be wasted, due to poor absorption of protein, or he may be obese with overabsorption of sugar, or he may show a combination of the two with weak muscles and unhealthy organs, but with excess fatty tissue. He may overeat or undereat, often alternating between the two. In any event he has lost touch with the internal signals which cue him to when food is needed and when he has had enough. The trusting relationship then, that should exist between the mind and the body, between the internal physiological signals and the psychological response, between the digestive tract and liver supplying energy and mental equilibrium is lost.

It becomes clear, then, that the liver is a strategic link between nutrition and the mind, serving as an intermediary through which they interact in many ways. Actually it may be involved even further in another intriguing way in this interaction: according to the teachings of traditional medicine in the East, the liver is affected by worry and rumination. In the terms of Ayurvedic theory, an obsessive concentration of energy in the intellectual sphere leaves the solar plexus and digestive system neglected and wanting. The healthy person, while capable of alertness and mental activity also has the flexibility to relax and allow the body to digest its food and carry out its eliminative processes. When one is too rigid and preoccupied to permit this to happen, however, then activation of digestive enzymes and the smooth functioning of the duodenal axis with its accessory organs, the liver, the pancreas, etc., becomes either diminished or unbalanced. The liver of necessity bears the brunt of such poorly regulated digestion and gradually begins to weaken. "Yond Cassius" who had the "lean and hungry look" because he "thought too much" probably suffered from a liver disorder.

When the digestive fire or *pitta* is properly regulated, energy is said to flow evenly and consistently from the solar plexus, giving one a feeling of vitality and well-being. When this fails, however, accessory organs of regulation which should normally be pushed into extra activity only in an emergency situation must take over. The adrenal glands, as we saw, may be activated, responding as though there is an emergency, sometimes contributing to a state of chronic tension and anxiety. The thyroid may also be called into play, and when it becomes overactive, another kind of nervousness and exhaustion is experienced.

INTERACTION BETWEEN NUTRITION AND THE MIND: A SPIRAL

It becomes apparent then that one's diet affects the mind and that the mind affects, in many ways, one's diet and nutrition. If, for example, one becomes more irritable and emotionally disturbed, his eating habits are very likely to become more erratic. Not only may he fail to take meals on time, skipping some entirely, but out of nervousness, restlessness, or simply a lack of awareness, he may overeat or he may eat too often. As the mind becomes disturbed, one loses touch with the subtle signals that cue him to what is appropriate to eat and when. Poor dietary regulation leads to poor intake of nutrients and deficiencies which in turn make one more irritable and mentally and emotionally disturbed. The result sounds like the classical "vicious circle."

Unfortunately, this cycle is not merely circular. A circular process would show no net change, for better or worse. Actually, however, there is often a gradual but definite worsening, a sort of building crescendo of emotion, unbalance and erratic living habits with poor dietary practices. The result, instead of a circle, is a downward-moving spiral.

As we have seen above, the interaction between the diet

and the mind may involve, as an intermediary step, effects on the liver. Of course other organs may also serve as the strategic link that mediates the primary interaction between the diet and the mind. The pancreas, as we have seen, is often involved. It may put out too much, too little, or poorly-timed insulin and it may do the same thing with glucagon, the hormone which releases stored glucose. Its production of digestive enzymes can also be affected, so that the tense, usually angry person who suffers from hypoglycemic spells may also have difficulty with digestion and absorption.

The stomach is also prone to be caught up in the spiral of interaction between diet and mind. Certain personality traits and attitudes toward the world such as suppressed hunger and dependency and a tendency to turn angry feelings inward may be reflected physiologically by increased gastric acid and the "eating away" of the stomach's lining.[7]   This often leads to overeating or snacking to keep the stomach full. When the extra foods are sweets, they may trigger a further secretion of acid.[8] On the other hand, hopelessness, depression and feelings of inadequacy may be related to an inadequate secretion of gastric acid[9] which weakens protein digestion, and drops the protective barrier against bacterial overgrowth in the small intestine, culminating in flatulence, indigestion, and again, an overloaded liver—the sum total of which clearly accentuates one's feelings of depression and inadequacy and completes one more turn of the downward spiral.

Mental states have a direct effect too, as we have seen, on the nature of the mucus secreted by the intestinal wall, which is probably the major factor tuning the interaction between intestinal bacteria and lining over the football field-sized surface involved.*

The colon is another site of interaction. Irritation of it tends to be associated with nervousness, fearfulness and a sense

* See Chapter 11, Elimination.

of overwhelming anxiety.[10] Developmental events and the design
of the autonomic nervous system are such that the proper
control of the colon is lost when one experiences the most
devastating kinds of fear. Large amounts of adrenalin paralyze
the muscles which hold the anus closed so that involuntary defecation is not only seen in terrified animals but is a primitive
response rooted in humans, too. The kind of fear expressed by
spasms and poor control of the large bowel is associated with
basic insecurities about one's existence. Once one is able to
externalize and verbalize such feelings they are often found to
be related to fears of annihilation that date back to earliest
infancy. Psychoanalysts have called this issue one of "basic
trust" or the fundamental ability to feel comfortable and secure
in the world, something which is ordinarily established in the
infant at a very early age.[11]

An irritable colon, such as that which results from constant diarrhea, interrupts the natural downward flow of the
excretory functions. This downward moving tendency of the
bowels and bladder is called in Ayurveda and yoga, *apana vayu*,
and it is said that when this downward course is disrupted it
tends to "move up," affecting the mind and causing it to become
"spacey," suspicious, and to lose touch with reality. This in turn
interrupts and interferes with the normal control of eating and
digestion which further aggravates the condition of the colon.

The interaction of nutrition and mind that results in
hypoglycemia and involves the pancreas and liver is perhaps the
most talked about at present and has been explored and studied
in most detail. But it seems that similar concepts can be used to
understand how stomach, colon or small intestine serve as points
of interaction in the way that the pancreas does in hypoglycemia.
We might wonder, too, if the difficulties experienced with sugar
and carbohydrate metabolism might not be mirrored by similar
difficulties with other macronutrients. Indeed, this is probably
true of fats, since those who have studied the person with the
"Type A" personality, who is more susceptible to heart attacks,

have found him to show different fat levels in the blood.[12] This may well be related to different ways of metabolizing fatty foods.

Fortunately, such downward-moving spirals as that occurring with disordered sugar metabolism can move in the other direction, too. If one becomes more alert and aware of the physical symptoms which guide toward the proper intake of nutrients and regulates his diet accordingly, then he will often find that his nervousness diminishes, his mental state improves, and he is able to think more clearly. This in turn allows him even finer and more successful regulation of his eating habits, which in turn again improves nutrition and his nervousness further. In other words, the cycle need not be vicious. It can move in a quite beneficial direction, toward balance. But when the spiral moves further and further away from balance and homeostasis, its downward course may carry one toward any number of chronic, degenerative and pathological conditions. The direction which one takes may hinge on many factors besides his physiological makeup which is actually, to a great extent, dependent upon other variables, such as the symbolic meaning that food holds for him and his past habits and experiences which have resulted in self-destructive tendencies and attitudes of which he may be only partially aware.

THE SYMBOLIC MEANING OF FOOD

After the initial breath of air, one's first contact with the world around him is the nipple and milk, which reassure him that he is loved, well taken care of and in contact with what is important. Eating remains thereafter a source of the most primal and basic pleasure. Food and air are the two essentials which man takes in from his environment. It is even true that the respiratory system is an offshoot, embryologically, of the digestive tract. The digestive tract is man's inside skin, i.e., it is his way of surrounding and internalizing a part of the world. It is, in a sense, his most intimate relatedness, his way of joining himself to the universe by taking a part of it and internalizing it. His attitude and his approach to food and air, then, is often one of the most fundamental indications of his way of relating to the rest of the universe.

Long before words and logic come along, food is already very important in the life of a child. Being of such a primal and basic importance, it is understandable that the relationship of one's mental and emotional life to nutritional habits is complex, but crucial. The most rational man is often known to leave his reason aside when he sits down to the table. It is commonplace that the most successful way of cultivating a business acquaintance is to provide him with a good meal. Most important rituals, either religious or political, revolve around food and drink. Every woman knows that "the best way to a man's heart is through his stomach."

Since attitudes toward food and the meanings that it holds may vary considerably from person to person, it is not surprising then that many of the most profound psychological disturbances manifest as disorders of eating or as strange and peculiar attitudes toward food. For example, a deeply rooted sense of aloneness and a profound craving for closeness and increased intimacy with the rest of the world may manifest in a bizarre way through overeating. This is bizarre in the sense that it does not, of course, lead to an increased relatedness either with the universe or with other people. In fact, the result is usually the opposite. One becomes insulated from the world and others by a thick layer of fat. As with most psychological disorders, there is an understandable but irrational attempt to resolve a basic problem. The problem, however, is translated to an absurdly physical and material level where its resolution cannot occur. The relatedness which is really needed on a more subtle mental, emotional or even spiritual level, is twisted into an attempt to secure closeness through physically incorporating material substance, i.e., food. Psychoanalysts call this "oral craving."

In some cases, the craving for closeness expressed through incorporating physically (food) may and often does involve an ambivalence. While one may wish to establish closeness and "surround the world," so to speak, he may at the same time, (and often does) have a distrust of those around him and of the material universe as a whole. The fact that this is so is not surprising since were this trustfulness present he would be better able to interrelate on the appropriate level, that is socially, mentally, emotionally or even spiritually. His distrust is one of the reasons that he resorts to attempts to interrelate through a physical means, that is, overeating. The anorexia nervosa patient dramatizes this ambivalence first by eating huge quantities and then throwing it up. Such cycles of overeating and vomiting often lead to a state of depletion and starvation and it is not unusual in the case of anorexia nervosa patients for this downward spiral to end with death. Of course the same stance in relationship to food and to the universe is often seen to a much less exaggerated degree in many "normal" people who are preoccupied with food and may have trouble maintaining their weight though this is a problem which is relatively rare compared to obesity.

OBESITY: EXTRICATING ONESELF FROM THE "FATTY SPIRAL"

The cycle of compulsive overeating alternating with guilt driven dieting and self-denial characterizes the eating pattern of many people who are overweight. Self-punitive "crash diets" may eliminate needed nutrients and can be harmful. This is especially true, as we have seen, in the case of fasting.* Besides, fasting is often undesirable for weight loss since it tends to perpetuate the obese person's preoccupation with food.

What is needed is an approach which will decrease the

* See Chapter 12, Fasting

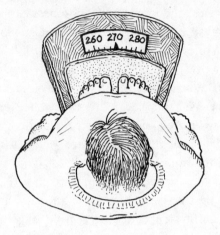

obsession with eating. This can be accomplished in a number of ways. First, it must be realized that some of the discomfort experienced by the overweight dieter is a result of nutritional needs that are not being met. Though he obviously doesn't need calories since he has enough fat stores to supply energy, the person who is overweight has other important requirements. Even though the preoccupation with food may be largely a psychological habit, craving for it can be drastically reduced. Once the proper nutrients are supplied, the body no longer has reason to send out so many frantic appetite signals.

Protein is one of the nutrients needed even when fat stores are providing calories. It is necessary for the manufacture of enzymes and the replacement of structural components in the cell. Moreover, when carbohydrate is absent from the diet, protein needs increase, since protein must be converted to carbohydrate to maintain blood sugar at adequate levels. If neither carbohydrate nor protein is supplied with the diet, then the body will begin to break down protein-based structures to convert their amino acids into glucose. This can result in serious damage to vital tissues. It may also leave one feeling weak and exhausted, aggravating a gnawing kind of appetite that is often beyond endurance. Obviously, it is difficult for one to cut through the obsession with food as long as there is such an overwhelming biological basis for it.

An understanding of this aspect of weight loss led to the development of the "protein sparing diet."*   Here, a small amount of carbohydrate is given in order to prevent the depletion of body protein. "Protein sparing" has also been used as a label for pre-digested protein diets, though technically speaking, this is a misuse of the term. Here the rationale is to provide the protein that is needed for body maintenance rather than for the purpose of preventing the use of tissue protein to keep up blood glucose. Liquid protein diets often supply no carbohydrate. For this reason, they may result in dramatic weight loss. But since fat stores cannot be converted to glucose to maintain blood sugar levels, then this liquid protein must be used for that purpose. As we noted previously, protein is not an ideal source of fuel. Not only does the conversion of amino acid to glucose use up as much energy as it will eventually supply, but the nitrogen based fragment of the amino acid that is eliminated in the production of sugar can be toxic. This may create an imbalance in the system of one who is dieting. A number of persons who remained on the liquid diet for a long period of time have developed inexplicable irregularities in the heart rhythm, some of which have proved fatal.[13, 14] Though the nature of this is not understood, it is suspected that either the complete lack of carbohydrate or the quality of the protein is in some way responsible.

Some of the liquid protein sold is even inadequate as a source of protein. This is especially true of those made of collagen, the tough, fibrous, connective tissue (such as tendons, ligaments and so forth) which are by-products of the meat packing industry. Ordinarily, these are not sold as food unless they are liquified to make gelatin. When treated further to

---

* See Chapter 6, Protein.

reduce them to their constituent amino acids, they are used as the basis of some liquid protein diets. Collagen, which has the same amino acid composition as gelatin, is deficient in methionine, one of the eight essential amino acids. This means that a protein food made from this source does not contain a balance of the most important amino acids and therefore does not serve as a complete protein. For this reason body protein must be broken down to supply the needed methionine, which of course, releases the other amino acids in corresponding amounts. The result is that the collagen-based food is of little use. Most of it must be converted to glucose. The best that can be said for it is that it has some protein-sparing action (since even poorly balanced amino acids can be converted to glucose) but it does not for the most part supply usable protein itself. In fact, the biological value of collagen (gelatin) is the lowest of any known protein[15] and the least suitable for one who is dieting. Though some protein *is* needed, collagen-based liquid protein diet foods fail to furnish it.*

The restlessness and discomfort that repeatedly bring the dieter's attention back to food may also be due to a lack of vitamins and minerals. As explained earlier, these nutrients are needed for the proper metabolism of the fat which is being burned. Fat deposits are rich in calories but almost devoid of vitamins and minerals. One of the most effective ways of easing the weight-loss process and of reducing the discomfort of going without food is to supply the dieter with frequent doses of fresh fruit and vegetable juices. These are extremely rich in vitamins and minerals, will usually supply enough carbohydrate to have a protein-sparing effect, and surprisingly enough, usually provide more than enough protein.†

* Such liquid proteins could be supplemented with methionine, but this would increase their expense as well as producing a bad flavor since methionine is strong and unpleasant in taste. It is apparently taste appeal and low price that have made collagen-based liquid protein preparations best sellers.

† See Chapter 6, Protein.

The kind of discomfort and craving that results from the overall lack of nutrients often seen in overweight people, especially when they are dieting, is quite different from what a healthier person calls hunger. Obese people, in fact, seem relatively insensitive to hunger. If no food is taken for some time, contractions of the stomach and reductions in blood sugar take place that would be interpreted by most people as hunger. In experimental situations, obese subjects, however, reported no feelings of hunger at that time.[16, 17] On the other hand, when snack foods were available, overweight persons who had just had a full meal ate more than a similar group with empty stomachs.[18]

Apparently people who tend to become overweight are insensitive to the inner cues that should let them know when food is needed and when it is not. Learning to tune in to internal states is probably an essential feature of any successful program for losing weight.

Though people who are overweight tend to ignore the internal signals that should regulate eating, they often respond to external signals. Besides being habituated to eating when food is present, they may respond to emotional situations by stuffing themselves with food. When put in a situation which aroused fear, a group of overweight persons did not "lose their appetites" as did those of normal weight. In fact, they ate more.[19] If one is to lose weight and keep it off, he must be involved in some systematic effort to learn new ways of handling stress and emotional upset. Methods of relaxation, breathing, biofeedback or meditation not only provide successful techniques for this purpose, but also promote the kind of body awareness that the obese person so badly needs to learn.[20]

Exercise fits this bill too. Not only does it help in diverting attention from food-oriented matters, but it also, obviously, burns up calories. In one study of a group of teenage girls, those who were overweight ate no more than their classmates, but they were much less active.[21] It has been estimated that a secretary who exchanges her manual typewriter for an electric one but keeps her diet and living habits otherwise the same, will gain four to six pounds a year. Without increasing the general level of physical activity, it is impossible for most people to lose weight. To maintain the reduction, it will be necessary to make physical activity a more prominent part of their lifestyle, even after weight is lost.

Regularity is part of this. If meals are erratic and un-planned, then scheduled exercise never comes off. Either one is about to eat and is not in the mood, or he has just eaten and can't exercise with a full stomach. Some experiments have shown that animals tend to gain less weight if allowed to eat when they're hungry.[22] A "nibbling" diet has been suggested, on this basis, for weight loss. This may be successful for the average person who only needs to lose a few pounds, since it helps him pay more attention to his internal signals. However, it will probably fail miserably for the majority of those who are seriously overweight since they have lost touch with their inner cues. For them, a regular schedule of meals is almost a necessity. If the diet is also rich in non-caloric nutrients which regularly satisfy genuine needs, it may be possible to gradually reestablish enough order in the internal chaos so that healthy and meaning-ful appetite signals can be perceived.

If carefully followed, a regular schedule of meals also does much to cut through one's obsession with food. If he knows, "Now I eat, now it is over. Nothing else until next meal," then the constant internal dialogue about whether to eat or whether to practice self-restraint can be eliminated. This frees up a great deal of energy which can be invested in other activities that gradually provide new fulfillment and open new horizons. It is also helpful for those who are losing weight to stick to a diet of foods that are plain, simple and relatively unseasoned. Research has demonstrated that fat people, who as we have seen, respond more to external stimuli, follow the same pattern with the food itself. If they find the taste appealing, they eat much more than they need and get fatter, but if they find it unattractive, they tend, even without trying, to eat less than they need to maintain their weight.[23]

But for some this may be the straw that breaks the camel's back. Those who live to eat rather than eating to live, find caloric restriction, uninteresting food and increased physical activity more than they're willing to bear. The cure becomes worse than the disease. They'd as soon stay fat. For this reason, it is essential that one who wishes to overcome obesity learn to find a sense of fulfillment in something other than eating. Otherwise, his efforts will be frustrated and his mental set and self-image will continue unaltered. He'll stay fat because he continues to "think fat." An overall program for successful and permanent weight loss must be one that leads to some significant psychological reorganization. Otherwise, it will be ineffective. This is probably why so many weight-loss approaches, from behavior therapy to Dr. Somebody or Other's Amazing, Fantastic Last Chance, Quick-Slim Crash Plan, have ultimately failed. Without any meaningful change, even fasting is not likely to be a successful approach to weight loss.

Cultivation of body awareness, learning techniques for handling emotional distress, finding new avenues for self-fulfillment and creativity along with establishing habits of physical activity and maintaining a balanced, simple, sensible diet especially rich in vitamins, minerals and high quality protein, can be successful. Such a program does not mechanistically or automatically remove weight from a fat person, but it does provide the conditions under which a fat person can sometimes "outgrow being fat."

Weight loss must be the by-product of personal evolution. The person who tackles the weight problem head-on, as though *it* is the basic issue, is doomed to fail. If one does not truly outgrow being fat, he will lose (and gain) tons in a long and unhappy career of dieting struggles.[24]

It must be remembered, too, that weight loss is a process

Reducing Diet

For those persons who are losing weight after having eaten poorly for some time, it is important to supplement a weight-loss diet with significant quantities of foods high in vitamins and minerals but extremely low in calories such as green salads, non-sweet fruits, and, especially important, freshly squeezed or extracted low-calorie vegetable and fruit juices such as grapefruit, celery, spinach, etc. Such a diet might look like this:

MORNING

Juice of 1½ grapefruits, fresh.
Scrambled tofu, 4 ounces.
1 rye crisp.

LUNCH

Tofu with vegetables, 1 cup.
Rice, 1 cup.
½ piece rye toast,
    or 1 ricecake,
    or 1 rye crisp.

LATE AFTERNOON

Vegetable juice (cucumber and
    grapefruit).
Fruit: 1 apple, 1 orange and 1/3
    cup cottage cheese.

LATE EVENING

Juice: carrot, celery, spin-
    ach, 6 ounces.

Total calories: 820
Fat: 8.0 (g)

Carbohydrate: 140 (g)
Protein: 47 (g)

Such a reducing diet maintains a balance of nutrients, supplies an extraordinary amount of vitamins and minerals from natural sources, and is surprisingly, even incredibly, low in calories. It should be remembered though, that no diet is suitable for every person. From this example, however, it should be clear that it is quite possible to create a balanced diet comprised of strictly vegetarian foods and milk products which is high in protein and low in calories.

of "uncovering." What emerges from the layers of fat during this process is not only a new, thinner person, but also the problems and conflicts that led to overeating. If one is prepared to come to terms with such issues as how he has closed the door on inner signals and feelings, how the tendency to be inactive relates to habits of thinking and feeling and what the self-image of "fat" means to him, he will become less burdened psychologically as well as physically.

When our attention becomes fixed on only the diet and its biochemical makeup, or on only the digestive system, pancreas, liver, etc., and their functioning or on only the mind and its conflicts, we see only part of the picture. Each of these affects the other in definite and strategic ways, and most nutritional problems can be unravelled and resolved only if we keep in view the entire interacting complex. To chide ourselves for overeating when we are starved for nutrients is an exercise in futility. The same is true of feeding ourselves vitamin pills when the problems are in our minds or emotions. Such an approach can lead us, as we are about to see, far astray.

Megavitamins and Food Allergies

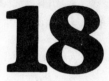

Do large amounts of vitamin C protect against stress? Is schizophrenia a biochemical disorder; can it be treated with megadoses of vitamin B_3 (niacin)? Do some people require higher doses of vitamin B_6 to function optimally? These are some of the controversial questions surrounding the issue of "megavitamins." There are ardent supporters of both sides, pro and con. Those who advocate using large quantities of vitamins insist that certain people are born with unusually high requirements for some of these nutrients. If they get only "normal" amounts, they will fall ill, in some cases mentally ill. Yet most experts in the field of mental illness ignore these claims, continuing the use of tranquilizers, or proceeding — often successfully—to treat such persons with psychological therapies. What is the answer? If we are to continue to untangle the knotted relationship between nutrition and the mind, we must confront such questions. Can vitamins really cure a mental disease? What, in fact, is the basic problem, is it psychological or biochemical?

Actually, as we shall see, the answers may not be so

difficult to find. Once all the data is assembled and examined it looks as though the solution is rather simple: how much we need of certain vitamins is due, at least in part, to how we function psychologically. Moreover, the principles of mind-body interaction that are involved here may well help us understand other puzzling problems such as food allergies.

VITAMIN DEFICIENCIES AND PSYCHOPATHOLOGY

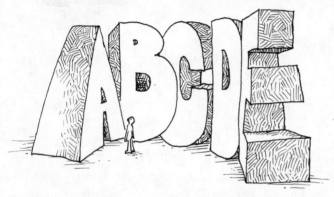

The most gross and obvious interrelationship between diet and the mind occurs when the diet is deficient in certain essential nutrients. The classic example involves deficiencies of the B vitamins. Thiamin, as we saw earlier, is found to be frequently deficient in people with neuropsychiatric disorders, and such persons become more disturbed when the amount of thiamin in the diet is lowered. Even when they had "recovered," their symptoms could be recreated by giving them a low thiamin diet. Vitamin B_3 (niacin) is another vitamin deficiencies of which classically produce symptoms of mental disorder. In the twenties and thirties, when pellagra was rampant in the Southeastern U.S.A., mental hospitals were filled with patients suffering from this disorder. Before the exact nutrient was isolated and made available in a form inexpensive enough to be used to reverse the condition on a large scale, the symptoms of pellagra were well-documented. It gradually became clear that the picture was very similar to that called "schizophrenia."

When niacin was finally isolated and used to treat patients with pellagra psychosis, the results were dramatic. Many patients were instantly cured who had been thought to be hopeless, doomed to the chronic wards.[1] Such success was to lead eventually to trials of niacin in other cases of psychosis where an association with pellagra was not so clear. The term "cerebral pellagra" was used for those patients treated with niacin who had many of the mental symptoms of the disease but without its typical physical signs.[2] Though some authorities have felt this is stretching the concept of pellagra beyond what is scientifically sound, this is not necessarily true. There is no reason to assume that the psychological disturbances resulting from niacin deficiency always have to be accompanied by the skin and intestinal problems. People vary and one might show one group of symptoms while another shows different ones. Though the physical symptoms may be more obvious and therefore harder to miss, it has long been suggested that the cerebral manifestations of pellagra might appear very early in the course of the disease. As long ago as 1817, Sir Henry Holland wrote about the "anxiety, watchfulness and moral depression" of the patient who later developed pellagra. These symptoms appeared early while the physical problems were slow to appear. He noted "The mania consequent upon pellagra is often of a very violent kind . . . where such affections occur the progress of the disease appears to be in some degree retarded and the strength less rapidly declines."[3]

In 1939 Dr. Tom Spies explicitly proposed that the cerebral manifestation of pellagra might be the first evidence of severe or complete depletion of niacin. He also described the mental symptoms and was the first to talk about "sub-clinical pellagra," those cases whose disease is mild enough so that it is not diagnosed or they do not seek help for it. He said, "Sub-clinical pellagrins are noted for the multiplicity of their complaints among which are many that are usually classed as neuraesthenic. The most common of these symptoms are fatigue, insomnia, anorexia, vertigo, burning sensations in various parts of the body, numbness, palpitations, nervousness, a feeling of unrest and anxiety, headache, forgetfulness, apprehension and distractibility. The conduct of the pellagrin may be normal but he feels incapable of mental or physical effort."[4]   Apparently niacin deficiency could look very much like what shows up in the typical psychiatrist's office.

In the 1940's, however, the second World War brought increased employment, a rise in wages, a reduction in poverty and an improvement in diet. Enrichment of flour and meal with nicotinamide was also instituted and soon thereafter, the severe and dramatic cases that could be easily recognized as pellagra had disappeared.

But the experience gained from treating pellagra was not forgotten. In 1951, as Doctors Osmond and Hoffer in Saskachewan were studying the biochemical aspects of schizophrenia, they were struck with the similarity between its symptoms and the delirium observed in pellagra. Recalling the work of Spies, which had shown that niacin deficiency could resemble psychiatric illness, and the fact that the mental symptoms of pellagra could come first, they wondered if thousands of the psychotic patients filling mental hospitals who had been diagnosed as schizophrenic might not in fact be suffering from a lack of niacin. Since most of the earlier treatments of chronic pellagra psychosis had involved high doses of niacin* they hypothesized that perhaps schizophrenics might simply be people who needed much larger amounts of this vitamin than normal. They began to treat such patients with huge doses (3,000 mg per day) of niacin and their results were encouraging. In 1952 they began an extensive controlled study, the results of which were reported to be positive.[5]

In 1956 Roger Williams published his book *Biochemical*

---

* In the 600 mg per day range compared to the 15 mg a day considered adequate for the average person.

Individuality, collecting vast amounts of evidence which indicated that there was a wide range of variability in the biochemical makeup and nutritional needs of different people. Even laboratory animals showed vastly different requirements for niacin, with some monkeys developing deficiency symptoms unless they were given five times what was required by others.[6] The rationale for giving certain patients extremely high doses of vitamins seemed to be gaining a firmer footing. The public began to hear about "megavitamin" therapy. Linus Pauling's work with large doses of vitamin C was leading in a similar direction. Doses incredibly large, by usual standards, seemed necessary for some people to ward off viral infections such as the common cold.

Pauling reasoned that the proper functioning of the nervous system must depend on the presence of precisely correct amounts of the necessary molecules, and that variations in biochemical functioning may cause some people to require relatively large amounts of a vitamin in order to deliver and maintain the necessary concentration in the brain. In 1968 he coined the term "Orthomolecular Psychiatry"* for the treatment of mental illness with large doses of nutrients.[7] If some people require more of certain nutrients than others, might it not be that those who require extremely large amounts of niacin would be unable to get them in an ordinary diet and would show the earliest signs of pellagra: depression, anxiety and eventually perhaps psychotic episodes?

Further experiences seemed to confirm this hypothesis. Dr. Hoffer who already had established some reputation for the use of high doses of nicotinic acid was approached in 1960 by a prominent Canadian who had been incarcerated during the second World War in a prison camp in Hong Kong. During the long stay of 44 months he had lost a tremendous amount of

---

* "Orthomolecular" meaning to straighten or correct the molecules in and around the brain cells.

weight and developed a combination of pellagra, beri-beri, scurvy and probably other deficiencies. After the war and upon returning to Canada he had been given what was considered then massive doses of vitamins but never seemed to fully recover though his weight returned to normal. While discussing with Dr. Hoffer the possibility of some research on niacin, he became interested in what it might do for him. He began, quite on his own, to take one gram of nicotinic acid three times a day. This is a huge dose—about 200 times the officially recommended daily intake of 15 mg! But in a few months he came back to say that he felt well for the first time since he had returned from the Hong Kong prison camp sixteen years earlier.[8] Since that time, Dr. Hoffer has had the opportunity to treat others of the veterans who were confined to the same prison camp with high doses of vitamins and reports further gratifying results. He feels that vitamin deprivation, such as that suffered by the Hong Kong prisoners can have permanent effects. This, he points out could be very relevant to the origins of schizophrenia.

"If all the vitamin B_3 were removed from our food everyone would become psychotic within one year. This pandemic psychosis would resemble pellagra and it would resemble schizophrenia." Most of the victims would recover within a few months, he says, if the vitamin B_3 were replaced in the diet. "But not everyone would recover with simple replacement. Many people would have been so severely damaged that only massive doses of B_3 would alleviate their symptoms and would be required for life . . . . This . . . illustrates vividly what does happen to one to two percent of our population."[9]

This notion that certain life experiences can so alter the metabolism that one requires thereafter extremely high doses of certain nutrients has become accepted by psychiatrists of the orthomolecular school, though so far the evidence for this is based only on conclusions drawn from such cases as that above. This condition has come to be called "acquired vitamin dependency."

This theory has been used increasingly as a rationale for the use of other megavitamin treatments such as vitamin B_6, B_{12} and vitamin C. Such treatment has received considerable publicity and has gained a good deal of popular support. Treatment centers using megavitamin therapy and orthomolecular treatment for psychiatric problems have sprung up around the country.

On the other hand, an impressive number of double-blind experiments by researchers who do not practice orthomolecular psychiatry have demonstrated no benefit from high doses of niacin in the treatment of schizophrenia.[10] As a result, the bulk of psychiatrists have not accepted this approach. A Task Force appointed by the American Psychiatric Association summarized the official attitude of the profession: while the claims of megavitamin therapists were "initially modest and supported by their own published data," more recently they have tended toward "categorical statements" made without adequate documentation.[11]   The bulk of experiments, they say, show no benefit from massive doses of vitamins like niacin.

Meanwhile, those who champion megavitamin treatment have offered sharp rebuttal to their critics.[12]   They point out that the Task Force was chaired by a man who had already taken a public stand against megavitamin treatment, and they claim that most of the negative research was designed in such a way as to necessarily get unfavorable results. A paper by Dr. Linus Pauling in the counter-report notes many inaccuracies and evidences of lack of understanding of biochemistry in the Task Force's statement. He observes that only niacin was mentioned, while the purpose of orthomolecular psychiatry is to create the proper molecular environment for brain cells by providing adequate concentrations of all the nutrients, not just niacin—even though it may be one that is unusually important. The controversy has spread from the profession into the press, especially to the health-oriented magazines, where megavitamin therapy is extolled as a deliverance from the evils of tranquilizers and their obvious side effects.   Unfortunately, in reality many, if not most, of the so-called "orthomolecular psychiatrists" use a combination of megavitamins and tranquilizers (claiming that the vitamins enable them to reduce the dosage of the drugs). Another school of psychiatric thought maintains that most schizophrenia is purely a psychological problem and should be treated with psychotherapy.   Those of this persuasion shun the use of tranquilizers as well as ignoring the claims of the mega-vitamin enthusiasts.

Though opinions vary widely, research continues.   In 1973 Dr. Linus Pauling and a group of his associates published a report of experiments done on schizophrenic patients whose urine was analyzed after they were given large doses of niacin, to see how much of it they "kept."   Compared to a group of normals, most of the schizophrenics excreted remarkably little of the niacin.   Apparently they were "using" more of it.   In-terestingly enough, however, there were a few of the schizo-phrenics who got rid of as much or more of the niacin than many of the normals.[13]   Obviously not all schizophrenics are alike.

When the evidence is finally in, we will probably have to conclude that some psychotic patients do respond to high doses of niacin while others don't.   Even some of the critics of mega-vitamin therapy are coming around to this point of view[14] and the work of several investigators has recently aimed at identifying the sub-groups who will respond to this form of treatment.[15, 16] If some persons do experience a clearing of their mental state when given huge amounts of niacin, the fact that some do and some don't must be due to a difference in the degree to which they absorb or use the vitamin.

The way one uses B vitamins is apparently related to the way his mind and emotions are functioning.   If one is very tense, nervous, constantly upset, on edge and anxious, then he will burn up many B vitamins.   Not only is niacin "used up" in this way, but probably others are too.   This may be one reason that some of the researchers failed to get positive results when testing vitamin therapy on the mentally disturbed. Not thinking in terms of the total "molecular environment of the brain cells," they did not consider other nutrients. They gave only niacin and found insignificant improvement. Psychiatrists accustomed to using megavitamin treatment often use a number of nutrients besides niacin, such as vitamin C, folic acid, B_{12}, zinc and vitamin B_6. When 800 psychiatric patients were tested, some were reported to need 80 times as much B_6 (pyridoxine) as that required by others.[17] B_6 which facilitates dream recall, is thought to be depleted in some people by stressful situations. One noted nutritionist has observed that when he is on a lecture tour, he must take more vitamin B_6 than usual in order to remember his dreams.[18] His particular way of reacting to such situations happens to involve physiological processes, perhaps increased muscle tension or autonomic arousal which use B_6 rapidly. Of course the point to be made is that one's basic problem here is how he uses his body—not a "deficiency" of B_6 or even, in fact, "unusual requirement" for the vitamin. The fact that one needs more if he uses more can hardly be considered "unusual!"

B_{12} SHOTS FOR TIREDNESS?

It has only recently been recognized that the depletion of other B vitamins can be related to psychiatric problems, too. Both folic acid and vitamin B_{12} are important here. It is now recognized by those who have studied this subject experimentally and clinically that low levels of B_{12} in the body are often accompanied by flagrant psychosis, and in many cases the mental symptoms may precede the classical pernicious anemia that is usually associated with lack of the vitamin.* While pernicious anemia is regarded as a completely distinct disease bearing no

---

* See section on vitamin B_{12}.

relation to those people who might have borderline levels of B_{12}, it may be more reasonable to think of their simply representing different degrees of the same problem. Roger Williams has pointed out that the occurrence of any extreme will usually indicate a spectrum of less severe but similar disorders which span the range from the normal to the glaringly abnormal.[19] Because of what we know about those who have pernicious anemia and their low levels of gastric acid and "intrinsic factor" (the substance in the stomach wall which helps with the absorption of B_{12}) we would expect to find that there are also many people who have borderline B_{12} levels due to moderate mental and emotional problems such as "nervousness" and "anxiety." Perhaps such persons would, if studied, be found to show mild to decreased levels of intrinsic factor and hydrochloric acid in the stomach.

Interestingly enough, it is thought that gastric acidity is reduced in patients with certain emotional disturbances. In fact, it is well established that during emotional upset the digestive juices in general are poorly regulated.[20] If the relationship between psychologic disorders and B_{12} absorption is further borne out by future research, we might expect that similar situations would exist with other nutrients, where emotional problems would lead to a decrease in absorption. Moreover, in the case of B_{12}, it is easy to see how psychological reorganization could lead to an improvement in the secretion of gastric acid with an increased ability to absorb B_{12}.*

While the psychologically and psychodynamically oriented psychiatrists scoff at those who administer vitamins for mental disease, the nutritionally-oriented psychiatrists are doing serum vitamin B_{12} levels and criticizing their colleagues for not giving B_{12} shots. The result is a perpetuation of the schism between mind and body which deprives the patients of an integrated and

---

*At least in those persons who have normal amounts of intrinsic factor. Whether the amount of intrinsic factor secreted is also a function of mental and emotional factors is another matter that deserves study.

holistic treatment.

There may well be persons whose absorption of B_{12} is normal but whose needs for the vitamin are increased. B_{12} is sometimes also used empirically for chronic fatigue. It was observed that some people "get a boost" from injections of the B_{12} even when they have none of the classic symptoms of deficiency. While most doctors are reluctant to give B_{12} when there is no evidence of anemia, and no good rationale for doing so, there are others who don't hesitate to use the injections for this purpose. They use it "because it works." Many exhausted, unhappy women go from doctor to doctor trying to find one who will give them B_{12} shots which they had felt sometime in the past had relieved their fatigue.

Such use of large doses of B_{12} was a controversial issue among physicians long before popular interest in taking mega-vitamins by mouth developed. But it is only recently that the effectiveness of this treatment has been researched. Twenty-eight patients suffering from chronic fatigue were given either B_{12} shots or a blank injection twice a week for two weeks. The doctors giving the medication didn't know which patient was getting what. After a two week rest period, the injections were resumed. Unbeknownst to the physicians, the B_{12} and blanks were exchanged so that each patient had two weeks on the B_{12} and two weeks off without knowing it. Symptoms were recorded daily. Almost every subject reported an increased "sense of well-being" while on the B_{12} and for some time afterward.[21]

Such research apparently confirms the belief that though some people do respond to high doses of vitamin B_{12}, what has not been explored is why. *How* they are using—or misusing—their bodies and nervous systems in such a way that large quantities of B_{12} are needed, is the crucial question. When B_{12} shots are given as a "boost" without also trying to understand what's wrong or how to change it, the patient is done a disservice. The vitamin injection may temporarily relieve the problem, but it is not solving it.

VITAMIN C AND STRESS

Next to niacin, vitamin C has probably been talked about most as a treatment for psychiatric disorders and nervous problems. As early as 1940 in Europe it was found that some schizophrenics excreted very little vitamin C in their urine, and when they were given large enough doses of it, half were soon well enough to go home.[22] It has been reported, on the basis of double-blind studies that some psychotics [23] respond to vitamin C, and Linus Pauling's test for urine excretion in such patients showed the same retention of vitamin C as it did for niacin.[24] Some researchers feel that the low vitamin C levels seen in hospitalized schizophrenics have to do with the poor diet that is usually available, rather than with the disease itself [25] but it has been shown that schizophrenics require up to 70,000 mg of vitamin C for complete saturation as opposed[26] to only 4,000 mg for other people. This would seem to be more than could be accounted for by having had a poor diet. The total body content of ascorbic acid in a normal person is only about 1,500 mg[27] and it is hard to believe that, even if this were totally depleted, 70,000 mg, nearly 50 times this amount, would be required for tissue saturation unless extraordinary amounts are being used. In fact, one researcher has concluded that on the average schizophrenics "burn up" ascorbic acid ten times as rapidly as do normal persons.[28]   It is generally thought that emotional stress and strain decrease body ascorbic acid levels when one responds to stress by becoming anxious.[29] For this reason, vitamin C is widely considered useful to prevent or ameliorate stress-related disorders ranging all the way from those due to physical overexertion or viral and bacterial infections* to those associated with emotional upset.

When we say that conditions of unusual stress result in the need for larger amounts of vitamin C, this simply amounts to

* See Chapter 7, Vitamins.

saying that when the individual functions in a certain way, there will be a tendency to some sort of biochemical breakdown which the presence of vitamin C in large quantities will help to alleviate. When we do not function in that particular way our vitamin C requirements are less. Even the British Naval physicians of two centuries ago observed that not all the sailors on the scurvy-struck ships came down with the disease. Some remained in good health despite the fact that their diets were exactly the same as those who fell ill. Obviously they were functioning in quite a different way from their sick mates. In view of the fact that large doses of vitamin C may provide some relief to those who suffer from anxiety and psychological disturbances, it is interesting to note that back in the 1700's, Dr. Lind made it a point to include not only lemon juice in his treatment of scurvy, but also the avoidance of tension and psychological stress.[30]   Clearly, there must be some difference in the way their metabolic machinery is functioning for one person to "use up" more of a nutrient than another does. Increased use of B vitamins and C must have something to do with an increased susceptibility to "stress."

Stress is produced by job pressures, fatigue, psychologic upsets, anxious situations and many other conditions. Stress is thought to "cause biochemical changes to take place in the body" and it has been said that "when animals on seemingly adequate diets are subjected to stress widespread damage occurs in their bodies.[31] Certain of the B vitamins and vitamin C are called the "anti-stress vitamins" and are taken increasingly to "combat stress." From this perspective one begins to feel that "stress" is a monster hovering overhead which can only be held at bay by eating large quantities of vitamin pills.

Though popular ideas of stress concentrate on environmental causes and assume that one necessarily reacts to them in a set, predetermined fashion, research has not borne this out. It has become increasingly evident that stress has little to do with external events. It is purely personal, a matter of how one responds to a situation, rather than the situation itself. It is our psychological stance that determines the amount of stress we experience.[32] What makes one person frightened or anxious or angry may simply amuse another person and perhaps even go unnoticed by a third. If the cause of stress lies more in one's attitude and patterns of thought than in the environmental circumstances that surround him, this probably explains why some people require more of certain vitamins, such as vitamin C, than others do. While some people tend to repeatedly and habitually interpret events and circumstances as stressful or disturbing, others consistently do the opposite. The result is a difference in modes of experiencing and a consequent difference in emotional tone and metabolic and biochemical functioning. Those who tend to be chronically anxious and find events around them upsetting will have higher levels of catecholamines in the urine, indicating that the adrenals, for example, are frequently responding to what is interpreted as "stress." Those who are able to remain more tranquil will maintain much lower urine levels of adrenalin-related substances.

In summary, then, it appears that we can conclude that the more chronically anxious person who tends to interpret events around him as disturbing will, as a result of the more frequent occurrences of those metabolic events that accompany his tense and anxious behavior, use up more of certain nutrients which are involved in his characteristic responses. It will generally be some combination of certain of the B vitamins and/or vitamin C* which are required in the most unusual quantities by those who tend to respond psychologically and physiologically with "anxiety." But there is no set proportion of B vitamins and C that is needed by every "stressed" person. Since people vary in the way they react to situations, it is not surprising that they also vary as far as which nutrients they use up most rapidly. Which

---

* The "stress tabs" now sold in many health food stores contain the B complex plus C with higher quantities of pantothenic acid which is thought to help the adrenals.

physiological processes are overworked will determine which nutrients are overused. If we were to study the matter carefully, we could probably learn to detect through psychological testing which vitamin a person would need in largest quantities, "predicting his deficiency" by his attitude and behavior.

Though one may draw some conclusions from all this about the relationship between "anxiety" and vitamin levels, the larger and more important concept which emerges is that one's mental attitude and habits of thought have a powerful effect on his vitamin requirements. This suggests that the resolution of psychological conflicts, the learning of techniques of relaxation and a reorientation in consciousness which allows one to become calmer and less susceptible to environmental stresses, will reduce requirements for unusually large amounts of B vitamins and perhaps vitamin C.

This does not in any way conflict with the observations of such workers as Dr. Hoffer, who found that the survivors of prisoner of war camps from World War II often had requirements for extremely large doses of niacin. The chronic disorders (nervousness and other vague complaints) which they had developed subsequent to their release often cleared up when large doses of the B vitamins, particularly niacin, were supplied. When the megavitamin doses were discontinued, the symptoms returned. From the above considerations it is possible to suggest an explanation for this "acquired vitamin dependency." Unresolved psychological problems resulting from the trauma of life in a prisoner of war camp might easily leave survivors with a mode of emotional and psychological functioning that keeps their metabolism continually geared in such a way that unusual demands for niacin result. While people generally vary widely in their psychological makeup—and within certain limits, their nutritional requirements—it would not be surprising if a psychological trauma as massive as that of war with long term imprisonment would deal a blow so severe and so impartially distributed that it could cut across individual differences and leave certain mental and physiological habits that would be common to the whole group. True recovery would have to be based on an emotional and psychological readjustment to the past trauma and an elimination of its effect on the mind, not on continual doses of niacin.

Nonetheless, this does not leave room for nutritional nihilism. It does not mean that one should be told "no more vitamin C, learn how to get along on less." Though it may be in the mental realm where changes can be made that will most profoundly affect vitamin needs, the use of supplements can be in the meantime a valuable expedient. The fact of the matter is that each of us must be seen in the context of his own personal growth and evolution. We each exist at different points along the pathway which leads toward realizing our full potential as human beings. In the meantime, there will be obvious limitations to what we can do at this time, at this place. These limitations are not only psychological, but also emotional, physiological, etc. These limitations characterize our present position along our personal path. In fact they characterize us as we exist at this moment. How we relate to situations around us, and the business and physiological chaos that we habitually create in the process, are part of our present stance and will take time to change.

Given these limitations, it would be foolish indeed for us to suffer unnecessarily, to exhaust our energy and fail to make progress or experience growth because of certain unusual and exaggerated nutritional requirements which we happen to have at this moment. Satisfying these nutritional requirements for the time being may be an important stop-gap measure. If it enables us to maximize our awareness and our ability to function, then it serves an important purpose and may give us the needed boost to outgrow this particular stage of development and move on to the next.

If one repeatedly relies on vitamins, however, he misses an opportunity to come to terms with the habits which have created the problem. The process of change that can modify one's mode of functioning so he doesn't require such large quantities of nutrients is essentially a psychotherapeutic one. This does not mean that psychological change cannot occur in one who takes vitamins. The two approaches are not mutually exclusive. It is certainly possible that there are times when psychotherapy could be promoted by the judicious administration of vitamin B_{12} injections without the physician suffering the delusion that either modality is the "only proper approach." The same principle applies to the common use of vitamins by mouth, and to the processes of growth that all of us are constantly undergoing as a result of life's experiences and what we learn from them, regardless of whether we are involved in formal "psychotherapy" or not.

If we rely on the added nutrients as a way of avoiding certain issues within ourselves, it can be an indication of stagnation and we may become dependent on vitamin supplements. Then we become, in effect, "vitamin junkies."

FOOD ALLERGY AND FOOD ADDICTION

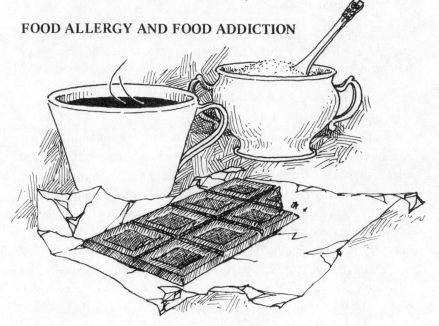

Apparently, some people have extremely strong reactions to certain substances in natural foods. Such a reaction is called a "food allergy," and some of them have been dramatic. Researchers in this area report full-blown psychotic episodes, for example, emerging almost instantly as a drop of an extract of the food to which the person is sensitive is placed under the tongue.

A demonstration of this has been filmed:

> After talking with a composed, pleasant young lady, the physician inserts a tube into her digestive tract by way of the nose so that, standing behind her, where she cannot see him or know what he's doing, he can introduce certain foods into the stomach. Various foods are given, including those to which the doctor suspects she may be allergic. After the first feeding is pushed through the tube by a syringe of water there is no change apparent. She chats calmly with the physician. After a few minutes he again steps behind her and injects a second food. This one is corn, a food to which at least three-fifths of people tested are said to show at least some slight reaction.[33]
>
> For a few moments little change is apparent. Then suddenly the young woman begins to scream and strike out at the doctor. Fighting the nurses, she tries to push her way to the door and escape, refusing to listen to what is being said to her. This psychotic state persists for four full days, after which she suddenly returns to normal, remembering very little of what had happened.

This patient had come to the doctor complaining of recurring psychotic episodes, and it was concluded that she had what is called a "cerebral allergy"—that is, an allergic reaction which is thought to affect the tissues of the brain primarily. Not all food allergies produce strange behavior, of course. Some affect other systems or organs, such as the skin, though they may be just as spectacular. One patient developed hives over the entire body after eating only a small amount of egg. Her head was swollen to the point that it appeared twice its normal size. Facial features were enlarged so much as to look like caricatures. Her tongue was also swollen alarmingly. In some such cases, airway obstruction can occur from the swelling and thickening of the linings of nose, mouth and throat. Allergic reactions are not always so dramatic. They may constitute only a mild feeling of unease, flushing, a runny nose, headache or any number of other miscellaneous aches and pains that seem to appear for no apparent reason. One need not go through the drama of having the food put through a stomach tube to test for food allergies. He can just as easily test himself at home by taking his pulse after he eats some food he suspects of causing trouble. If the pulse is markedly elevated[34] then one knows he is sensitive to the food in question. Physicians usually don't use a nasogastric tube for testing anyway; they most often simply use drops of extracts which they put under the tongue.*

Such reactions are sometimes reversible by using a weaker concentration of the same substance as an antidote.† There is also, paradoxically, some evidence that the adverse effects of foods to which one is sensitive can be dulled to some extent when one eats more and more of the same thing. Chocolate, for example, produces nervousness and emotional upset in people sensitive to it, but they are able to fend off these feelings to a certain degree if they eat chocolate again. This sometimes leads to a vicious circle (or rather, downward spiral) in which the more one eats of a food, the more he feels compelled to eat. One physician describes a patient of his who, restraining herself as long as she could, would dash out of her house in the evening at the time the stores were due to close, grab a taxi and speed to the nearest quick-stop market in search of a chocolate cake. This

---

* Skin tests, where possible allergens are injected just under the skin are virtually useless in testing for food allergies, since one may be sensitive to a material introduced into the skin but experience no ill effects from it when it is taken by mouth.

† This is worthy of note since it amounts to a crude form of homeopathy and it is the more sophisticated use of homeopathy which is major treatment that offers at least the possibility of permanently overcoming (rather than simply avoiding those things which trigger) food allergies.

she would purchase and consume enroute as the taxi driver searched the city for another late night store or dining spot where she could buy a second cake. Often she would go from one restaurant to another buying whole cakes, but paying for them by the slice. Having exhausted all possibilities, she would return home with one last chocolate cake which she would consume in its entirety before she turned in for the night. The next day she would be in a deep depression which lasted until evening, when she would again go off her diet, have more chocolate and recapture once more a temporary feeling of well-being.[35] Another patient, treated by the present author, who has similar problems with chocolate, describes a feeling of emptiness that precedes the craving and observes that when she's very upset nothing will calm her except eating sweets. Such behavior has led to the term "addiction" for cases where the craving has become an obsession.

How frequently this plays a role in emotional problems is not known. Some researchers claim that 92.8% of all schizophrenics suffer from allergies.[36] Others report that when institutionalized adolescents with behavioral and emotional problems were tested for food and other allergies and were kept away from those substances to which they reacted, average time before discharge was reduced from 26 months to nine months.[37]

THE TREATMENT OF FOOD ALLERGIES

Physicians who have studied such problems call themselves clinical ecologists. By identifying which foods cause the reaction, they are able to eliminate them. On careful testing, however, a patient is seldom found to be allergic to only one food.[38] Commonly, problems are caused by such foods as wheat, corn, eggs and milk. To eliminate several of these from the diet, however, is not practical for most people. In children this can be especially true, since by avoiding many of the available nutritious foods they can miss important nutrients and become seriously malnourished. Fortunately, by eating small quantities of a food that causes some reaction, one can usually build a tolerance for it, whereas taking large amounts alone can aggravate the condition.   Moreover, the substances in foods to which one becomes allergic are proteins and cooking often denatures such a protein so it loses its power to trigger allergic reactions.   Thus a person sensitive to raw milk or even pasteurized milk may suffer no ill effects from milk that is boiled.

Even pinning down exactly which foods are the culprits may not be so easy. Immediate reactions can be picked up by the sublingual tests, but the delayed reactions which are thought to occur days later are very difficult to identify. One may be mistaking a delayed reaction to a food taken yesterday for an immediate reaction to something just eaten. Sometimes a total fast is carried out for several days to a week or more, then gradually foods are added, one at a time, to observe their effects. This has occasionally been dramatically helpful, bringing disturbed children or adults back to equilibrium and then revealing which foods were most upsetting for them. But usually this is carried out in a hospital where all conditions can be controlled and it is, unfortunately, both expensive and time-consuming. Moreover, it doesn't always provide a permanent solution since food allergies can shift. One may cease to be allergic to the first food and suddenly develop reactions to a second. The approach of clinical ecology is to look at other factors in the environment besides food that might cause trouble. Dust and mold are often offenders, and to eliminate them may require special carpets, draperies, etc. Though some persons find themselves allergic to one discrete substance and by simply eliminating it obtain some relief, usually it is a combination of things that must be avoided. The whole program can become very complicated and awkward:

> Mrs. G saw a well-known clinical ecologist for a stuffy nose. As a test for allergies she was fasted and then given large amounts of the food suspected of causing trouble. On the day she ate six scrambled eggs she felt very ill. Similar

reactions resulted from other foods such as wheat and milk products. She was counseled to avoid all these foods and to be careful to use only organically grown produce. Finding the foods she could eat became quite difficult. This was especially true since she was found to react adversely to exhaust fumes and so couldn't drive an automobile. She would spend her day on the phone locating usable items and then her husband would go in his time off work to purchase them. He began to tire of this and to suspect that she did it to provoke him. The situation between them was worsened when, because of pollens and dust, they were advised to move to a different town. Though he gave in, foods continued to upset her and the doctor insisted that anything which caused any negative reaction should be avoided. Since by now almost any food seemed to cause her to feel giddy or sluggish, she ate very little. She lost weight, her skin became discolored and she developed strange and uncontrollable cravings. On one occasion she ate 1½ pounds of honey at a sitting, and "felt a great sense of relief and well-being." At this point a glucose tolerance test showed hypoglycemia, so she put herself on a high protein diet, but that made her feel dull. She tried the climate in the Southwest, but the water in the hotel was chlorinated, which gave her a bad reaction. After one frightening weekend when she couldn't get anyone to bring her water by automobile, she fled, terrified, feeling herself a fugitive from the world.

Another patient had ended up after 18 years of treatment on a diet of only wild game:

Her prescribed menu was as follows: venison on Mondays (2 or 3 meals of it, but no other foods), pheasant on Tuesdays, shrimp on Wednesdays and bear, moose, squab or antelope on each of the following days of the week. This diet presented obvious practical problems and though she felt reasonably well on it, she found herself craving other foods such as fruits. She was also so sensitive to airborne chemicals that she carried an extra purse with her that contained an air filter. From this protruded a plastic tube and she puffed on it between sentences, as she talked.

The allergist calls this perspective "exogenous," i.e., the cause of illness or distress is seen as external to the person.[39] This

means, of course, that correction of the problem requires alterations in the environment and in the food supply rather than in
the person himself. Not only is this cumbersome and unwieldy,
but it does little to help the patient outgrow and overcome his
problems. It may be more useful to adopt a different viewpoint
and ask what it is internally that sets the stage for such a reaction.

FOOD ALLERGIES AND THE MIND

Allergic reactions are a result of malfunctioning of the
immunologic system. The immunologic system is one of the
body's first lines of defense. It manufactures antibodies to
"foreign" materials, those that "don't belong" in the body.
It "recognizes" them as foreign and prepares antibodies which
attach to them and help in their destruction and elimination
from the body. This is the way that the body rids itself of
bacteria and viruses, as well as many other useless and potentially harmful protein substances.

Occasionally, however, things go haywire. The body
"recognizes as foreign" a protein molecule that is actually
familiar and customarily present—such as one of those found in
commonly eaten food. Such is the basis of food allergies. In
extreme cases one's own tissues may be treated as "foreign"
and antibodies manufactured that attack them. This results in
a class of diseases called "autoimmune."

On the other side of the coin, when the body fails to
recognize as foreign a material that is, then infections can run
rampant, or cells that are abnormal are not properly destroyed
and eliminated. Certain unhealthy cells appear periodically that
function poorly in the tissue, but multiply rapidly when the
immunologic system fails to "recognize" these as "foreign";
they are given free reign and may invade and destroy healthy
tissue. The result, which we call cancer, is therefore, in a sense,
a disease of poorly regulated immune mechanisms. But what
regulates immune mechanisms?

Recent research has begun to turn up some interesting information about the control of immune responses. In experimental animals, when certain small areas of the brain are destroyed, antibody production is affected.[40] Significantly, it is precisely those areas which are most closely involved with emotional states where tissue destruction disrupts immune responses. This particular point in the brain, called the hypothalamus, is both part of the "circuit" that is active when one is anxious or upset, as well as a bridge to the pituitary gland that regulates the secretion of hormones. Certain hormones are thought to play a role in the regulation of antibody production too, and it is thought that mental and emotional states affect the way one reacts to a foreign substance by means of this complicated network.[41] This is probably particularly true in the case of those reactions we call "allergic."[42]

If future research bears this out, we may find that the "diagnosis" of food allergy, and the attention and anxiety it arouses in the patient may actually do more to aggravate the situation than it does to help it. Certainly in most cases it is true that a balanced, healthful diet of wholesome foods, along with a well-designed program of relaxation, breathing exercises and other techniques to improve one's ability to handle stressful situations will enable most persons with "food allergies" to eventually overcome them. In fact children, who are often subject to food allergies, but who are fluid and flexible and everchanging are constantly outgrowing such reactions and usually by age five, have left most of their food allergies behind for good.*

The same principles that apply to the understanding of megavitamins also probably apply to food allergies. Behind the allergy will usually lie a complex of problems and difficulties of a psychological nature. To invest one's energy in a continual

---

* At this age allergies to dust, pollen or animal hair may arise, though they are usually outgrown later too.[43]

quest for everchanging "permissable" foods and in a constant struggle to avoid dust, animals, or pollens, is similar to taking refuge in vitamin supplements. It is an attempt to escape the work that faces one and to retreat into an uncomfortable status quo.

It seems likely that we have hardly begun to appreciate our capacity for overcoming difficulties with certain foods or special needs for nutrients. Not only may one be able to outgrow food allergies or "vitamin dependencies," he may even have the potential for getting along with less of certain essential nutrients than we ordinarily consider the bare minimum, as we have already seen in the case of certain of the B vitamins.*

Even more surprising is the possibility that we may have some capacity for manufacturing some of the very nutrients that are usually regarded as essential. Though it had been widely accepted for some time that man is unable to synthesize vitamin C, this may not be a hard and fast rule. Research scientists in India have discovered, for example, that women who were breast feeding their infants regularly put out in their milk and in their urine quantities of vitamin C that far exceeded their dietary intake.[44] This could only be explained by acknowledging that a physiological "law" was being broken. Apparently these women had actually manufactured vitamin C. Further evidence that this is possible emerged when it was shown that vitamin C is also synthesized in the human placenta.[45]

Just as superhuman feats of strength accomplished in an emergency give us a glimpse of what we are capable of, so may such a synthesis of vitamin C by a nursing mother tell us much about our untapped physiological powers. The degree to which we develop our ability to function smoothly and creatively, even in the face of a less than ideal environment and a less than perfect diet will depend to a great extent on how well we come to terms with the psychological aspects of our dietary habits and tendencies.

* See Chapter 7, Vitamins on thiamin and riboflavin.

Food Sadhana

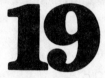

In previous chapters we have seen the complexity of the variables which affect the nutritive value of what one eats. Vitamin and mineral and even protein content varies not only from food to food but from foods grown in one area to those grown in another. The value of protein also depends on the way in which various foods are combined, and the amount of carbohydrate one needs depends on his activity and his way of life. Moreover, each person's needs vary according to his individual makeup, his personality and his way of reacting to situations around him, so that some people have higher requirements for one vitamin and lower requirements for another. The amount of food assimilated from that which is taken in depends to a great extent on the functioning of the digestive system. This also varies from person to person, but it may vary from day to day or even hour to hour as well, depending on one's emotional or mental state. One may secrete more enzymes or less depending on his state of mind, and on his attitude toward the food, what it might mean to him, or whether it looks and tastes appealing.

Climatic and seasonal variables also enter into the picture, having an effect on one's requirements.

If we all vary in our psychological makeup, and because of this, use our bodies in different ways so that our nutritional requirements vary, how then does one go about finding out which diet is a good one for him? Faced with the complexity of choices in diet, biochemical individuality and the unpredictability of daily needs, it becomes quite apparent that one can't calculate mathematically what his requirements are.

Clearly, the optimal selection of food for an individual is a matter that defies his intellectual capacity. No amount of education and training prepares him to consider all these multiple variables in himself and in the food before him. One must therefore rely on taste, appetite, instincts, feelings, impulses and intuition. After we have learned to recognize what is wholesome and what is not, we must then make from the best available foods a selection that is based on our inner promptings.

Experiential criteria as a basis for nutritional understanding and the personal devising of a diet by-passes many difficulties. No longer is it necessary to try to analyze from the outside one's physiology, biochemistry and metabolic needs. Nor is it any longer necessary to analyze from the outside each food (which is, as we have noted before, extremely difficult in any case since one tomato varies from the next, and so forth). Of course it is an intuitive or subjective process of selection that we ordinarily use every meal, every day. But most of us have not examined this process to see how it might be sharpened and refined.

Once one has begun to approach the subject of nutrition from a personal, experiential point of view new horizons open. For instance, if one makes a careful study of the effects of different foods on oneself, he will begin to find that he can classify them into different categories. What's more, he will begin to learn interesting things about himself—his feelings, his desires, his conflicts. In the East there are many systems which provide the framework within which one can do this, such as the Ayurvedic system which we discussed earlier. The same is probably true of other ancient cultures, but much of their knowledge has been lost when there is not the continuous, living tradition found in countries like India, Tibet and China.

Developing one's fullest capacity for studying himself in relationship to his food calls on the best of contemporary scientific data on nutrition and physiology combined with the essence of ancient traditions of organizing the experiential data of self-observation. But the rewards are worthwhile, both in terms of improved nutrition and personal growth.

MAKING ONESELF A NUTRITIONAL LABORATORY

Studying nutrition from an experiential approach requires that one prepare himself. If the outcome of an experiment is to be clear and intelligible, it must be carried out where conditions are stable and predictable. The laboratory must be in good order. One can't do productive research in the midst of confusion and chaos. The setting must be quiet, calm and constant. In other words, a laboratory is a place where one can keep constant most things that would affect an experiment, focussing on only one. Then it is changed so that the results can be studied. Whatever happens must have been due to the change that was made, since everything else remained the same. But this only works when conditions in the laboratory are well under control.

In working with the body and diet, if one's system is functioning smoothly it becomes a suitable laboratory. After eating something different, if the body reacts strangely, or the mind becomes fuzzy, it is possible to have some idea of what caused it.

So there are several steps that are preliminary to beginning to discover the proper foods. They clear the field, so to speak, so that one's experiments are not obscured. The first is to adjust the quantity of food eaten. If a lot of food is piled into the system then it is going to be clogged. As we saw in chapter ten, it is possible to overwhelm the capacity for the digestion of food. The enzymes are limited in amount and they can only handle so much. Charak says, " one must eat in proper measure and the proper measure of food is determined by the strength of one's gastric fire,"[1] and in a later verse, "The self-controlled man always feeds his gastric fire with the fuel of wholesome food and drink, mindful of the consideration of measure and time."[2] If too much is put in, it piles up, bacteria begin to grow in it and the result is wastes and contaminants that mess up the internal laboratory. Trying to learn about diet in such a situation would be like trying to work in a lab where huge boxes of supplies were piled, things that should have been refrigerated and hadn't been so had spoiled, where containers were knocked over and spilling on the floor so that everywhere one turned there was found another collection of garbage. In the midst of all that, it would be impossible to do a successful experiment.

So the first order of business is to be sensible about the quantity of food eaten. This helps provide a cleaner place to work in. If a reasonable amount of food is put into the body, a lot of digestive problems disappear and the system begins to function in a quieter, less confused way.

The next matter of importance is *when one eats*. It is often necessary at first to get on a fairly regular schedule, eating at set intervals. If one skips two out of three meals on one day, and then eats six times on the next, his system will be upset regardless of whether he is eating the best food or the worst.

Scheduling should be such that there is more or less the same pattern each day. For most people, two meals a day are enough. If one feels more comfortable with three, then the schedule should include three. But to have four or five or six feedings a day is almost always unnecessary, (even in those who are susceptible to hypoglycemic episodes). If the digestive tract is full of food and, before it even begins to be processed and digested, more is dumped in, how can one know what is the effect of what? It becomes difficult if not impossible to know whether the feelings one experiences are due to the juice he drank at eight o'clock, the granola and bananas he had at nine, or the "mid-morning snack" at eleven.

If, on the contrary, one eats one meal and then waits five hours or six hours before eating another meal, the digestive system has time to finish what it is doing before it starts over. This is important not only to facilitate self-study, but, as we saw in Part III, the "machine" doesn't work well otherwise. It's not designed to have a constant input. Whenever something is put in the mouth, digestive juices are secreted and a definite series of processes is triggered. The stomach secretes acid, the intestines get ready to secrete digestive enzymes. Like a computer, it has a set program. Once it is cranked up, it runs until it's finished.

If one has breakfast at eight o'clock in the morning the whole system is set into motion. Food goes through your intestines, juices are secreted in each place and digestion is completed. Once the process is over, there is a "clean-up," after which the digestive tract is ready for another dose of food. That may be at one or two o'clock in the afternoon.

Therefore the first and most obvious step toward establishing the conditions that will enable one to learn more about the effects of food is to apply these common sense principles to the use of the digestive system. Once these simple matters are in order, one can begin then to discover which specific foods are best for him. It is only necessary to take the food in question, and observe the results. If the effects of the experiment are not immediately obvious, then it may be necessary to take the food once or twice a day for several days to see the changes it makes. Is there more gas? Does the stomach always feel full? Is there a feeling of heaviness and fatigue? Is the mind sluggish? These, of course, are indications that what was eaten doesn't agree. An excess of mucus is another indication, as is a bad taste in the morning or offensive breath.

Eating fourteen pieces of pizza doesn't really qualify as an experiment. Blasting the gastrointestinal system with a handful of hot chilis may produce a slightly different variety of stomach ache from that following a whole loaf of bread but nothing very valuable is learned from either. Violent actions produce violent reactions, but understanding of the subtler aspects of oneself and his diet comes when a slight change is made in a calm setting so that the results can stand out in clear relief.

Dietary changes should be made gradually. Becoming vegetarian on Tuesday after having a half chicken on Sunday and a jumbo sirloin on Monday is not helpful. Drastic changes will yield no useful information. They may produce reactions— sometimes dramatic ones—but this usually provides little understanding. Overzealous and self-righteous "reforms" in diet are ill-advised.

In the *Charak Samhita* it is written:

> By degrees the wise man should free himself of unwholesome habits; also, by degrees he should develop wholesome ones. The acquisition of the new good habits and the giving-up of the old bad ones should be achieved by regular quarter-steps of decrease at orderly intervals of one, two and three days.[3]

This allows one to settle gradually into a new eating pattern. Not only is this approach more likely to establish lasting changes, it provides more opportunity for observation. It is said that Gandhi changed his diet regularly to learn of how it affected him. That is true, but he changed it only every four months. Thus he was able to conduct meaningful experiments. Though one's "research" on himself may not allow him to draw statistically supported conclusions, it does open new realms of self-awareness.

If living habits are reasonably regular and sane, one will begin to notice that he has certain impulses or feelings that one food or another is not suitable or is "just what he needs." Such a subjective sense of what is right can be a valuable guide. Even experimental animals distinguish between a mixture containing all the essential amino acids and an otherwise identical mixture which lacks one of them. Horses will choose the feed with the most minerals and cows will graze bare a strip of pasture grown organically leaving the chemically fertilized grass standing around it.[4] Moreover, in the case of man, this intuitive sense of what is best, or what is needed at the moment, can be sharpened and refined.

DIET AND SELF-REGULATION

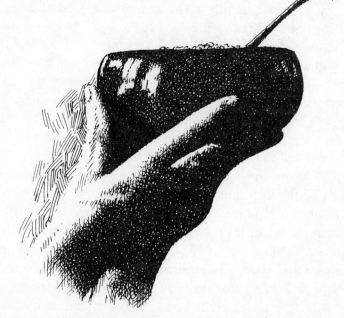

As one begins to tune in to inner cues, he encounters a variety of urgings and impulses. Some are based on habit and past conditioning whereas others are based more on current and realistic needs. To sift and sort through these requires a lack of distraction, ample time and a process of retraining oneself. If one has lost touch with these inner cues and is trying to re-establish contact and awareness, he will at first find conversation, noise, a tight schedule and other distractions a great hindrance. According to the Ayurvedic scriptures, where experiential awareness of diet played a central part, certain suggestions were laid down for the practice of eating.

1.   Eat alone.   At least at the beginning of reeducating oneself and one's attitudes toward food, it is often helpful to be alone during meals.   This allows one time to pay attention to the taste of the food, its texture, and the way it affects one's body. It allows one time to tune in and consult his body asking, "Do I need more?   Have I had enough?   Do I need some of this or some of that?"

2.   Chew carefully.   The scriptures suggest chewing each bite thirty-two times, "once for each tooth." Prolonged chewing makes one more aware of the food which he is eating.   It also allows him to digest it more properly.   One will find that the taste of food varies during the full process of chewing.   The full spectrum of tastes that occurs during the proper chewing of a bite of food allows one's body to assess its properties and develop a feeling about what such food supplies, how much more is needed and so forth.

3.   Amount.   It is helpful to serve oneself the amount which he thinks is appropriate, to go off alone, eat it, and then be finished.   This removes the tendency to overeat or undereat and allows one to learn to gauge how much he needs.   Another approach is to eat only one food at a time, chewing thoroughly and pausing between bites, eating that food until one has had enough and then going on to what seems to be appealing next. If this is done thoughtfully and with full attention, if one offers himself only wholesome foods from which to choose, and if foods are selected according to what seems to be needed rather than what might taste interesting, then surprisingly enough, one does not overeat.   In fact, this approach has been successfully used for weight loss.[5]

4. Which foods. Other more complex guidelines to food selection are provided by the Ayurvedic principles briefly outlined in Chapter 15, which specify which foods could be expected to be appropriate during which seasons for which sort of people,

at what time of day and so forth.

The guidelines which have been laid down for helping one who is attempting to learn how to select his food properly are not to be followed slavishly, in a mechanical or rigid way. No one can determine what is right for another person to eat. Although a nutritionist may make general statements about what the average person needs, he may have much more trouble determining exactly what is right for himself.

In the ancient cultures of the East one was trained in self-observation, and rules for sane living were regarded as valuable aids in establishing the conditions that permitted one to experiment. Inner experimentation became a way of life. Though to the modern urban dweller who keeps strange hours, eats a hodge-podge of processed and semi-artificial foods and rushes around in his polluted environment, the ancient Indian would appear regimented and unimaginative, the truth may be different.

Regularity of living was valued not as an escape from variety and change, but as providing the freedom to experience it. In India rules are generally followed but widely regarded as made to be broken. A self-regulatory approach to diet requires constant experimentation and exploration. The proof of the pudding is in the eating. Sometimes what is right is what seems to be most contrary to all the rules.

The story is told of an Irishman lying on his deathbed who was asked by his physician whether he had a last wish. Rallying enough to reply, the dying man responded, "Yes. I would like a cold pork pie and a bottle of stout." His wife shuddered, sure that it would kill him, but the doctor took her aside and gently reminded her that since her husband could not, in any case, recover it would be best to let him have this last wish fulfilled. So a friend was dispatched to the corner pub and soon returned with the pie and stout. The patient swallowed it down almost in one gulp whereup he stood up looking much improved. He then proceeded to make a rapid recovery.

The rules are not hard and fast. There are times they

should be broken—if for no other reason, simply to see what happens when they are. They are not really rules at all, in the usual sense of the word, but guidelines to help in establishing conditions which will facilitate inner experimentation.

Learning to be aware of one's real needs and taking in what will satisfy them is not the easiest of challenges to meet. Habits often lead us to eat when we're not hungry or to eat things for which our bodies have no use. There are many signals and urges one will encounter experientially. Some are based on taste appeal and associations with past experiences. Others are based on genuine physiological needs. To sift and sort through these requires much attention, thoughtfulness and sensitivity. A Spartan approach and an attitude of self-denial is of no help. To the extent that one can tune in to his physiological cues and select his food appropriately, he will feel clearer, more alert and more comfortable and content. What we know about the biochemistry of nutrition (vitamins, minerals, fats, carbohydrate, protein) and of digestive physiology, along with what we have learned of more traditional ideas about nutrition, plus our perception of our internal signals, leads upon each encounter with food or appetite to a hypothesis: "I think I need *this*, and it will probably make me feel *that* way." Then we are ready to proceed with the experiment (eating) so we can collect the data (see what happens). But it is the internal cue that gives the whole experiment meaning, since it ties it to subjective experience in a way that allows us to gradually sharpen and come to trust our urges and impulses.

When properly trained, appetite, tastes and bodily cues can be a very accurate and dependable source of information about what one needs nutritionally. Moreover, they change from moment to moment and keep one current as to what is needed and what's not. If we're emotionally upset we lose our appetites. This is the way our physiology has of advising us that digestion would be difficult at this time. Unfortunately, these cues are not always acknowledged or recognized. Too often the small, still voice of our inner urgings is overwhelmed by the noise around us, the force of our habits, the pressure of peer groups and the curiosity to try things for which we have no real appetite. Too often we eat according to our schedules and according to what is convenient rather than according to our needs.

There is a story told in the East of two fakirs who had spent years in seclusion studying yoga, having learned extraordinary feats of physical and mental control and mastery of their minds and bodies. Standing on the banks of the Ganges they fell into one another's company, and in the course of their conversation one of them happened to imply that he had developed the ability to do more miraculous things than most, probably including his companion.

The other fakir, a bit older and perhaps a bit wiser, rebuked him gently, wondering whether he might not be carried away by a moment's boastfulness. But his newfound friend bristled with pride and volunteered to demonstrate what he could do.

The older man agreed to this. "Go ahead, " he said.

The younger proceeded, "See the man across the river? I will make appear on a piece of paper in his hand the name of a friend whom he has long forgotten."

The older man smiled, "Is that really the sort of thing you do? That's nothing."

The younger fakir replied, now with some heat, "Oh, really! That's nothing? Well, please tell me, what sort of miraculous feats do *you* accomplish?"

The first fakir looked at him calmly and his eyes twinkled, "I eat when I'm hungry and drink when I'm thirsty."

If one can eat only when hungry and yet, at the same time take his meals with reasonable regularity and at proper intervals, he will have met one of the greatest challenges of good nutrition.

MAKING SENSE OF EXPERIENTIAL DATA

From what has been said, it should be clear that the

schools of nutrition that have grown up in ancient civilizations are based more on experiential data than experimental data. By that is meant that their understanding of what is appropriate food for each person is based more on the information that each person will have at his immediate disposal: his feelings, his sensations, his ideas, his sense of himself. They tend not to be based on the kind of particularistic, mechanistic, molecular analysis that must be carried out in a specially equipped laboratory. This is partially, of course, because the technology required for this latter kind of external, material study was not available in the older civilizations. In any event, interest was focused more on the interface between man and food, a field of data that can best be apprehended by an inward turning of attention, an experiential self-observation of internal events that precede, accompany and follow the intake of food.

But he also had to come to terms with what he observed. It was necessary to have some systematic way to conceptualize experience. Of course one can say, "After I ate that I felt bad," or "after this, good." But a more sophisticated system of evaluating of responses was evolved in some traditions.

THE THREE GUNAS

In Indian philosophy, all phenomena of the universe are classified according to different properties or "gunas." Some properties are specific and reflect an appreciation of detail such as lightness/heaviness or dryness/oiliness. As mentioned when discussing pharmacology, there are twenty-two such gunas which figure prominently in Ayurvedic medicine. For non-technical use, however, there is a more common and universally understood three-fold classification. It is simpler than the elaborate principles of Ayurvedic taste pharmacology* but a bit more complex than the *yin* and *yang* of Chinese philosophy.

* See Chapter 15, Ayurvedic Nutrition.

In categorizing foods into these three gunas, it is further understood that food must be seen as more than simply matter. It has an existence on different levels, that is, food nourishes many different aspects of a person at the same time.

Tamas

Those foods which are "dead," which are partly spoiled, which have been processed a great deal, which have been preserved in some way, which have no spark of life about them, which lack the vitality of food that is alive or has been recently cooked are called *tamasic*. Such foods create a feeling of heaviness, of lethargy; they nourish only the grossest aspects of the body. If the diet is consistently comprised of tamasic food, then the person can continue to live but he may gain weight so that the body will become heavier, or else functioning will be sluggish, and diseases of degeneration and accumulation of excessive matter are likely to occur (obesity, arthritis, hardening of the arteries, and so forth.) The matter of the body may be added to, but its energy, vitality, and its consciousness is not increased through the use of such food.

Tamasic foods cause irritability. They motivate or activate but not in a constructive or enjoyable manner. Because of the feeling of restlessness and lack of ease, one may be likely to act in a cruel or thoughtless way. Tamasic food can lead to a tyrannical, oppressive kind of disposition.

When food is spoiled its chemical structure breaks down. Because of the acidity that results some nutrients are destroyed. Rather than being present in usable form they may break down into products which can't be used by the body but must be excreted. In the meantime, they're in the circulation and may act as irritants to the nervous system as well as other cells, tissues and organs. Eating tamasic foods makes one less alert. Concentration, attention or meditation may be very difficult. One may vacillate between an irascible restlessness and a tendency to fall asleep.

The experience that led to the ancient Indian writings on diet did not include taking a diet containing preservatives, insecticides, emulsifiers, artificial colorings and other chemicals that contemporary foods contain. Such substances do, however, have the potential for acting as irritants and would most likely from the traditional point of view be considered tamasic.

Alcoholic drinks, especially the poorer quality alcoholic preparations, are tamasic in nature. Fermentation is essentially a process of decomposition, especially when it is poorly controlled and overdone. Meat is also likely to be tamasic especially when it is not fresh. Most meat marketed is not freshly slaughtered and in some cases must be "cured" to destroy toxic substances or to improve taste. Again, unless this is carefully and knowledgeably controlled, the result is likely to be undesirable. Once animal cells die, the process of degeneration and decay begins. Meat tends to have a tamasic effect for this reason, though the way in which an animal lives and grows may also affect its properties. Animals that are sluggish, heavy and unhealthy are more likely to yield meat that has a tamasic effect.

Wild game and fish, freshly killed and properly prepared, was not considered by the ancient Indians to be detrimental. On the contrary, in many cases, it was considered appropriate depending on the person who was eating and the effects desired. In general, however, meat was considered to be rajasic.

Rajas

Food which is cooked a great deal to increase its taste appeal, that which stimulates the nervous system, speeds up metabolism and activates is called *rajasic*. Such foods as coffee, tea and tobacco are usually considered rajasic. Rajasic foods will energize, but not in the sense of lending a clear, balanced energy. Rather they tend to stimulate and push the organism to increase its speed and to indulge more in physical activity, sensual pleasure and "creature comforts." Rajasic food is the fare of the *bon vivant* and of the epicure. Spiced and cooked to perfection with gobs of rich sauces, it tempts one to eat more and leads the attention into the savor of the food and away from internal signals.

Rajasic food is of good quality and fresh. Green chili peppers are considered rajasic while the dried red ones tend to be more irritating and tamasic. Rajasic food is in no way inferior. It is well cooked and "fit for a king."

In fact, "raja" means "king" or royalty and it is recognized that a pushing, aggressive, worldly kind of activity is appropriate for rulers, for the military forces and for those who concern themselves with matters political—who deal in the area of domination, forcefulness and warfare. In fact, in some of the Indian traditions, the caste which filled such roles—the *rajput*—(literally "son of the king") was expressly permitted to take meat and wine, whereas the brahmin, who is not a ruler but a scholar, teacher and spiritual seeker, has always been forbidden these rajasic foods. In fact, as in most oriental systems of medicine and nutrition, the purpose of the classification is not to distinguish between what is "good" and what is "bad," nor even what is "healthy" and "unhealthy," but rather to help one to see the difference in the effects of various foods. What is best will, of course, depend on the person eating, his makeup, what activity he wishes to involve himself in after eating, what he is trying to learn by this experience, etc.

Sattva

By contrast to the above two categories, those foods which are fresh, whole, natural, of good quality yet mild, neither over nor undercooked, are experienced as lending a calm alertness and at the same time a state of quiet energy. Such foods are called *sattvic*. They are said to "nourish the consciousness." They not only provide nourishment for the body, but they do not adversely affect the overall energy state. They add vitality to the total system by bringing a perfect, harmonious balance of energy states in the food itself. They don't *pull* energy from the body, they don't *weigh* it down, they don't *make* it heavier; neither do they irritate it nor push it beyond its capacity. Rather, they provide a precise balance of nourishment and create no undue waste. These foods are the ones which are most likely to be experienced as sattvic. They are the ones which are likely to give the body lightness, alertness, energy and create a keener consciousness.

Sattvic foods give strength from within as contrasted with rajasic foods which supply strength to the muscles and give one a feeling that his energy is coming from the food he has eaten. Such sattvic food as fresh fruit and the fresh milk of the cow are considered the epitome of sattvic food. Raw milk just drawn from the cow is considered ideal. If, however, it has sat for some time, then it is brought to a boil before it is taken. Milk of the water buffalo is considered more rajasic since it is heavier and more fattening. Any milk which becomes sour or spoiled of course tends to acquire a tamasic property.

Although the three gunas are based on philosophical concepts that seem to be extremely far from the practical concerns of daily life, they are actually taught as a way of organizing personal, everyday experience. They are seen by the Indian people as a very practical and down to earth way of dealing with the phenomena which make up one's life. When life is seen as a process of expanding consciousness, of increasing and deepening one's awareness of himself and the universe, then such a threefold classification of inner experience and reactions is very helpful: That which is tamasic will cloud consciousness and create lethargy or cruelty and ill temper; that which is rajasic will leave one busy, restless and even confused; that which is sattvic will create a feeling of calmness, alertness and will assist in the expansion of consciousness and the attainment of tranquility and inner peace.

Moreover, this concept of the three gunas is used not only to organize one's experience with food, but also to organize his experience in other areas of life: the kind of physical activity he engages in, the kind of music he listens to, even the sort of thoughts he thinks. Each of these can be seen as promoting an effect that tends toward cruelty and lethargy (tamasic), frenetic "busyness" (rajasic) or calm alertness (sattvic). This then is a system not only for organizing but also for integrating experience. An extraordinarily rajasic state need not be blamed entirely on the cup of coffee one had, but can also be seen to be partly a result of the rush, frantic state of mind that preceded it. Similarly, one need not mistakenly attribute a heavy tamasic feeling to the meal he ate when he realizes he's been sleeping longer than usual and has had no exercise.

AUTOPSYCHOTHERAPEUTIC FOOD HABITS

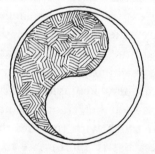

Somewhere in the conflicting impulses and urges that arise into our awareness when we think of eating is the data which we need to guide us to the food that our bodies require. These internal indicators have to be patiently retrained, however. What is often referred to as hunger, for example, is not really hunger at all but the socially or psychologically conditioned urge to eat. One has to filter out all other connections involved with food, tuning in to the correct signals and tuning out the static. This is not always easy, but as one learns from experience which signals are reliable and which aren't, he gradually gains facility in distinguishing those which will not mislead him, and these gradually become clearer and more easy to perceive. The result is a cooperative effort between one's mind and his body which provides the information one needs in order to select the food which is most appropriate for him at a given time. One well known writer on health has called this "biofoodback," agreeing that despite all the elaborate information which is available on the biochemistry of nutrition, the cues provided by one's own system are the most reliable guide.

The goal then, of any successful nutritional approach is for one to become more sensitive to himself, more aware of the choices that he has, and more attuned to how they affect him. It matters not whether this is conceptualized in terms of *yin* and *yang*, in terms of the three *gunas* mentioned above, or in terms of *tridosha*. The important point is that self-awareness be allowed to grow and that one's experience with food become part of an ongoing experiment in an inner laboratory. In this way, nutrition study takes its place alongside other methods of self-examination and inner searching such as the various forms of psychotherapy and meditation. Here, an awareness of and sensitivity to diet can play a complementary role to one's awareness and study of his thoughts, emotions and the use of his body.

By getting in touch with the cues that one's body offers him, he can decide what is appropriate to eat and what is not. Through sharpening his awareness of himself and his reactions to foods over a period of time, one can evolve dietary habits and practices that seem comfortable, natural and conducive to health. The use of this approach to nutrition lends flexibility and the capability for constant change. One no longer needs to establish a plateau of nutritional status. He need not settle into a rut. Instead, he is free to go through a process of evolution. As his body and mind change and evolve, he is also able to reorganize his dietary habits so that at each stage of transition, they shift to meet his new needs, and can continue to contribute to creating states of greater health and alertness.

Moreover, in his struggle to cope with old habits, to increase his sensitivity to himself, and to open his eyes to ways in which he has misused his digestive system and body, one will learn much. Not only will he learn about nutrition, but he will also gain important insights into the emotional and physiological aspects of his nature. It has long been known that many of one's deepest psychological problems and most serious emotional conflicts show up most clearly in his dietary habits. Such frank abuse is often covered up by the most amazing blindness, and it is not uncommon to have a patient who has undergone some treatment with training in nutrition and dietary awareness remark, "I never realized what I was doing to myself!"

Learning to deal with food and what it means to oneself becomes, then, an autopsychotherapeutic process. Mixed in with those signals and cues which reflect a true need for certain nutrients are many other impulses and associations which have to do with one's past. The sight or smell or taste of a certain dish may bring back memories or associations of a pleasant experience or of someone who was loved and with whom a certain food was shared. Sometimes these memories may not come fully into awareness, and one may feel an inexplicable urge to eat something for which his body has no use at the time. Food may symbolize many things which give them attraction quite apart from their nutritional value. Eating certain foods with another person may be a way of feeling closer while eating other foods may provide a stimulation or mask an allergy.*

Sorting out the signals and becoming aware of one's non-nutritional reasons for eating results in more than simply getting a good diet. It is really a process of self-study, a continuing adventure in self-exploration, a progressive untangling of past memories and conflicts, and a way of coming to terms with them. Working out and overcoming one's cravings often involves

---

* See Chapter 18, Megavitamins and Food Allergies.

working out and overcoming deep-seated psychological conflicts. This work with the food, the schedule and the eating, then, is the battleground on which such conflicts may be resolved. Their resolution in terms of food may in many cases amount to their psychological resolution, and thus, this process of working through can be therapeutic in a total sense rather than being merely an improvement in one's diet.

Only those who have struggled sincerely with their eating habits can appreciate the profundity of this concept. It is said in the East that "he who would attain enlightenment must first conquer the palate." Diet, like any other area of one's life, if approached in the right spirit, can become a means to growth and personal unfoldment. For this reason, a quiet, persistent approach to diet involving self-study and a cultivation of increased self-awareness might properly be called "food *sadhana*." "Sadhana" is a Sanskrit word meaning "pathway" and is often used to denote that particular practice by means of which one works toward personal unfoldment and spiritual evolution.

From the ancient Eastern perspective, consciousness is potentially much more capable of influencing the way the body functions and the way it handles food than is the food itself. Yet it is curious that while the Eastern point of view relegates diet to an inferior place in the scheme of variables affecting the human being, it is in the East where diet is managed in the most sane and healthful fashion. The Westerner, whose philosophy would suggest that his material being is of utmost importance and that, moreover, "he is what he eats," tends constantly to violate all the rules that he has acknowledged lead to good health. Even from an Eastern perspective, this is a serious spending of all our time chasing after organic produce and counting milligrams of vitamins to the point that we become harried and flustered and require more of the nutrients we're trying to get! Though food may be relatively unimportant compared to one's state of mind in determining the overall nutritional picture, it still plays a role. It is wise to recall the cyclic or spiral-like interaction between what we eat and our consciousness. Though the mind affects nutrition in numerous and complex ways, what was eaten today can also affect one's clarity of consciousness. As we struggle to become more aware of ourselves and what food does to us, our diet itself may, at the same time, be one of the most potent means of assistance we have.

It has been found, for example, that both human infants and laboratory animals, when allowed to select freely what they will eat, chose more wisely and did much better if they had been well nourished up to the time that they were put on their own.[6] Those who had been on a poor diet for some time seemed confused and unable to select the foods they needed. Good nutrition fosters the development of "body wisdom," we might say, just as sensitivity to body cues fosters good nutrition.

Of course it remains true that what we can learn intellectually about the rational selection of food and the deliberate design of diet is probably inferior to a highly developed intuitive sense of what we need. Yet it may be precisely that contrived diet and schedule which bring enough regularity and sanity to our eating habits to clear our heads and enable us to begin to reawaken and cultivate our innate sense of what is appropriate and right for us.

A NEW PERSPECTIVE

Clearly in the course of this book our emphasis has shifted. We began discussing the soil and then looked at how the biochemical constituents of food both arose from the soil and air and water, and contributed to the body's nutrition. Then we found digestion and cooking—both "cooking" in a sense—were crucial to the way the food affected the body.

In the last part of the book, we have seen how the mind is involved in nutrition, and discovered in fact that it may be more important than the body and more important than the food itself in determining our nutritional status. Moreover, in this chapter we have looked at some reasons for thinking that working to improve one's diet might have its most important impact on the mind and on the evolution of awareness rather than merely on one's ability to get more or less of certain biochemical compounds.   This constitutes a real revolution in nutrition, shifting its focus away from the purely material.   Unfortunately our contemporary science of nutrition is ill-equipped to assimilate such ideas.   Why this is so and what may be done about it will become more apparent as we re-examine the philosophical biases and premises on which current nutritional science is based.

The Philosophy
of Nutrition

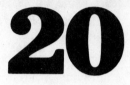

In view of what we have discussed in the last three chapters, it is apparent that nutrition cannot be limited to the study of food. The digestive system is important and the mind is even more so, playing a crucial and probably even the major, role in nutrition. Yet our established science of nutrition, which has discovered so much, is not geared to dealing with the mental-nutritional interplay. Like a huge, unresponsive machine, it grinds on, turning out biochemical and physiological data, oblivious to the possibility of setting its sights in a new direction. The minority opinion—the "natural foods" reaction against materialistic molecular science and its processed foods, while valid to a point, is in essence more negative than positive. Part of a recurring tendency to "return to nature," it constitutes an understandable reaction to the mechanized and sterile aspects of modern Western civilization. Yet its emphasis is still external. Its answers to nutritional problems have more to do with the quality of the food than of the consciousness of the person who eats it. Little attention is paid to one's potential for regulating himself in such a way that nutritional needs are altered. It is limited too often to the naive implication that we should crawl back into a cave—or at least return to the jungle. The role of the mind and the potential of consciousness are still neglected.

Of course, most schools of nutritional thought pay at least some lip service to holism. The natural food enthusiasts would insist that wholesome foods make one mentally more alert and healthier. A whole host of new books on trace elements, hypoglycemia and megavitamins and psychiatry suggest a growing awareness among more conventional physicians and scientists that nutrition can have important effects upon the mind and mental functioning. But this is still chemistry first, consciousness second. The mind is still affected *by* diet, rather than vice versa.

There has been an increasing tendency to concentrate on the physical, pharmacological and material measures which alter mental functioning. Of course, from the time of Descartes and even earlier, the mind and body were regarded as largely separate and independent. In recent decades, however, the mind has come to be thought of as nothing more than a product of the brain. This is in turn considered simply a complicated computer whose functioning can be affected by altering its molecular structure and environment, whether this is done through ortho-molecular psychiatry or drugs.

The work with tranquilizers led the way, fueling the idea that the mind could be brought under biochemical control. Recent successes using trace elements and megavitamin therapy in psychiatric problems, and work on hypoglycemia have accentuated the tendency to view the mind as a mere outcome of material and physical events. While this may lead to a better recognition of the importance of certain nutrients such as copper and zinc, it threatens to perpetuate an already overmechanistic and materialistic approach to the human being. Nutritional treatment is degenerating to a computer-analyzed, computer-prescribed program regimen. This approach totally ignores the importance of the mind and the effect of one's mental and emotional habits on nutritional requirements (as we saw in Chapter 18 with niacin and vitamin C). It also overlooks other important aspects of nutrition, such as one's ability to sense, discriminate, select and create himself anew through an exploratory, experiential approach to diet which emphasizes personal awareness and choice.

Here is where the Eastern perspective on medicine and nutrition serves to counterbalance the Western extreme. From the point of view of Ayurvedic medicine, as we have seen, though what is in the food is considered important, it is never considered primary. Although diet is acknowledged as an important influence on the mind, the mind is seen as a much more powerful influence on nutrition. One always has the power to step outside the causal chain and restructure his diet or even alter the way in which he digests or processes the food. Here we are not speaking of any extraordinary exercise of yogic self-control, though such feats have been well documented in those specially trained. What we are speaking of is the ability of the mind, one's attitude and psychological state, to affect the way in which he absorbs and metabolizes food or even the way in which he strings together molecules to form his own nutrients.

An example of this is the apparent synthesis of vitamin C by lactating mothers,* a fact altogether surprising in view of the previously well-accepted and apparently well-documented inability of the human being to synthesize this vitamin. In some way, perhaps through a synthesis of Eastern perspectives and Western science, one must try to establish a philosophical base that provides for the difference between the machine with its metal parts or the test tube with its inorganic compounds, where mechanistic concepts are generally adequate, and living tissue where they aren't.

---

* See Chapter 18, Megavitamins and Food Allergies.

ENTROPY VERSUS LIFE

For better or for worse, contemporary nutritional science is based on chemistry, and chemistry is based on models that are essentially mechanical. The sticks and balls and atoms and bonds that we use to represent our idea of what happens on the level of body chemistry are carry-overs from Newtonion physics, the physics of mechanics and machines. There is much more to the chemistry of biological systems than one isolated atom sidling up to another with which it establishes a "chemical bond." Not only do atoms seldom move singly, forming instead parts of complex molecules, but these are not isolated either. Each molecule is arranged in contact with hundreds of others that surround it, and its relationship to each of them is important.

Tinker Toys and Water Bags

Historically, we came to study the molecular events inside the cell after having studied simpler chemical reactions in the laboratory. Our theories and models for thinking about bio-chemistry come from the test tube and are based on our experience with "inorganic" or non-biological compounds reacting primarily in water solutions; thus our tendency to carry this way of thinking into our study of living protoplasm. If our notions of molecular structure are like tinker toys, our thinking about the cell tends to picture it as a little bag filled with water within which certain particles float about and undergo chemical reactions.

While it is reasonable to conceptualize molecules as being held together by relatively stable and identifiable "chemical bonds," it is unfortunate that up until recently biological science has largely ignored the importance of the "weaker" bonds that exist between various molecules which are neither so rigid nor so stable. The various components of the cell are not, in fact, piled up randomly like so many tinker toys thrown into a box, or so many little particles floating in water. They do not rattle around or shift aimlessly when we move. Instead, the huge variety of compounds that make up the inside of the cell are arranged in definite and meaningful juxtaposition. Each molecule relates not only to another with which it is "having a chemical reaction," but to all the others in the vicinity. To single out and study one molecule in living protoplasm would be like exploring the relationship of one person in a crowded room where all the others are friends and relatives. The subtlety and intricacy of interactions that shift and change as he moves through the people, speaking to one, forgetting another, offending a third, is impressive. Such, too, is the case of the individual molecule circulating through the busy interior of a living cell.

As we begin to understand that the cell is not really a spherical membrane full of a water solution with simple compounds dissolved in it, we can see that it is the interrelationship of various force fields which causes molecules to slip and slide over one another, reshaping themselves in ways that produce the "metabolic processes" taking place within the cell. Because the cell is a complex layering of intricate, coiled and folded molecules, each intimately related to those around it the slightest change in their relative position has extraordinarily important ramifications. As a molecule shifts or changes place, its energy relationship to other molecules shifts and changes, and the biological reactions of living matter thereby occur.

Though water molecules make up the major part of the protoplasm of the cell, we cannot assume that the water itself is inert or uniform. In fact, much evidence has accumulated that a molecule can leave an imprint in water solution through the way that the water molecules shape themselves around it and that this imprint itself can carry important information and serve important biological functions.[1]

When we think of the atom and the molecules made up of them as complex interactions of "energy fields," then we begin to realize that the cell itself is something quite different from what we had thought. It is not a phenomenon easily dealt with in terms of "nutrients" like vitamins, minerals, proteins, fats and carbohydrates. Even a careful study of the "non-nutritional" substances in the cells of food, such as the pharmacologically active compounds discussed in Chapter 13, will not throw any light on the subtle and delicate properties of living matter that we are discussing here. Our particularistic way of splitting up the components of the cell and dealing with them in nutritional science must eventually turn out to be inadequate.

To study the intricacy of the interrelationships between one given molecule and its neighbors and to trace the shifts and modifications in these relationships as that molecule moves one-millionth of a millimeter would be sufficient subject matter to occupy an entire doctoral dissertation. In fact, volumes could be written on it. We begin to feel the futility of trying to discuss intelligently the molecular events that go on in living protoplasm. Yet it is precisely this intricacy, this very purposeful and meaningful interrelationship that exists between each molecule and each of its neighbors that surround it, that makes for the quality of protoplasm that we call "life." Without this web of intricate interactions, the movements, responsiveness and self-perpetuation that we find characteristic of living matter would not be possible.

Unfortunately since our model for chemistry is based on the study of non-living systems, it does not take into account such properties which are unique to living systems. Chemical reactions which occur in a test tube are based on the principle of entropy which stipulates that a loss of energy results as one approaches a more stable but more disorganized state. Chemicals dissolve, they react, but they do not interact to form more evolved and complex substances. Living matter, however, is based on the opposite principle. The tendency of life is to become more organized, not to become disorganized or drift into chaos.

There are two basically different principles operating here, and they have been related to the concepts of *yin* and *yang*. *Yin* is that which moves outward and dissipates while *yang* is that which pulls together and organizes. (This is also very similar to Freud's idea of the death instinct and the life instinct.) There is the tendency in the material universe to move toward disorganization, and that is what we see in chemical reactions and test tubes and that tendency is what is called entropy. But when chemical reactions occur in living matter, they are not governed by entropy. In fact, biologists have coined the term "negative entropy," which simply means that entropy is not in operation, that something opposite of entropy is in force. This other principle moves toward higher organization, toward life and toward intelligence. While this idea is not new, it is only recently that we can point to discrete biological events that dramatize it so clearly. Especially impressive is work done with minerals since their measurement is simpler and more reliable than that of the complex and delicate molecules that make up the bulk of living matter. One can always burn a plant or animal tissue and analyze its ash for minerals, since they are not destroyed by the fire. Other nutrients which are more easily damaged do not survive many attempts at measurement. Moreover, technological advances have increased our analytic precision, opening new realms of understanding.

BIOLOGICAL TRANSMUTATIONS[2]

As a child, Louis Kervran, a French scientist and biophysicist, lived on a farm in Brittany. The soil of the region was derived from granite; there was no calcium in it. Nevertheless, the family kept hens who regularly produced eggs with good, firm shells, despite the fact that they were supplied no significant source of calcium in their feed. Though it never really quite occurred to young Kervran to wonder how the hens could lay almost daily an egg with a complete calcified shell, something else caught his eye. The hens were attracted, it seemed, to the bits of mica scattered through the sand in the barnyard. They picked out the sparkling fragments of the potassium compound by preference, leaving the other pebbles and sand. No one could explain to the curious child why the hens ate the shiny mica. Yet he observed that when his mother prepared a hen for cooking, the gizzard contained grains of sand, tiny rocks, but never the mica he'd seen them eat. Where did it go, he wondered. Such things stick in the minds of children, and sometimes stay there long after they've grown up.

Later, as an adult, Kervran made a practice in the course of his work to take note of such observations which did not fit one's expectations. One example was an experiment performed in 1875 by a Dr. Herzeele. He germinated seeds under a bell jar where the air was pure and used only distilled water. He took half the seeds and measured the calcium in them. Then he took the other half and germinated them. After germinating them with nothing but the mineral-frée water, he found that the amount of calcium in them increased. But he could not determine where this extra calcium came from.[3]   Almost seven decades after this, one of the researchers in the Organic Chemistry Laboratory of L'Ecole Polytechnique in Paris decided to repeat this experiment because it intrigued him, too. He followed the same routine only this time he double-distilled the water, used filtered air, and executed the experiment with all the scientific rigor of the modern laboratory. He had statisticians analyze the results carefully, but the outcome was the same: there was more calcium after germination than there was before.[4] Where did it come from?

A number of similar inexplicable observations came to his attention but in 1955 a more pressing problem arose. His work required that he investigate three deaths occurring in different factories a few months apart. In each case there were high blood levels of carbon monoxide. Of course industrial deaths due to carbon monoxide fumes are not unheard of. Yet there was no apparent source of carbon monoxide in any of the three cases. Though each of the deceased had been working with welding equipment or white hot sheet metal, there was no carbon monoxide detectable in the air coming from them either. This problem fascinated Kervran because of another puzzle he remembered from his youth. During the cold of winter in the little rural schoolhouse he attended, the pot-belly stove used for heating was often stoked till it became red hot. At that point, everyone complained of headaches. The teacher said that this was because carbon monoxide was formed. He told the young students that it resulted from incomplete combustion of the fuel. But young Kervran was skeptical. He observed that the headaches always occurred when the fire was drawing best. If the teacher's explanations were correct, one would expect the opposite to be true. He had remained puzzled.

Now he saw the same situation: poisoning in someone near red hot metal, but this time it was well established that there was no carbon monoxide in the air. Remembering the formulae of nitrogen as it occurs in the air (N_2) and of carbon monixide, (CO), he was struck by an idea: The two molecules are so similar. The only difference between the two is the location of one proton. If the molecule of N_2 were excited and made unstable by energy from the intense heat of the glowing metal, might not one proton "jump" from the nucleus of one nitrogen to that of the other? This would transform both the atoms, yielding one carbon and one oxygen. Though this clearly did not happen in the air, perhaps it happened when the nitrogen hit the tissues in the lung.

This might solve the calcium question, too, as well as the appetite of the chickens for shiny bits of mica. Experiments with hens were conducted to see if the theory could be confirmed. Kept where they had access only to clayey soil and given no source of limestone, their eggs became soft and pliable after a few days. At this point purified mica was given. The hens dived into it, rolling about, tossing it in the air, and gobbling it up with great relish. The next day, in 20 hours, they laid eggs

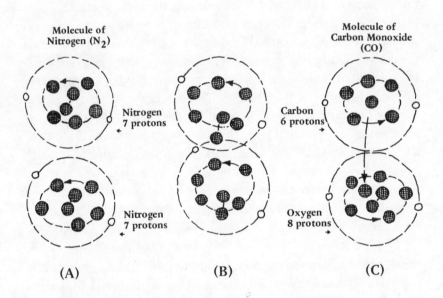

Intermolecular Exchange of a Proton[12]

Carbon atoms contain 6 protons; Nitrogen 7; and Oxygen 8. A molecule of Nitrogen is excited (A), the vibration frequency of its protons increases, and it is possible for one of the protons to jump (B) from one atom to another. When this occurs, a new molecule—Carbon Monoxide (C) will be formed.

with normal hard shells.

Though mica contains no calcium, it does contain potassium. The addition of only one proton (hydrogen ion) to the nucleus of a potassium atom would change it to calcium:

$$_{19}K + {}_1H \rightarrow {}_{20}CA$$

Though there was no glowing metal here to "energize" the atoms, perhaps the same function could be accomplished by enzymes which are known to facilitate transformations that can be effected outside living tissue only through exposure to tremendous levels of energy.[5]

When Kervran went back and looked through the scientific literature he found many such unexplained phenomena in mineral metabolism that could only be accounted for in this fashion. He called them "aberrant observations." Unfortunately what had usually happened was that they had been thrown out because the experimenter couldn't make any sense of them and they couldn't be integrated into current thinking.* The aberrant observations dated back as far as 1799 when a French chemist had found that hens put out, through feces and in eggs, five times as much calcium as they took in through the diet.

The list was long. It had been known that fish eggs, which contain no calcium, hatch to produce tiny fishes with complete and well-calcified skeletons, which they develop while inside the egg. The same is true of certain birds. Both had been considered inexplicable.

Kervran had himself observed on the plaster wall at his seaside house the usual formation of a sort of excrescence of saltpeter, a potassium compound, which occurs in damp areas. He doubted that the plaster contained such quantities of potassium since he had regularly removed the deposits for 11 years! The $K \rightarrow Ca$ transformation was obviously reversible. In this case the process was apparently facilitated by bacteria growing on the damp wall.[6]

The evidence in the case of nitrogen was particularly compelling. In 1950 another French scientist had collected a number of unexplained observations on nitrogen metabolism. When detached leaves of a plant are kept in a controlled environment until they die, about 10 days later, total nitrogen content increases by 70%.[7] In another experiment a rat had been enclosed for two months in a sealed tube. At the end of that time, the nitrogen content of the air had decreased considerably, while the oxygen increased.

---

* Science acknowledges and integrates data only to the extent that it is able to make sense of them and only to the extent that it is able to contribute to an orderly and constructive growth of scientific thinking in the area in question.

Moreover, it had long been known that Spanish moss was able to thrive on a wire—with no apparent nourishment except what came from the air. What is especially striking is the iron content of the moss, which is ample even when the plant is grown on a copper wire under controlled conditions in a greenhouse. Apparently copper is transformed into iron by the plant.

It would seem that our ideas of the immutability of our "elements" is not correct. The more one looks the more he finds examples that support this conclusion. Kervran quotes G.B.Shaw who commented wryly that once we decide to change our ideas, we discover not only that there are plenty of reasons to do so, but that they've been staring us in the face for a long time!

Kervran began the intensive investigation of what he called biological transmutations, a project that has extended over 20 years and established him as a respected scientist around the world. His work has provided answers to some of the more perplexing problems of physiology and medicine. Recent work in America, for example, had shown that during hot weather many people lose potassium in the perspiration rather than sodium. Yet it remains a time-honored practice to take table salt (sodium chloride) when one is to be exposed to heat. Could the traditional salt tablet simply be a big mistake?

Kervran did some revealing research on human physiology in intense heat. In the Sahara he studied a team of oil workers who stayed out in the broiling sun for long periods. If the human has the capacity to function in unusual ways one might expect to find it used under such extreme conditions. Over a six month period of observation he found that on the average each man put out about four liters a day of perspiration. This is sufficient to absorb only 2,200 calories of heat each day. But when he looked at the heat that was generated through each man's work he found an average of 4,000 calories a day.[8] Therefore they should have been retaining 1,800 calories a day, which means that their temperature should have risen each day, and they should have died of overheating. Yet they remained quite well. In an effort to explain this, Kervran then studied their mineral metabolism. He found that the workers ate tremendous amounts of salt (sodium chloride). Some of this was lost in perspiration and some in the feces, but a lot of it simply "disappeared." He also found that the men put out huge amounts of potassium through the sweat glands although their diet was very low in potassium. Later experiments have demonstrated that the conversion of sodium to potassium takes up energy. It is an endothermic process. This provides an explanation of how the extra heat produced in the oil workers could be removed from their bodies. It also explains how potassium can be found in perspiration during very hot weather even though salt (sodium chloride) tablets are taken.

Kervran also found that the Sahara workers excreted ten to twenty milligrams more calcium every day than they ingested, and yet after the six months, their bones showed no signs of decalcification. The sea salt which the workers were taking, however, was very high in magnesium, and tests showed that the magnesium "disappeared" faster as calcium excretion increased during the hottest months. This suggests the transmutation of magnesium into calcium, another endothermic "reaction."

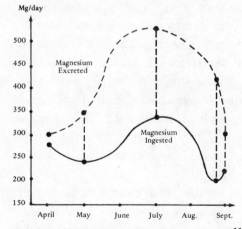

Variation of Magnesium in Workers in the Sahara[11]

Such a process is not a chemical reaction, but a nuclear reaction. For example, the nuclei of one sodium and one oxygen, fuse to create a potassium atom. It is not merely an alteration in the shells of the electrons, which is what occurs in chemical reactions. There's something much more profound going on here. The nucleus itself is changed. Of course, it has been known for some time that such changes can be effected at tremendously high temperatures such as those in a reactor designed for atomic fusion. But in most of the cases described by Kervran the transformation is occurring at body temperature or less. Thus Kervran's use of the term "biological transmutation." Such reactions are possible in the body, he suggests, because of the work of the enzymes. We have long known that our tissues "burn" carbohydrate—oxidizing it to produce energy. Yet we are not burnt, since the reaction at low energy level can be accomplished by the action of enzymes. The intricate enzyme molecule has the power to gently manipulate atoms so that they merge without the brute force of a massive input of energy.

TRANSMUTATIONS VERSUS ENTROPY

The subject of biological transmutations is very important because it demonstrates that in living matter, higher levels of organization are able to completely transform lower levels. Animals and plants can change one element into another. Stone can be brought to life, so to speak. With the clear documentation that living systems have the ability to completely change one form of matter into another the field of nutrition is drastically altered.

While Louis Kervran's work indicates that the human being has the potential to create, at least in part, the minerals which are missing from his diet, it is clear that many of us do not do this. This may partially explain why it is that one person's calcium requirements can be so much higher than another's. Many people remain deficient in certain minerals because they apparently do not use the inherent potential they have for producing them. We might say, in fact, that this "unwillingness" to create the needed cogs for the metabolic machine is the true essence of a state of imbalance, ill health or sickness. Exactly which cogs are not supplied will vary with the individual. Though our research has yet to fully explore such sophisticated issues, it seems increasingly clear from what we have learned that the exact minerals and vitamins used which the body does not supply itself either through selection, absorption or even transmutation add up to a sort of profile. If interpreted properly, this profile might tell us much about both the physiological and psychological makeup of the person in question. This, of course, doesn't mean that deficiencies due to poor or inadequate food can't occur. They can, but with the affluence of the majority of people, and the choices of food generally available, even in winter, deficiencies are more commonly psychological in origin.

Our increasingly complex and precise instruments for measuring such things as trace elements are permitting us to look in more and more detail at the makeup of each person's body. Furthermore, in recent years, a great deal of research has been done with trace mineral analyses of hair and nails since they furnish a sort of historical record of one's mineral metabolism. It is thought that minerals are deposited in the hair as it grows, so that a length of hair one inch long reflects an average of what was going on over a period of a month or two.

Exactly how to interpret this information has not been well understood, however. Zinc deficiency, for example, will usually show certain clinical signs in the skin and nails, as well as low zinc levels in the hair, and there may be overall improvement when dietary zinc is increased. But sometimes the signs and symptoms are there while zinc in the hair is very high—and there may still be improvement in zinc supplementation. Some writers have suggested that this means zinc is "utilized poorly," so it is "excreted" in the hair. In any event, the question is important, since high hair zinc may mean one is getting too much zinc.

Even more baffling is the presence of certain toxic minerals. Lead, for example, is sometimes found to be elevated in the hair of persons who have had no apparent exposure to the metal. Copper is frequently high in those who are emotionally upset, even though a careful search shows no apparent source of it in water, food, etc. Though the writings on biological transmutations have, to date, concentrated on the lighter elements which occur early in the periodic table* with the idea that living systems tend to transmute only the lighter elements, one might wonder whether in sickness this process could be diverted in an unhealthy direction toward the production of the heavier elements that ordinarily make up lifeless substances such as metal and stone.

Possibly some of the puzzles encountered in trying to understand trace element levels in body tissues are due to such biological transmutation, an issue that researchers in the field have not really explored. In any case, our use of this data is primarily limited at this point by our inability to conceptualize its significance, and it is clear that they are not merely a reflection of one's eating habits. Their significance is not even limited to individual variations in absorption or to "metabolic requirements."

Of course all of the more obvious variables will affect the mineral levels found in blood, hair, etc., but there is apparently the other more intriguing and as yet largely unacknowledged variable, the hierarchy of intelligent, organizational levels which govern the functioning of living matter. In man this includes the endocrine system, the autonomic nervous system, and quite likely, the unconscious mind. All of these must play some role in the way that a person supplies himself, fails to supply himself or over-supplies himself, through biological transmutations, with

* See Chapter 8, Minerals.

one mineral or another. Variations in trace mineral analysis suggest that this is a highly personal matter and that probably each person is unique in the particular pattern of elements he tends to augment or decrease. We seem to be moving toward the realization that the chemical profiles that we measure in a person's blood, tissue and hair are really a complex but potentially decipherable message by means of which the person tells us what he is really like psychologically as well as physically. It seems likely that when we look at a trace mineral analysis, we are looking at a reflection of how a person "creates himself." Though it may sound like medical science fiction at this point, the day may well come when chemical tests are regarded as the most reliable reflection of personality makeup.

That man's mind affects his eating habits is recognized even by the rank and file of nutritionists and dieticians. That his emotional and mental makeup might affect his digestion, his absorption, and even the character of his metabolism is recognized by only a minority of physicians though it is an area of growing interest as evidenced by a series of new books on stress, biofeedback and "body work."* That the unconscious, as well as conscious mind may tune the metabolic machinery to change vitamin requirements, or even to create certain vitamins or, more amazingly, yet, to transmute one element into another, is understood only by a handful of biophysicists and is beyond the capacity of even the most sincerely motivated practitioners of medicine or nutrition to comprehend.

Because of their stubborn clinging to the idea that the phenomenon of consciousness must arise out of a material base, Western scientists are hard put to digest the data collected by such researchers as Kervran. It will require a revolution in philosophical thinking for Western science to apprehend that the physical elements of which living matter is made are the product of intelligence rather than the origin of intelligence.

* See Pelletier, K.R., *Mind as Healer, Mind as Slayer*, B. Brown, *Stress and the Art of Biofeedback*, Dychtwald, K., *Bodymind*.

As Kervran says:

> The entire genesis and evolution of our planet needs to be restudied in light of transmutation, which opens new horizons to geologists and philosophers, as well as to metaphysicians. The latter can find grounds for meditation in the fact that the vital phenomenon of life is not chemistry alone.[9]

What will be necessary, then, is a reorientation along lines similar to those of Eastern philosophy where the major schools of thought insist that the world of material phenomena is but a manifestation of that which is subtler. Obviously this opens up vast horizons for the practice of medicine since it becomes possible that the reshaping of consciousness, i.e., work with the psyche and work with meditation, is potentially, if done skillfully, the most powerful tool we have for altering the functioning of the human body.

In the East the perspective that Kervran's discoveries thrust upon us is not considered uncomfortable at all. It is consonant with the traditional philosophy that consciousness is able to alter matter, and it is widely regarded as proven that certain famous spiritual masters were able to exist without food for years. Kervran's work makes clear for the first time how this might be true, how all the essential elements can be derived, if one has sufficient mastery over himself to allow it to happen, from the air which he breathes.

Moreover, the work of Kervran brings up the possibility that some of those physicians and philosophers who called themselves alchemists were possessed of more understanding and wisdom than is generally thought today. A study of the metals and their transmutations, something which has been considered in the twentieth century to be superstition and fantasy, suddenly becomes intriguing and pregnant with possibilities. If a certain mode of functioning psychophysiologically and metabolically enables one to transmute one element to produce more of another, then we begin to grasp the important relationship between the appearance of elevated levels of certain minerals in the body and the overall psychophysiological functioning of that human being. A certain character structure, for instance, going through a certain kind of personal, emotional and psychological change, may well manifest this by subtle shifts in the trace element balance in the body, resulting from the change in potential for transmuting one or another of these trace elements. At crucial points in human growth, especially, it would not be unlikely that transition from one state of mind or consciousness to another would be linked in some essential and profound way with the ability or tendency to transmute a certain element into another. This might then provide some key to unlocking the mystery of the alchemist's physical/spiritual discipline and to understand why it was that he labored so with the physical element externally, claiming all the while that by so doing he could help bring into being an internal transmutation.

It should be noted that perhaps the greatest of the alchemists, and certainly one of the greatest physicians of the Middle Ages, Paracelsus, was said by his biographers to have spent many years wandering in the East, apparently passing a long period in India. It was when he returned that he demonstrated the ability to heal so many difficult patients and wrote some of his most revered and yet obscure treatises. India has a long tradition and vast lore describing the transformation of minerals and metals.*

Such a correspondence between the physical or external and consciousness, which by comparison is "internal," goes far beyond our usual simplistic concepts of "mind influences

* Related to this is the ancient and elaborate procedure known in Ayurveda as the making of a *bhasma*. Beginning in the 1800's, the homeopaths, following the lead of Paracelsus, concentrated on similar laborious, step-wise methods of preparation and transmutation of medicinal substances in an attempt to render them capable of acting on higher levels of organization. This science has survived on a small scale and continued to evolve, especially in India. When it is properly applied, the result is the restoration of balance in metabolic functioning, in some cases where nutrition is less than ideal.

hypothalamus which influences the autonomic nervous system, which influences the organs," etc., or "nutrition affects brain chemistry which affects . . . " and so on. While thinking in terms of such causal chains may be simplistic, it is not very practical. It becomes impossibly awkward and cumbersome when we try to conceptualize what is going on in such situations as we have described in the last few chapters. When mind influences nutrition through a multitude of pathways, and nutrition influences the mind, in equally complex ways, then our cause and effect, reductionistic thinking becomes as outmoded as the use of 19th century physics for dealing with space travel.

To deal intelligently with the complexities of mind/body/food interactions, we need a way of thinking that cuts across the conventional categories. We need a conceptual scheme that won't land us in the middle of tangled chains of cause and effect, such as the mind-brain, autonomic nervous system tissue fiasco, where too many of the links remain poorly defined and many are only hypothetical. Though such causal relationships can, and should, (and probably eventually will) be clarified, they serve us poorly when it comes to getting a manageable, usable idea of what is happening overall. When all the detailed information is in, it is sure to be so complex and so variable from person to person as to be of little use in discussions of *this* individual, with *this* personality, confronted by *that* food.

It seems increasingly likely, then, that if we are to find a philosophical framework that will accommodate all we have learned that is relevant to nutrition, if we are to develop a base on which we can build a more comprehensive and holistic science of nutrition, we should probe into the philosophical systems of the East, especially those traditions in India that nurtured the development of Ayurvedic medicine, yoga and meditation, disciplines where the emphasis has always been on personal experience and an integrated understanding of all facets of human nature.

THE FIVE GREAT ELEMENTS

Long before Western science reached its present level of sophistication, and long before the technological tools were available to study material phenomena in such detail, thoughtful minds in ancient cultures were searching for ways to conceptualize man and his place in the universe. In a fashion that presaged and even went beyond our present emphasis on ecology and our view of man as one part of a larger whole, Eastern philosophers were struggling with a way of expressing the profound understandings of human nature that had come from intensive contemplative study.

It was their goal to find a system of classifying not only the material phenomena of the world around them, but also of the "world within": their observations of their own bodies, of their reactions to food and drink, and of their emotions, minds and spiritual experiences and the complex interactions of all of these. To capture their perspective and make it useful for those who were trying to learn, they sought to reduce it to the simplest terms possible. What emerged was a categorization—but not one that was limited to material phenomena. Instead phenomena of all types—physical, emotional, psychological were broken down into "elements." These elements were in some ways reminiscent of the elements we have discussed like carbon, nitrogen, hydrogen, etc., but were less tied to the material world and more universal in their application. They were the elements of which a rock, or tree or plant were made, but they were also the elements of which a thought or emotion were made.

The first element of this system, and the one which is probably the easiest to understand is the one that is called *prithivi*. It is translated "earth" because it is the more solid, substantial and tangible aspect of the universe and it is the earth, *terra firma*, that most aptly symbolizes this element. Things which can be felt and touched and measured, cut up and dissected and examined under a microscope—these things are largely *prithivi* or earth-like. They are material and solid in a familiar and obvious way. The concept of *prithivi*, however, is broader than this. It extends beyond those simple, material things which we can easily touch and identify. Thoughts, for example, may also be comprised partly of *prithivi*. This is true at least of those thoughts which have a solid, substantial nature which tend to be centering, grounding, common sensical kinds of mental activity. Thus we see that this element of "earth" (*prithivi*) is something quite distinct from the solid material earth or soil or stone which is the sum total of our usual concept of earth. The puzzlement we experience when trying to grasp such a different way of thinking has been portrayed in a short story where a "certain Chinese encyclopedia" is discovered, the first page of which begins:

> animals can be categorized as follows: a) those which belong to the Emperor, b) the embalmed, c) the tame, d) suckling pigs, e) mermaids, f) animals in fables, g) free-running dogs, h) those included in the present classification, i) those which act like fools, j) the innumerable, k) those sketched with a very fine camel's hair brush, l) et cetera, m) those which have just broken the pitcher, n) those which from a distance resemble flies.

A respected anthropologist, commenting on this passage, remarked: "What becomes most obvious to us, as we regard the fascinating absurdity of this panorama is precisely how limited our own vision is, the stark impossibility of thinking *that!*"[10]

The categories are beyond us. They in no way parallel our own conceptual schemes so they leave us feeling disoriented. So are the Eastern philosophical concepts of the elements to the Western man who has no familiarity with them. The five elements differ in one important way from the storyteller's fictional Chinese encyclopedia, however, for they have a redeeming appeal. This stems from their inherent ability to pull together and bring into one satisfying schema the whole spectrum of human experience.

The second element, for example, is something that is not quite so solid, not quite as dense or crude or gross, but which is more fluid and movable and active. It is called *apas*. This is often translated as water, though it does not literally mean water. It is certainly true that water is the most apt symbol for it. It is that which has the nature of water: it is liquid, it is fluid, it is movable. If we return to our view of the surface of the earth, we are talking about something now that is related to the hydrosphere, one of the strata of the physical world. The hydrosphere includes all the bodies of water—lakes, rivers, oceans. The atmosphere is the layer of air that overlies both this and the lithosphere, which is the solid, mineral crust of the earth. Inhabiting and growing out of these three is the biosphere, which includes all forms of life.

The lithosphere is similar to *prithivi*, that which is earth-like, while the hydrosphere corresponds to *apas*, yet in both cases the Eastern philosophical concept is broader and deeper than the biophysical one. Thoughts that are fluid and the flow of the voice suggest an element of *apas*, and *apas* is traditionally associated with the sense of taste which as we now know is based on water soluble substances. This distinguishes it from the sense of smell, which registers tiny amounts of airborne solids and in the ancient scheme is limited to *prithivi*.

This way of conceptualizing the world cuts across our Western concepts. Ordinarily we categorize the phenomena of our existence in a very horizontal way. Our elements are those of the physical world, carbon, nitrogen, oxygen, etc., and are merely divisions of physical matter. We momentarily forget that we have a mind or that we have some kind of capacity for higher consciousness, or that there are energy phenomena that we can't see but which make the lights burn, our bodies move, etc. We maintain each of these levels separately in our thinking. There are elements in the physical world and there are elements in the mental world, such as memories, perceptions and cognitive functions, but our conventional categories don't extend across these horizontal strata. The *mahabhuttas* do, however. They are "elements" that are not limited to any stratum or sphere. Rather they cut across all of them.

The third element in Eastern philosophy is called *agni* or *tejas*. It is no longer material. It can't be put on a scale and weighed. It's not even possible to take hold of it with the hand. Though it can be seen, it is not quite material. It is often translated "fire." It is not simply fire, of course. Electricity also has that quality of *agni*, as does light, and the element *agni* is related to vision. That which gives light, such as a flame, for example, is primarily energy. We can see what it is doing, and we can certainly see its effects. Yet we can't quite weigh it or cut it apart. It is not that material. It is *almost* material, but not quite. That is similar to what Einstein talks about when he talks about energy. Something less dense, less material. But still a definite phenomena that is observable and falls into the realm of physics.

These categories are more than simply quaint concepts dragged out of a dusty tomb by the archeologists of the philosophical world. They are neither dependent on, nor invalidated by, modern laboratory research. Rather they offer an independent, enduring and timeless perspective which may help us tie together our scattered observations about nutrition and the mind.

The next element is called *vayu*. The Western rendition of the term is wind or air. *Vayu* is something that can't be seen, can't be measured and can't be grasped, though one can sometimes feel it touch the skin. All that can be seen, however, is the evidence of it. It is never, itself, seen. Though both are quick-moving, it doesn't have any heat like *agni*. The window opens and things move. What makes them move? It is "convection currents," we say. But that's only one way of looking at it. From an Eastern perspective it is *vayu* making things move. One must break free from the mentality of a mechanistic science if he is to see things from a significantly different point

of view.   That doesn't mean that such science isn't valid, for
study and work of certain kinds, but it means that it is only
one perspective and not nearly so absolute as one may tend to
think.

Beyond *vayu* there is one more element and it is called
akasha.   That one is difficult even to conceptualize.   Whatever
exists, exists in *akasha*.   *Akasha* is what would be there if everything else were taken away.   Sometimes it is called "space" but
that can be misleading since ordinarily we use the term "space"
to refer to areas beyond the atmosphere where there is no
gaseous matter present.   *Akasha*, however, also refers to the
space within which tangible, earthly things exist.

Sometimes it is called "the ether."   Physicists have on
occasion talked about "the ether" when they were in a pinch
and didn't know what else to say.   This ether was said to be
that through which light moved.   Sounds were said by scientists
to move through air because the molecules vibrate.   But what
does light move through when it goes through the sun to the
earth?   Apparently it doesn't go through anything.   The question then, from the point of view of physics, was how is it
transmitted?

The physicist answered rather sheepishly, "Well, it is
transmitted through the ether."

But, what is "the ether"?   Well, it really isn't anything.
But it was a concept that became necessary in physics.   And so
physicists have on occasion talked about "the ether," though
for the most part they would prefer not to do so.   Actually it
is a bit embarassing.   It sounds a dissonant note in a materialistic science. Such a concept only became necessary when physicists
departed the simple world of the mechanical interaction of physical bodies and began to study light, which is primarily *agni.* An
Eastern philosopher would say, "Well, you never even really
studied material objects completely because besides their purely
physical aspects, the presence of the earth-like and water-like
elements, there are also subtler elements admixed—fire, air, etc."

Fortunately for the materialistic scientist these were present in small enough degree that his "laws" were not far off, and were generally satisfactory. But when the modern scientist turned his attention to light, something primarily of the element *agni* (fire-like) he suddenly departed the physical world and his concepts were ill suited to this new type of phenomenon—then he began to have to talk in such awkward and "unscientific" terms as "the ether."* In the East the concept is not embarrassing. *Akasha* is the void, the emptiness, space, but it has an essence and it is one of the elements and behaves similarly. It can be mixed with some degree of the other elements to make recognizable objects or experiences. And all the things of which we are aware in the universe, both internally and externally, are various mixtures of these different elements.

Man is made up to a great extent of this *akasha*. If this is especially pronounced he may have the quality of being "spacey," unpredictable, or strange and may drift off into weird states of mind.† Lower animals are more characterized by the lower elements. Plants are also largely comprised of these last two elements, the water-like *(apas)* and earth-like *(prithivi)*. The surface of the earth, of course, is almost entirely characterized by the *prithivi* element except, of course, for the most superficial layer, the soil, which is alive. So higher life partakes increasingly of the higher elements.

The spectrum of phenomena that makes up the universe, then, is broken down in traditional Indian philosophy into five levels or strata of phenomena which are called *bhutas* or *mahabhutas*. Though they sound quaint to modern ears, the symbols of earth, air, fire and water echo through the history of human

---

* Actually in classic Indian philosophy there are five "ethers"—each of which transmits input to one of the five senses. The luminiferous ether transmits light—but this is not *akasha*. The latter transmits sound. The vibration of physical molecules is just the *prithivi* aspect of this phenomenon.

† This is obviously, as we shall see below, related to the *vatta* of Ayurveda (see Chapter 15, Ayurvedic Nutrition).

thought, recurring as profound representations of meaningful categories at times when civilizations have attained peaks of understanding and insight.

　　This is not a system that is separate from or unrelated to Ayurveda.　It is, in fact, the philosophic grounding on which Ayurveda is built.　The three doshas relate in a very systematic and common-sensical way to these five elements. *Vatta* encompasses that which is lightest and most subtle—namely space or ether *(akasha)* and air *(vayu)*. *Pitta,* of course, relates in a simple and straightforward way to fire *(agni).† Kaph* is the psychophysiological manifestation of earthy and watery elements in the system.

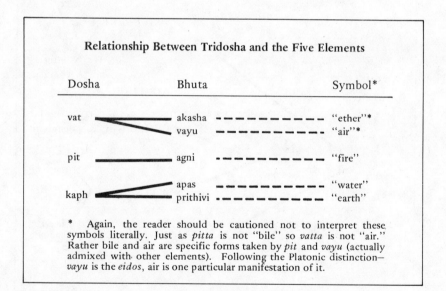

Relationship Between Tridosha and the Five Elements

Dosha	Bhuta		Symbol*
vat	akasha	– – – – – – – –	"ether"*
	vayu	– – – – – – – –	"air"*
pit	agni	– – – – – – –	"fire"
kaph	apas	– – – – – – –	"water"
	prithivi	– – – – – – –	"earth"

*　Again, the reader should be cautioned not to interpret these symbols literally. Just as *pitta* is not "bile" so *vatta* is not "air." Rather bile and air are specific forms taken by *pit* and *vayu* (actually admixed with other elements). Following the Platonic distinction— *vayu* is the *eidos*, air is one particular manifestation of it.

Perhaps partly because of the unwieldiness of conceptualizing five elements, the effects of foods and natural medicines

---

† The words can almost be regarded as synonymous, though in this context *agni* has a broader meaning: all the instances of this principle in the universe, whereas *pitta* is microcosmic in signification, that about the human being which is *agni*. In fact, *pitta* has five subdivisions or "agnis"—*jata, agni,* etc.

are usually expressed in terms of the effects on the three doshas.

Other qualities (*gunas*) of foods and medicines can like-wise be better understood in the light of the foundation for them provided by the elements (*bhutas*). Each of the six basic tastes, for example, discussed in Chapters 10 and 15 bears a definite relationship to two or more of these elements. That is, according to Ayurvedic tradition, the presence of a certain taste reflects the tendency of the substance (food or drug) to affect the psycho-physiological complex in a certain way: to increase the preponderance of those particular elements.

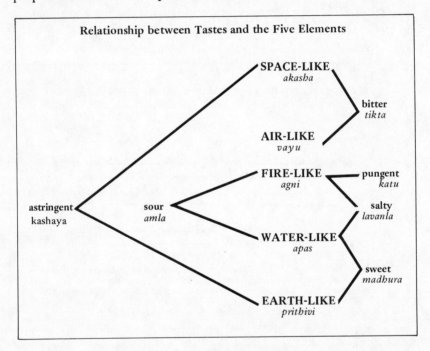

Relationship between Tastes and the Five Elements

SPACE-LIKE
akasha

bitter
tikta

AIR-LIKE
vayu

FIRE-LIKE
agni

pungent
katu

astringent
kashaya

sour
amla

salty
lavanla

WATER-LIKE
apas

sweet
madhura

EARTH-LIKE
prithivi

Thus, for example, that which is bitter increases the elements of air and ether (which together make up the Ayurvedic dosha *vatta*. It will make a person lighter and more mobile. It was the custom in Europe less than a century ago to take bitters with heavy meals.

That which is *kashaya* (astringent) has a drawing together

effect—pulling earth and air together, and this explains why it dries up liquid discharges.

That which is sour increases fire and heat as well as solidity (as we have seen in the case of increased gastric acidity increasing protein digestion and absorption) but will not increase fluid in the body. Salty tasting substances, on the other hand, are notorious for causing thirst and the retention of water. This explains why some tastes which are said to "increase *kaph*" increase primarily liquid, while other *kaphic* foods, such as sour ones, increase solids more.* Sweet things, of course, increase both solid and liquid and are therefore the most strongly *kaphic* (since *kaph* is earth and water together). That which is sweet, then, is the strongest representation of the grossest and most material aspects of existence. It is the epitome of the *rajasic* energy food. It gives energy from outside yet if the sweet food is not burned through exercise, if the material fuel is not transformed into energy, it remains material and is stored as fat.

From the point of view of Eastern philosophy, it is man's desire for and attachment to the material world that determines his existence on that level. If consciousness is not fixed on the material world, it will have the freedom to separate itself from physical phenomena. Foods which have a sweet taste have a special significance and the language is filled with expressions of endearment and affection which relate to sweetness. The same is true of fat, another *kaphic* food, so that luxurious living is living off the fat of the land, and the best of anything is "the cream of the crop." The use of fat in the diet ranks even above that of sweets as a common problem. The average American takes 40 to 45% of his calories as fat compared to only 20 to 25% as sugar.

It is perhaps a natural tendency of human nature to try to extract for oneself that which is gratifying. So it is that the

* See Chapter 15, Ayurvedic Nutrition.

essence of material existence, the most tempting inducements to deepening involvement in the physical world, would be condensed, concentrated, and eaten with single-minded delight. Our snack and junk foods, which are universally acknowledged as health hazards, such as pastries, candies, etc., are predominantly fat and sugar. They tend, like a heavy weight, to pull us downward in the spiral that characterizes the interaction between mind and nutrition. Their *kaphic* nature, their predominance of elements that are symbolized by earth and water, make it clear that from the perspective of Eastern philosophy they would be expected to bind us ever more closely to the more material and less conscious strata of existence. This is seen not only in the endless cycle of craving and binding that characterizes a diet heavy in those foods made primarily of fats and sugars, but also in the substance, either under the skin as fat deposits or inside the arteries as the fat-like plaques of cholesterol that drags one down from a feeling of lightness and a clarity of consciousness.

It is true that growth-producing *kaphic* food is more likely to "create mucus" especially when it is of poor quality *(tamasic)*. But even very wholesome, fresh food which is *kaph*-producing may have this effect. It is our desire for, and ingestion of, food and drink which anchors us to the physical world. *Kaph* is the building material of the physical body which is made of food. When we reject its assimilation, we cart it off as waste—"mucus." This is a minor protest against life, and the "other-worldly" person may become not only thin and ectomorphic but even obsessed with a revulsion toward mucus and the food which produces it. A case in point is Arnold Ehret, who in the last century became convinced that the cause of all disease was mucus, and that this problem could be relieved by eliminating all mucus-causing foods, but mucus continued to form. He progressively omitted each food which was *kaphic*, i.e., that had the power to build substance and fuel work. Ultimately his diet reached the extreme of only raw foods—mostly fruits and vegetables. He became more and more ethereal and "light," sometimes taking only a little fruit and walking miles. He died of tuberculosis as a young man.

Somewhere on the fringes of nutrition there are always to be found certain standard departures from a sane balance. One of these is 100% raw foods, one is no carbohydrate (all meats and salads) one is only grains, one is repeated water fasts to cure any disease. This doesn't mean it's not possible to live on a markedly reduced intake of food. Research on biological transmutations gives us a glimpse of what our potential in this direction might be. To by-pass ordinary nutritional requirements demands, however, a high degree of mastery of physiological processes. One who attempts this should be able to supply what his body needs and not to suffer ill effects from eating less. One who, unprepared, attempts such a feat is foolish and vain and will end, like Ehret, by ruining his health. This throws new light on some common problems and puts them in new perspective.

Over-involvement with the physical world can lead to obesity, while an ambivalent relationship can lead to disorders such as anorexia nervosa where there's overeating and vomiting. A clear-cut rejection of the physical world can lead to malnutrition and susceptibility to infections, while the infatuation with a distorted fantasy of the world can lead to the near exclusive intake of refined and artificial foods. Neither their taste nor their composition suggests they are suitable for nourishing a physical body that will fit harmoniously into the ecological balance of the material world. Their effect on the mind is even more dissonant and less in keeping with an evolutionary movement toward higher consciousness. Repeated use leads inevitably to a subsequent and corresponding distortion of the body through birth defects and degenerative diseases.

A balanced, healthy attitude toward life and earthly existence leads to a well-modulated use of *kaphic* elements (*apas* and *prithivi*) and a well-constituted, healthy body, as well as well-modulated, solid, well-grounded thoughts on which spiritual growth can be built.

It is from such considerations that we realize that it is impossible to discuss the basis of traditional Eastern medicine and nutrition without becoming deeply involved in a struggle to grasp that philosophy and world view out of which it has emerged. This is not a task to be mastered in a few moments of reading. The possibilities it offers seem unlimited and an understanding of it grows with us. Our attempt to comprehend, however, is not without its rewards, since this philosophical system and its child, the psychosomatic conceptual scheme *tridosha*, have proved to be remarkably accommodating. They are inclusive and extensive enough to integrate physiological, psychological and emotional phenomena as well as higher states of consciousness. If our science of nutrition is to mature enough to bring together its diverse data—from research on vitamins and intestinal microbes to information on psychological aspects of digestion and biological transmutations, then it may need to look to the perennial wisdom of such an ancient system of philosophy. It may be this which can free us from the narrowness that leads to counterproductive conflicts and which will permit us to see how we can integrate our hard-won information into one complete vision of man and his diet.

References

1. *Nat. Restaurant Assn. Washington Report 20* (29): 5, 1977
2. *Nat. Restaurant Assn. 20* (45): 4, 1977
3. Wilson, Ewen, Dir. of Econ. and Stats., Am. Meat Inst., Wash., D.C. (personal communication), Feb 1978
4. *Nat. Restaurant Assn. Washington Report 20* (29): 6, 1977
5. Lerza, C., and Jacobson, M., Eds. *Food for People, Not for Profit.* New York: Ballantine Books, 1975, p 165
6. *Ibid*
7. Garard, I. *The Story of Food.* Westport, Ct: AVI Publ. Co., 1974, p 194
8. Jacobson, M. *Eater's Digest.* Garden City, Ny: Doubleday & Co., 1972, p 4
9. Labuza, T. and Sloan, E. *Food for Thought.* Westport, Ct: AVI Publ, Co., 1977, p 150
10. McCarrison, Sir Robert and Sinclair, H. *Nutrition and Health.* 3rd ed., London: Faber, 1964
11. Price, W. *Nutrition and Physical Degeneration.* La Mesa, Ca: Price-Pottenger Foundation, 1972
12. Comm. on Nutr. and Human Needs, U.S. Senate, *Dietary Goals for the United States,* Washington, D.C.: U.S. Gov't Ptg. Office, Feb 1977, p 1
13. *Summary Report of the National Commission on the Cost of Medical Care,* Max Parrott, Chairman, A.M.A., Dec 1977 pp 3, 9
14. Knowles, J., Ed. *Doing Better and Feeling Worse—Health in the United States,* New York: W.W. Norton, 1977, p 2
15. Lerza, C. and Jacobson, M. *op cit,* p 48
16. Braidwood, R. The agricultural revolution. *Sci Am,* Sept 1960
17. Adams, R. The origin of cities. *Sci Am,* Sept 1960
18. Braidwood, R. *op cit,* p 10
19. Walters, A. *Ecology, Food and Civilization.* London: Charles Knight, 1973, p 25
20. Price, W. *op cit,* p 26

CHAPTER 2

1. Eckholm. E. *Losing Ground.* New York: W. W. Norton, 1976, p 35
2. Albrecht, Wm. Our teeth and our soils. *Ann Dentistry 6*: 209, 1947
3. Tompkins, P. and Bird, C. *The Secret Life of Plants.* New York: Harper & Row, 1973, pp 240-241

4.   Ermolenko, N. *Trace Elements and Colloids in Soils.* 2nd ed., Israel Program for Scientific Translations, 1972, p 80

5.   *Ibid*, pp 97, 100

6.   *Ibid*, p 78

7.   *Ibid*, p 96

8.   *Ibid*, p 86

9.   *Ibid*, p 87

10.   Buchele, W. Mechanization of soil erosion control principles, *Tillage for Greater Crop Production.* (Conf. Proc.) St. Joseph, Mi: Am. Soc. Agr. Engl, 1967, p 76

11.   Taylor, Leland. Was it drought? *Acres, USA, A Voice of Eco-Agriculture,* March 1977, p 1

12.   Burnett, J. *Fundamentals of Mycology.* London: Edward Arnold, 1968, pp 339-42

13.   Hutner, S. Inorganic nutrition. *Ann Rev. Microbiol 26*: 313-38, 1972

14.   Burnett, J. *op cit*, pp 344-45

15.   Albrecht, Wm. Mycorrhiza VII: Proteins, amino acids and benzene rings. *Let's Live,* Oct 1964, p 42

16.   Albrecht, Wm. Mycorrhiza V: Parasite or symbiont according to soil as nutrition. *Let's Live,* June 1964, pp 38-39

17.   Albrecht, Wm. Mycorrhiza VI: Some field observations. *Let's Live,* Aug 1964, p 40

18.   Sauchelli, V. *Trace Elements in Agriculture.* New York: Van Nostrand Reinhold, 1969, pp 45-52

19.   Albrecht, Wm. *Let's Live,* Aug 1964, p 41

20.   Lerza, C. and Jacobson, M. *Food for People Not for Profit.* New York: Ballantine Books, 1975, pp 74-82

21.   Taylor, L. *op cit*, p 29

22.   *To Protect Tomorrow's Food Supply, Soil Conservation Needs Priority Attention.* Report to Congress by Comt. Gen., U.S. Dept. of Agr., CED-77-30, Feb. 14, 1977, p 3

23.   Pimentel, D., *et al.* Land degradation: effects on food and energy resources. *Science 194*: 49-55, 1976

24.   *Ibid*, p 30

25.   *Alternative Futures for U.S. Agriculture; Minimum Tillage.* U.S. Dept. of Agr., Washington, D.C.: U.S. Govt. Ptg. Ofc., 1975, p 79

26.   Nelissen, T. The Zen of natural agriculture. *East West 7*: 60-63, 1977

27.   Price, W. *Nutrition and Physical Degeneration.* La Mesa, Ca: The Price-Pottenger Foundation, 1972, p 26

28.   Corbett, T. *Cancer and Chemicals.* Chicago: Nelson-Hall, 1977, p 113

29.   *Ibid*, p 120

CHAPTER 4

1.   Shroeder, Henry A. *The Trace Elements and Man.* Old Greenwich, Ct: Devin Adair, 1973, p 59

2.   Davidson, Sir Stanley, *et al. Human Nutrition and Dietetics* . 6th ed.,

New York: Churchill Livingstone, 1975, p 216

3. Lamont, N. M. Effect of vitamin C supplementation on black mine-workers. *S A Med J 50*: 198, 1976 (letter)

4. Osborn. T., Noriskin, J. and Staz, J. A comparison of crude and re-fined sugar and cereals in their ability to produce in vitro decalcifica-tion of teeth. *J Dent Res 16*: 165-171, 1937

5. Fox, F. and Noriskin, J. Does raw sugar cane juice protect against dental caries? *S A Med J 50*: 760, 1976 (letter)

6. Campbell, G. Diabetes in Asians and Africans in and around Durban. *S A Med J 37*: 1195-1207, 1963

7. Cleave, T. *The Saccharine Disease*. New Canaan, Ct: Keats Publ., 1975, p 89

8. *Ibid*, p 7

9. *Nutrition Action*, Aug 1977, p 8

10. Life Sci Res Ofc, Fed. of Am. Soc. for Exp. Biol. *Evaluation of the Health Aspects of Sucrose as a Food Ingredient.* Springfield, Va: Nat. Tech. Info. Service, U.S. Dept. Commerce, 1976

11. Roberts, A. Effects of a sucrose free diet on the serum-lipid levels of men in Antarctica. *Lancet*, June 2, 1973, pp 1201-1204

12. Harper, H. *Review of Physiological Chemistry*. Los Altos, Ca: Lange, 1971, p 433

13. Ganong, Wm. *Review of Medical Physiology*. 7th ed., Los Altos, Ca: Lange, 1975, p 350

14. Palm J. *Diet Away Your Stress, Tension, Anxiety*. New York: Pocket Books, 1977

15. Michaelson, O. and Makdani, D. Factors affecting nutrient metabolism in *Nutritional Evaluation of Food Processing.* 2nd ed., Edited by Harris, R. and Karmas, E., Westport, Ct: AVI Publ., 1975, p 633

16. Davidson, S. *op cit*, p 217

17. Cleave, T. *op cit*, pp 106-118

18. Heaton, K. Fiber, blood lipids, and heart disease. *Am J Cl Nutr 29*: 125-6, 1976

19. Trowell, H. Ischemic heart disease and dietary fiber. *Am J Cl Nutr 25*: 926-932, 1972

20. Heaton, K. and Pompare, E. *Lancet* Jan 1974, pp 49-50

21. Newbold, H. *Mega-Nutrients for Your Nerves*. New York: Peter H. Wyden, 1975, p 102

22. Cleave, T. *op cit*, p 21

23. Aykroyd, W. and Doughty, J. *Wheat in Human Nutrition*. Rome: FAO of the U.N., 1970, pp 25, 36

24. *Ibid*, pp 18-19

25. The Farm *The Farm Vegetarian Cook Book*. Summertown, Tn: The Book Publ., 1975, p 58

26. Dohan, *et al*. Cereal-free diet in relapsed schizophrenics. *Fed Proc 27*: 219, 1968

27. Aykroyd, W. *op cit*, pp 21-26

28. *Ibid*, p 93

29. *Ibid*, p 87

30. Reinhold, J. Phytate destruction by yeast fermentation in whole

wheat meals. *J Am Diet Assn 66*: 38-41, 1975

31. Mellanby, E. *A Story of Nutritional Research*. Baltimore, Md:Williams and Wilkins, 1950, pp 207-411
32. Rheinhold, J. *op cit*, p 38
33. Davidson, S. *op cit,* p 114
34. Shroeder, H. *op cit*, p 104
35. *Ibid*, pp 53, 55
36. Pleasants, J. Our daily bread. *Integrity*, Mar 1949, p 38 (Reprint no. 44, Lee Found. for Nutr. Res., Milwaukee, Wis)
37. Schroeder, H. *op cit*, p 55
38. Aykroyd, W. *op cit*, p 32
39. Davidson, S. *et al, op cit*, p 206
40. Aykroyd, W. *op cit*, p 22
41. Aykroyd, W. *op cit*, p 97
42. Williams, Roger. Should the science-based food industry be expected to advance? in *Orthomolecular Psychiatry*. Edited by Hawkins, D. and Pauling, L., San Francisco, Ca: W. H. Freeman, 1973, p 317
43. *Consumer Reports*. You can't judge a loaf by its color. May 1976, pp 256-260
44. Inglett, G. Effects of refining operations on the composition of foods. in *Nutritional Evaluation of Food Processing*. 2nd ed., Edited by Harris R. and Karmas, E., Westport, Ct: AVI Publ., 1975, p 148
45. Cullumbine, H. Nitrogen balance studies on rice diets. *Brit J Nutr 4*: 129-134, 1950
46. Jensen, L. *Man's Foods*. Champaign, Il: Garrard Press, 1953, p 81
47. Inglett, G. *op cit*, p 151
48. Cleave, T. *op cit*, p 169
49. Jensen, L. *op cit*, p 81
50. Davidson, S. *op cit*, p 336
51. Kempner, W. *et al.* Effect of rice diet on diabetes mellitus associated with vascular disease. *Postgrad Med 24*: 359-371, 1958
52. Crapo, P. *et al.* Plasma, glucose and insulin response to orally administered simple and complex carbohydrates. *Diabetes 25*: 741-747, 1976
53. *Charaka Samhita*. Jamnagar, India: Shree Gulabkunverba Ayurvedic Society, 1949, Sutrastana 27: 8-15, Vol II, pp 447-479
54. F.A.O. Nutritional Studies (no 9) *Maize and Maize Diets, A Nutritional Survey*. Rome: FAO of the U.N., 1953, p 14
55. Roe, D. *A Plague of Corn*. Ithaca, Ny: Cornell University Press, 1973, pp 158-166
56. *Maize and Maize Diets. op cit*, p 56
57. Hackler, L. In vitro indices in *Evaluation of Proteins for Humans*. Edited by Bodwell, C.E., Westport, Ct: AVI Publ., 1977, p 60
58. Inglett, G. *op cit*, p 152

CHAPTER 5

1. Ganong, Wm. *Review of Medical Physiology*. 7th ed., Los Altos, Ca:

Lange, 1973, p 226

2. Miettinen, M. Prevention of coronary heart disease by cholesterol lowering diet. *Postgrad Med J 51*: 47-51, 1975

3. Riepma, S. *The Story of Margarine*. Washington, D.C.: Public Affairs Press, 1970, p 109

4. Thomas, L. Mortality from arteriosclerotic disease and consumption of hydrogenated oils and fats. *Brit J Prev Soc Med 29*: 82-90, 1975

5. Riepma, S. *op cit*, p 55

6. Sauer, H. The enigma of the Southeast. in *Trace Substances in Environmental Health IX*. Edited by Hemphill, D., Columbia, Mo: University of Mo., 1975, p 3

7. Gattereau, A. and Delisle, H. The unsettled question: butter or margarine? *Canad Med Assn J 103*: 268-271, 1970

8. Miettinen, M. *op cit*

9. Pinckney, E. The potential toxicity of excessive polyunsaturates. *Am Heart J 85*: 723-725, 1973

10. West, C. and Redgrave, T. Reservations on the use of polyunsaturated fats in human nutrition. *Am Lab* Jan 1975, pp 24-25

11. Williams, R.J. *Nutrition Against Disease*. New York: Bantam Books, 1971, p 85

12. Pinckney, E. *op cit*, pp 723-726

13. Pearce, M. and Dayton, S. Incidence of cancer in men on a diet high in polyunsaturated fat. *Lancet*, March 1971, pp 464-467

14. Mackie, B. Malignant melanoma and diet. *Med J Australia*, May 1974, p 810 (letter)

15. West, C. and Redgrave, T. *op cit*, p 28

16. Pryor, Wm. Free radical pathology. *Chem Eng News*, June 7, 1971, pp 34-51

17. Mead, J. Dietary polyunsaturated fatty acids as potential toxic factors. *Chemtech 2*: 70-71, 1972

18. Pinckney, E. and Pinckney, C. *The Cholesterol Controversy*. Los Angeles, Ca: Sherbourne Press, 1973, p 130

19. Williams, R. J. *op cit*, pp 296-298

20. *Ibid*

21. Kritchensky, D. and Tepper, S. Cholesterol vehicle in experimental atherosclerosis. *Atheroscler Res 7*: 647-51, 1967

22. *Ibid*

23. Bordia, A. *et al*. Effects of the essential oils of garlic and onion on alimentary hyperlipenia. *Arterscler 21*: 15-19, 1975

24. Vesselinovitch, D. *et al*. Arteriosclerosis in the rhesus monkey fed three food fats. *Arterioscler 30*: 303-321, 1974

25. Hunter, Beatrice T. *Consumer Beware!* New York: Bantam Books, 1972, pp 209-210

26. Cleave, T. *The Saccharine Disease*. New Canaan, Ct: Keats Publ, 1975, pp 103-104

27. Thomas, L. *op cit*, pp 82-90

28. Pinckney, E. *The Cholesterol Controversy*. p 41

29. *Charaka Samhita*. Jamnagar, India: Shree Gulabkunverva Ayurvedic

Society, 1949, Sutrastana 27: 293, Vol II, p 545

30. Pinckney, E. The potential toxicity of excessive polyunsaturates. p 723-726

31. Mead, J. *op cit*, pp 70-71

32. Pryor, Wm. *op cit*, pp 34-51

33. Horwitt, M. Vitamin E: a reexamination. *Am J Clin Nutr 29*: 572-573, 1976

34. West, C. and Redgrave. T. *op cit*, p 28

35. Simons, L. *et al. Austr N Z J Med 7*: 262-266, 1977

36. Bordia, A *op cit*, pp 15-19

37. Miettenen, M. *op cit*, pp 47-51

38. Nichols, A. *et al.* Independence of serum-lipid levels and dietary habits. *JAMA 236:* 1948, 1976

39. Pinckney, E. and Pinckney, C. *The Cholesterol Controversy*. pp 19-27

40. Mann, S. Diet-heart: end of an era. *New Eng J Med 297*: 644-650, 1976

41. Williams, R.J. *op cit*, pp 83-84

42. Malhotra, S. Epidemiology of ischemic heart disease in India with special reference to causation. *Brit Heart J 29*: 902, 1967

43. Wrench, G. *The Wheel of Health.* New York: Schocken Books, 1972, p 33

44. Williams, R.J. *op cit*, pp 298-302

45. Davidson, Sir Stanley *et al. Human Nutrition and Dietetics*, 6th ed., New York: Churchill Livingstone, 1975, p 88

46. *Medical World News*, Oct. 17, 1977, p 82

47. Moore, W. and Holdeman, L. Discussion of current bacteriological investigations. *Cancer Res 35*: 3418-3420, 1975

48. Reddy, B. *et al.* Further leads on metabolic epidemiology of large bowel cancer. *Cancer Res 35*: 3404-3406, 1975

49. *Ibid*

50. *Current Prescribing,* Can diet cause cancer? Jan 1977, pp 35-57

51. Davidson, S. *op cit*, pp 88-89

52. Wissler, R and Vesselinovitch, D. Regression of atherosclerosis in experimental animals and man. *Mod Concepts Cardiovasc Dis 46*: 28-29, 1977

CHAPTER 6

1. Ghadimi, H. The silent emergency: iatrogenically enhanced substrate deficiency in premature infants. *Am J Clin Nutr 30*: 1147-52, 1977

2. Register, V. and Sonnenberg, L. The vegetarian diet. *J Am Diet Assn 62*: 253-261, 1973

3. Hegsted, D. quoted in Register, V. and Sonnenberg, L. *J Am Diet Assn 62*: 254, 1973

4. Register, V. and Sonnenberg, L. *op cit*, p 254

5. Hardinge, M. and Stare, F. Nutritional studies of vegetarians, part I, nutritional, physical, and laboratory studies. *Am J Clin Nutr 2*: 73-82, 1954

6. Crosby, Wm. Can a vegetarian be well nourished?   *JAMA 233*:

898, 1975

7. Vegetarian diets. *Am J Clin Nutr 27*: 1095-1096, 1974

8. Labuza, T. *Food and Your Well-Being.* New York: West Publ., 1977, p 177

9. Ruys, J. and Hickle, J. Serum-cholesterol and triglyceride levels in Australian adolescent vegetarians. *Brit Med J 2*: 87, 1976

10. West, R. and Hayes, O. A comparison between vegetarians and non-vegetarians in a Seventh-Day Adventist group. *Am J Clin Nutr 21*: 853-562, 1968

11. Sacks, F. *et al.* Plasma lipids, and lipoproteins in vegetarians and controls. *New Eng J Med 292*: 1148-51, 1975

12. Williams, R. J. *Nutrition Against Disease.* New York: Bantam Books, 1971, p 260

13. Wynder, E. *et al.* Cancer and coronary artery disease among Seventh-Day Adventists. *Cancer 12*: 1016-28, 1959

14. Armstrong, B. *et al.* Blood pressure in Seventh-Day Adventist vegetarians. *Am J Epidem 105*: 444-9, 1977

15. Sacks, F. Rosner, B. and Kass, E. Blood pressure in vegetarians. *Am J Epidem 100*: 390-398, 1974

16. Ellis, F. *et al.* Incidence of osteoporosis in vegetarians and omnivores. *Am J Clin Nutr 25*: 555-558, 1972

17. Mendeloff, A. A critique of fiber deficiency. *Dig Dis 21*: 103-111, 1976

18. Diet, intestinal flora, and colon cancer. *Nutr Rev 33*: 136-137, 1975

19. Hardinge, M. *et al.* Nutritional studies of vegetarians, part III. *Am J Clin Nutr 6*: 523-525, 1958

20. Painter, N. and Burkitt, D. Diverticular disease of the colon: a deficiency disease of western civilization. *Brit Med J 2*: 450-454, 1971

21. Trowell, H. Ischemic heart disease and dietary fiber. *Am J Clin Nutr 25*: 926-932, 1972

22. Ershoff, B. Antitoxic effects of plant fiber. *Am J Clin Nutr 27*: 1395-1398, 1974

23. McClure, J. *Meat Eaters are Threatened.* New York: Pyramid Books, 1973, pp 103-105

24. Hunter, Beatrice T. *Consumer Beware!* New York: Bantam Books, 1971, pp 99-135

25. McClure, J. *op cit*, pp 40-65

26. Mayer, J. *A Diet for Living.* New York: David McKay Co, 1975, p 198

27. Hayes, W. in *Chemical and Biological Hazards in Food.* Edited by Ayres, J. *et al.* New York: Hafner Publ, 1969, p 144

28. Bieler, H. *Food is Your Best Medicine.* New York: Vintage Books, 1973, p 165

29. Mayer, J. *op cit*, pp 197-198

30. Hunter, B. T., *op cit*, p 112

31. Corbett, T. *Cancer and Chemicals.* Chicago, Il: Nelson-Hall, 1977, p 81

32. Ayres, J. *et al. Chemical and Biological Hazards in Food.* New York:

Hafner Publ, 1969, p 144
33. Corbett, T. *op cit*, p 81-86
34. Ershoff, B. *op cit*, pp 1395-1309
35. Shakman, R. Nutritional influences on the toxicity of environmental pollutants. *Arch Environ Health 28*: 105-113, 1974
36. Hunter, B. T. *op cit*, p 104
37. Hall, R. *Food for Naught*. New York: Vintage Books, 1976, pp 89,97
38. *Ibid*
39. Hunter, B. T. *op cit*, pp 177-118
40. Hunter, J. *Memoirs of a Captivity Among the Indians of North America*. London: Longman, Hurst, Orme, Brown and Green, 1824. (Reprinted by the Lee Foundation for Nutr. Res. 1964)
41. Childe, V. quoted in Jensen, L. *Man's Foods*. Champaign, Il: The Garrard Press, 1953, p 39
42. Lappe, F. *Diet for a Small Planet*. New York: Ballantine Books, 1971, pp 7-8
43. *Organic Gardening and Farming*, Sept 1977, p 44
44. Wrench, G. *The Wheel of Health*. New York: Schocken Books, 1972, p 49
45. Cunningham, A. Morbidity in breast-fed and artificially fed infants. *J Ped 90*: 726-29, 1977
46. Kretchmer, N. Lactose and lactase. *Sci Am 227*: 70-78, 1972
47. Paige, D. *et al*. Lactose malabsorption in preschool black children. *Am J Clin Nutr 30*: 1018-1022, 1977
48. Woodruff, C. Milk intolerances in *Present Knowledge in Nutrition*. New York: Nutrition Foundation, 1976, pp 478-487
49. Kretchmer, N. *op cit*
50. Lund, B. Effects of Heat Processing on Nutrients. in *Nutritional Evaluation of Food Processing*, 2nd ed., Edited by Harris, R. and Karmas, E. Westport, Ct: AVI Publ, 1975, p 206
51. Rodale, J. *Complete Book of Food and Nutrition*. Emmaus, Pa: Rodale Books, 1972, p 145
52. Daniels, A. and Stearns, G. cited in Wrench, G. *The Wheel of Health*, New York: Schocken Books, 1972, p 100
53. Davidson, S. *et al. Human Nutrition and Dietetics*. 6th ed., New York: Churchill Livingstone, 1975, p 240
54. Wolf, W. Effects of refining operations on legumes. in *Nutritional Evaluation of Food Processing*, pp 169-170
55. Lappe, F. *op cit*, pp 51-52
56. *Life and Health*, Spec. Suppl. Nutr Faculty, Loma Linda Med Sch, Washington, D.C.: Review and Herald Publ Assn, p 30
57. Geiger, E. The role of the time factor in feeding supplementary proteins. *J Nutr 36*: 813-819, 1948
58. Bressani, R. Protein supplementation and complementation. in *Evaluation of Proteins for Humans*. Edited by Bodwell, C., Westport, Ct: AVI Publ, 1977, pp 216-218
59. *Life and Health. op cit*, p 33
60. Grande, F., Anderson, J. and Keys, A. Effect of carbohydrates of

leguminous seeds, wheat, and potatoes on serum cholesterol concentration in man. *J Nutr 86*: 313-317, 1965

61. Mathur, K., Khan, M., Sharma, R. Hypocholesterolaemic effect of Bengal gram: a long-term study in man. *Brit Med J 1*: 30-31, 1968

62. Moore, M. Guzman, M., Schilling, P. and Strong, J. Dietary-atherosclerosis study on deceased persons. *J Am Diet Assn 68*: 216-223, 1976

63. Rackis, J. *et al*. Soybean factors relating to gas production by intestinal bacteria. *J Food Sci 35*: 634, 1970

64. Rackis, J. Flatulence problems associated with soy products. Paper presented at: World Soybean Res Conf, Champaign-Urbana, Il, Aug 1975, pp 5-7

65. Wolf, W. Flavor and oligosaccharides as limiting factors in soy consumption. Paper presented at: First Latin Am Soy Protein Conf, Mexico City, 1975

66. Aykroyd, W. and Doughty, J. *Legumes in Human Nutrition*. Rome: FAO of the U.N., 1964, p 54

67. Liener, I. Protease inhibitors and hemagglutinins of legumes. in *Evaluation of Proteins for Humans*. Edited by Bodwell, C., Westport, Ct: AVI Publ, 1977, pp 296-299

68. Vaughn, D. Processing effects. in *Evaluation of Proteins for Humans*. pp 257-258

69. Aykroyd, W. and Doughty, J. *Wheat in Human Nutrition*. Rome: FAO of the U.N., 1970, p 19

70. *Ibid*

71. Lappe, F. *op cit*, p 88

72. Albrecht, Wm. *The Albrecht Papers*. Edited by Walter, C. Raytown, Mo: Acres, U.S.A., 1975, pp 293-302

73. Chen, P. *Soybeans for Health, Longevity, and Economy*. St. Catherines, Ontario: Provoker Press, 1970, p 99

74. Lappe, F. *op cit*, p 28

75. Davis, Adelle. *Let's Eat Right to Keep Fit*. New York: New American Library, 1954, p 39

76. Newbold, H. *Meganutrients for Your Nerves*. New York: Peter H. Wyden, 1975, p 110

77. Mayer, J. *op cit*, p 16

78. Register, V. and Sonnenberg, L. *op cit*, pp 253-261

79. Bender, A. in *Proteins in Human Nutrition*. Edited by Porter, J. and Rolls, B. New York: Academic Press, 1973, pp 167-178

80. Crim M. and Munro, H. Protein in *Present Knowledge in Nutrition*, 4th ed., New York: Nutrition Foundation, 1976, p 49

81. Rand, Wm. Determination of protein allowances in human adults from nitrogen balance data. *Am J Clin Nutr 30*: 1129-1134, 1977

82. Grieve, J. Prevention of gestational failure by high protein diet. *J Reprod Med 13*: 170-174, 1974

83. Keys, A. *et al. The Biology of Human Starvation Vol II*. Minneapolis, Mi: Univ. of Minn. Press, 1950, pp 976-978

84. Payne, P. The relative importance of protein and energy as causal

factors in malnutrition. *Am J Clin Nutr 28*: 281-6, 1975

85. Young, V. and Scrimshaw, N. Human protein requirements in *Evaluation of Proteins for Humans,* p 28

CHAPTER 7

1. Roddis, L. *James Lind: Founder of Nautical Medicine.* New York: Henry Schuman, 1950, p 44
2. Wrench, G. *The Wheel of Health.* New York: Schocken Books, 1972, p 68
3. Davidson, Sir Stanley *et al. Human Nutrition and Dietetics.* 6th ed., New York: Churchill Livingstone, 1975, p 145
4. *Ibid*
5. U. S. Dept. of HEW. *Ten-State Nutrition Survey, 1968-1970.* HEW Publ No (HSM) 72-8132, V: 233
6. Cohen, B. *et al.* Vitamin A-induced nonspecific resistance to infection. *J Infect Dis 129*: 597-99, 1974
7. Sivakumar, B. and Reddy, V. Absorption of labelled vitamin A in children during infection. *J Nutr 27*: 299-304, 1972
8. Wrench, G. *op cit,* p 71
9. Smith, J. *et al.* Zinc: a trace element essential in vitamin A metabolism. *Science 181*: 954-5, 1973
10. Michaelsson, G., Juhlin, L. and Vahlquist, A. Effects of oral zinc and vitamin A in acne. *Arch Derm 113*: 31-34, 1977
11. Cone, M. and Nettesheim, P. Effects of vitamin A on 3-methycholan-threne-induced squamous metaplasias and early tumors in the respiratory tract of rats. *J Natl Cancer Inst 50*: 1599-1603, 1973
12. Bjelke, E. Dietary vitamin A and human lung cancer. *Int J Cancer 15*: 561-65, 1975
13. Vitamin A and cancer prophylaxis. *Brit Med J*, July 3, 1976, p 2
14. Williams, Roger *Physician's Handbook of Nutritional Science.* Springfield, Il: Charles C. Thomas, 1975, pp 48, 94
15. Davidson, S. *et al.* p 146
16. Rao, C. and Rao, B. Absorption of dietary carotenes in human subjects. *Am J Clin Nutr 23*: 105-109, 1970
17. Davidson, S *op cit,* p 144
18. Bray, W. Leaf-protein concentrate as a source of vitamins. *Proceedings Nutr Soc*, May 1976, p 7A
19. Stimson, Wm. Vitamin A intoxication in adults. *New Eng J Med 265*: 369-373, 1961
20. Pease, C. Focal retardation and arrestment of growth of bones due to vitamin A intoxication. *JAMA 182*: 980-985, 1962
21. White, A., Handler, P. and Smith, E. *Principles of Biochemistry.* 4th ed., New York: McGraw-Hill, 1968, p 1019
22. Edozien, J. Udo, U., Young, V. and Scrimshaw, N. Effects of high levels of yeast feeding on uric acid metabolism of young men. *Nature 228*: 180, 1970
23. Davidson, S. *op cit,* p 208

24. Clarke, A. Beriberi in Bethnal Green. *Brit Med J 2*: 278, 1971 (letter)
25. Williams, Ray D. *et al.* Induced thiamin (vitamin B₁) deficiency and the thiamin requirement of man. *Arch Intern Med 69*: 721-738, 1942
26. Williams, Roger, *Biochemical Individuality.* Austin, Tx: Univ Texas Press, 1956, p 149-152
27. Najar, V. and Holt, E. The biosynthesis of thiamin in man. *JAMA 123*: 683, 1943
28. Aykroyd, W. and Doughty, J. *Wheat in Human Nutrition.* Rome: FAO of the U.N., 1970, p 36
29. Najra. V. *et al*, The biosynthesis of riboflavin in man. *JAMA 126*: 357-8, 1944
30. *Ten-State Nutrition Survey, 1968-1970*, p 217
31. Davidson, S. *op cit*, p 170
32. Steir, M. *et al.* Riboflavin deficiency in infants and children with heart disease. *Am Heart J 92*: 139-143, 1976
33. Davis, Adelle. *Let's Eat Right to Keep Fit.* New York: New American Library, 1970, pp 90-91
34. Sydenstricker, V. *et al.* The ocular manifestations of ariboflavinosis. *JAMA 114*: 2437-2445, 1940
35. Rodale, J. *The Complete Book of Food and Nutrition.* Emmaus, Pa: Rodale Books, 1961, p 488
36. Calloway, D., Giauque, R. and Costa, F. The superior mineral content of some American Indian foods in comparison to federally donated counterpart commodities. *Ecol Food Nutr 3*: 203-211, 1974
37. Laguna, J. and Carpenter, K. Raw versus processed corn in niacin-deficient diets. *J Nutr 45*: 21-28, 1951
38. Christianson, D. D. *et al.* Nutritionally unavailable niacin in corn; isolation and biological activity. *J Agr Food Chem 16*: 100-104, 1968
39. Parsons, Wm. Reduction of serum cholesterol levels and beta-lipoprotein cholesterol levels by nicotinic acid. *Arch Intern Med 103*: 783-90, 1959
40. *Ibid*
41. Altschul, R. Niacin in vascular disorders and hyperlipemia. Springfield, Il: Charles C. Thomas, 1964, p 259
42. *Ibid*, p 294
43. Pfeiffer, C. *Mental and Elemental Nutrients.* New Canaan, Ct: Keats Publ, 1975, p 119
44. Davis, A. *op cit*, p 110
45. Herbert, V. Destruction of vitamin B₁₂ by ascorbic acid. *JAMA 230*: 241-2, 1974
46. White, P. Megavitamin this and megavitamin that. *JAMA 233*: 538-0 1975
47. Pfeiffer, C. *op cit*, p 122
48. Altschul, R. *op cit*, p 70
49. Davidson, S. *op cit,* p 349
50. Reinken, I., and Gant, H. Vitamin B₆ nutrition in women with hyper-

emesis granidarum during the first trimester of pregnancy. *Clin Chem Acta 55*: 101, 1974

51. Heller, S. *et al*, Vitamin B6 status in pregnancy. *A J Clin Nutr 26*: 1339-1348, 1973

52. Wachstein, M. and Graffeo, L. Influence of vitamin B6 on the incidence of preeclampsia. *Obs Gyn 8*: 180-1956

53. Bennick, H., Coelingh and Schreurs, W. Improvement of oral glucose tolerance in gestational diabetes by syridoxine. *Brit Med J 5*: 13-15, 1975

54. Ekelund, H. *et al*, Apparent response of imparied mental development, minor motor epilepsy and ataxia to pyridaxine. *Acta paediat Acand 58*: 572-576, 1969

55. Schroeder, H. Is aterosclerosis a conditioned pyridaxal deficiency? *J Chron Dis 2*: 28-41, 1955

56. *Ibid*

57. Davidson, S. *op cit*, p 180

58. Adams, P. *et al*. Effect of pyridaxine hydrochloride (vitamin B6) upon depression associated with oral contraception. *Lancet*, Apr 1973, pp 897-904

59. Gleeson, M. and Graves, P. Complications of dietary deficiency of vitamin B12 in young caucasians. *Postgrad Med J 50*: 462-464, 1974

60. Strachan, R. and Henderson, J. Psychiatric syndromes due to avitaminosis B12 with normal blood and marrow. *Quart J Med 34*: 303-316, 1965

61. Williams, Roger, *Nutrition Against Disease*. New York: Bantam Books, 1971, p 61

62. Folates and the fetus. *Lancet*, Feb 26, 1977, p 462

63. Stone, M. *et al*, Folic acid metabolism in pregnancy. *Am J Obs Gyn 99*: 638-648, 1967

64. Davis, A. *op cit*, p 78

65. Streiff, R. Folate deficiency and oral contraceptives. *JAMA 214*: 105-108, 1970

66. Hunter, R. *et al*, Serum B12 and folate concentrations in mental patients. *Brit J Psychiat 113*: 1291-1295, 1967

67. Shulman, R. A survey of vitamin B12 deficiency in an elderly psychiatric population. *Brit J Psychiat 113*: 241-251, 1967

68. Pfeiffer, C., *op cit*, p 164

69. Davidson, S. *op cit*, p 178

70. *Ibid*, p 180

71. Cohenour, S. and Calloway, D. Blood, urine and dietary pantothenic acid levels of pregnant teenagers. *Am J Clin Nutr 25*: 512-517, 1972

72. Ishiguro, K. Pantothenic acid and age. *Tohoky J Exper Med 75*: 137-150, 1961

73. Williams, Roger, *op cit*, pp 146-147

74. Davis, A. *op cit*, p 81

75. Davidson, S. *op cit*, pp 181-182

76. Zarafonetis, C. Darkening of gray hair during para-amino-benzoic acid therapy. *J Invest Derm 15*: 399-410, 1950

77. Krebs, E. Vitamin B15 (Pangamic Acid) properties, functions and use. Sci Publ House, Moscow, USSR: McNaughton Foundation Sponsoring Independent Research. Reprinted by Cancer Book House Cancer Control Society, Los Angeles, Ca, 1965

78. Taylor, T. *et al*, Ascorbic acid supplementation in the treatment of pressure-sores. *Lancet*, Sept 7, 1974, p 544

79. Gerson, C. and Fabraye, E. Ascorbic acid deficiency and fistula formation in regional enteritis. *Gastroent 67*: 428-433, 1974

80. Buzina, R. Brodarec, A. Jusic, M. *et al*, Epidemiology of angular stomatitis and bleeding gums. *Int J Vit Nutr Res 43*: 401-415, 1973

81. Walker, G. *et al*, Trial of ascorbic acid in prevention of colds. *Brit Med J 1*: 603-06, 1967

82. Tebrock, H. *et al*. Usefulness of bioflavonoids and ascorbic acid in treatment of common cold. *JAMA 162*: 1227-1233, 1956

83. Pauling, L. *Vitamin C and the Common Cold.* San Francisco, Ca: W. H. Freeman, 1970, pp 99-102

84. Anderson, T. *et al*, Vitamin C. and the common cold: a double-blind trial. *Canad Med J 107*: 503-508, 1972

85. Tebrock, H. *op cit*, pp 1227-1233

86. Miller, J. *et al*, Therapeutic effect of vitamin C. *JAMA 237*: 248-251, 1977

87. Coulehan, J. *et al*, Vitamin C and acute illness in Navajo school children. *New Eng J Med 295*: 973-977, 1976

88. Anderson, T. *et al*, Winter illness and vitamin C: the effect of relatively low doses. *Canad Med J 112*: 823-826, 1975

89. Stone, I. *The Healing Factor—Vitamin C Against Disease*. New York: Grosset & Dunlap, 1972, p 60

90. Dahl, H. and Degre, M. The effect of ascorbic acid on production of human interferon and the antiviral activity in vitro. *Acta Path Microbio Scand 84 (Sect B)*: 280-84, 1976

91. Stone, S. *op cit*, p 79

92. Wilson, C. Vitamin C. tissue saturation, metabolism and desaturation. *Practitioner 212*: 481-492, 1974

93. Shilotri, P. and Bhat, K. Effect of mega doses of vitamin C on bactericidal activity of leukocytes. *Am J Clin Nutr 30*: 1077-81, 1977

94. Klenner, F. Observations on the dose and administration of ascorbic acid when employed beyond the range of a vitamin in human pathology. *J Appl Nutr 23*: 61-87, 1971

95. Stone, I. Humans, the mammalian mutants. *Am Lab* Apr 1974, pp 32-39

96. Zuskin, E. *et al*, Inhibition of histamine-induced airway constriction by ascorbic acid. *J Aller Clin Immunol 51*: 218-226, 1973

97. Pelletier, O. Vitamin C and cigarette smokers. *NY Acad Sci Ann 258*: 156-168, 1975

98. Cameron, E. and Campbell, A. The orthomolecular treatment of cancer. II Clinical trial of high dose ascorbic acid supplements in advanced human cancer. *Chem Bio Interact 9*: 285-315, 1974

99. Klenner, F. *op cit*, pp 61-87

100. Spittle, C. Atherosclerosis and vitamin C *Lancet*, Dec 1971, p 1280-1281
101. Hindson, T. *et al*, Ascorbic acid for prickly heat. *Lancet*, June 1968, pp 1347-8
102. Lai, Hsiao-Ya *et al*, Effect of ascorbic acid on rectal polyps and fecal steroids. *Fed Proc 36*: 1061, 1977
103. Herjanic, M. Treatment of schizophrenia in *Orthomolecular Psychiatry*. Edited by Hawkins D. and Pauling, L. San Francisco, Ca: W. H. Freeman, 1973, pp 303-315
104. Holmes, H. Campbell, K. Amberg, E. The effect of vitamin C on lead poisoning. *J Lab Clin Med 24*: 1119-1127, 1939
105. Chatterjee, G. *et al*, Cadmium administration an L=ascorbic acid metabolism in rats: effect of L-ascorbic acid supplementation. *Int J Vit Nutr Res 43*: 370-377, 1973
106. Fox, M. Spivey and Fry, B. Cadmium toxicity decreased by dietary ascorbic acid supplements. *Science 169*: 989-991, 1970
107. Rivers, J. and Devine, M. Plasma ascorbic acid and concentrations and oral contraceptives. *Am J Clin Nutr 25*: 684-689, 1972
108. Coffey, G. and Wilson, C. Ascorbic acid deficiency and aspirin induced haematemesis. *Brit Med J 1*: 208, 1975
109. Singh, G. Usefulness of ascorbic acid (vitamin C) in treatment of industrial chemical toxicity. *Ind J Med Sci 28*: 219-223, 1974
110. Nitrosamines look more like human cancer villains and new studies illuminate chemistry of nitrosamines. *JAMA 238*: 15, 19-20, 1977
111. Brown, R. Possible problems of large intakes of ascorbic acid. *JAMA Med Assn 2249*: 1529-30, 1973
112. Vitamin C and oxalate stones *JAMA 237*: 768, 1977 (letter)
113. Briggs, M. *et al*, Urinary oxalate and vitamin C supplements. *Lancet*, July 1973, p 201
114. *Ibid*
115. Loomis, W. Skin pigment regulation of vitamin D biosynthesis in man. *Science 157*: 501-506, 1967
116. *Ibid*
117. Davis, Adelle *op cit*, pp 140, 117
118. Deluca, H. Active compounds in *The Vitamins* Edited by Sebrell, W. and Harris, R. New York: Academic Press, 1971, pp 203-230
119. Davidson, S. *op cit*, p 324
120. Davis, A. *op cit*, p 139
121. Helmer, A. and Jansen, C. Vitamin D precursors removed from human skin by washing. *Stud Inst Divi Thom*, 1937, pp 207-216
122. Reinertson, R. and Wheatley, V. Studies on the Chemical Composition of Human Epidermal Lipids. *J Invest Derm 32*: 49-57, 1959
123. Olson, R. Vitamin E and its relation to heart disease. *Circ 48*: 179-84, 1973
124. Farrell, P. *et al*, Megavitamin E supplementation in man *Am J Clin Nutr 28*: 1380-6, 1975
125. Anderson, T. and Reid, Wm. A double-blind trial of vitamin E in angina pectoris. *Am J Clin Nutr 27*: 1174-1178, 1974
126. Rinzler, S. *et al*, Failure of alpha tocopherol to influence chest pain

in patients with heart disease. *Circ 1*: 288, 1950

127. Makinson, D. *et al*, Vitamin E in angina pectoris. *Lancet 254*: 102, 1948
128. Schute, W. *The Complete Updated Vitamin E Book.* New Canaan, Ct: Keats Publ, 1975, p 65.
129. Vogelsang, A. Twenty-four years using α-tocopherol in degenerative cardiovascular disease. *Angiol 21*: 275-279, 1970
130. Olson, R. *op cit*, pp 178-84, 1973
131. Haeger, K. Long-time treatment of intermittent claudication with vitamin E. *Am J Clin Nutr 27*: 1179-1181, 1974
132. Marx, W. *et al*. Effects of the administration of a vitamin E concentrate and of cholesterol and bile salt on the aorta of the rat. *Arch Pathol 47*: 440-5, 1949
133. Steiner, M. and Anastasi, J. Vitamin E an inhibitor of the platelet release reaction. *J Clin Invest 57*: 732-737, 1976
134. Horwitt, M. Vitamin E: a reexamination. *Am J Clin Nutr 29*: 569-578, 1976
135. Vogelsang, A. *op cit*, p 275
136. Melhorn, D. and Gross, S. Relationships between iron-dextran and vitamin E in iron deficiency in children. *J Lab Clin Med 74*: 789-802, 1969
137. Vitamin E in clinical medicine. *Lancet*, Feb. 9, 1974, p 220
138. Bieri, J. Vitamin C. *Nutrition Reviews 33*: 161-166, 1975
139. Cohen, H. *New Eng J Med 289*: 980, 1973
140. Hillman, R. Tocopherol excess in man. Creatinuria associated with prolonged ingestion. *Am J Clin Nutr 5*: 597-600, 1957
141. Williams, Roger, *Physician's Handbook of Nutritional Science*, pp 53-50
142. Mustafa, M. Influence of dietary vitamin E on lung cellular sensitivity to ozone in rats. *Nutr Reports Int 2*: 473-75, 1975
143. Roehm, J. Hadley, J., Menzel, D. Antioxidants versus lung disease. *Arch Intern Med 128* 88-93, 1971
144. Shakman, R. Nutritional influences on toxicity of environmental pollutants *Arch Environ Hlth 28*: 105-13, 1974
145. Pryor, Wm. Free radical pathology. *Chem Eng News*, June 1971, pp 34-51
146. Horwitt, M. *op cit*, pp 569-578
147. Bieri, J. and Evarts, R. Tocopherols and fatty acids in American diets. *J Am Diet Assn 62*: 147-51, 1973
148. Hodges, R. Vitamin E and coronary heart disease. *J Am Diet Assn 62*: 638-642, 1973
149. Williams, Roger, *Nutrition Against Disease*. p. 276
150. Dietary Goals for the United States, prepared by Comm. on Nutr and Human Needs, U.S. Senate, Feb. 1977
151. Vitamin P, its properties and uses. from *Vitamin Sources and Their Utilization*, Collection 4. Akademiya Nauk SSSR. Translated from Russian Pub. for Nat Sci Found. Washington, D.C. and Dept of Agr, Israel Program for Scientific Tranlation, Jerusalem: 1977

152. Merkel, R. The use of menadione bisulfate and ascorbic acid in the treatment of nausea and vomiting of pregnancy. *Am J Ob Gyn 64*: 416-418, 1952

153. Gamball, D. and Quackenbush, F. Effects of cholesterol and other substances on essential fatty acid deficiencies. *J Nutr 70*: 497-501, 1960

154. Hart, J. and Cooper, Wm Vitamin F in the treatment of prostatic hypertrophy. Milwaukee, Wi: Lee Foundation for *Nutr Res Report no 1*, Nov 1941, pp 1-8

155. Mayer, J. *Diet for Living*. New York: David McKay, 1975, p 59

156. Antar, M. *et al*, Changes in retail market food supplies in the United States in the last seventy years in relation to the incidence of coronary heart disease, with special reference to dietary carbohydrates and essential fatty acids. *Am J Cl Nutr 14*: 169, 1964

CHAPTER 8

1. Nordin. B. Clinical significance and pathogenesis of osteoporosis. Brit Med J 1: 571-576, 1971

2. Albanese, A. Problems of bone health in elderly *NY State J Med* Feb 1975, pp 326-336

3. Underwood, E. *Trace Elements in Human and Animal Nutrition* 4th ed., New York: Academic Press, 1977, p 176

4. *Ibid*

5. Ashmead, D. The need for chelated trace minerals. *Vet Med* Apr 1974, pp 467-468

6. Ellis, F. *et al*. Incidence of osteoporosis in vegetarians and omnivores. *Am J Clin Nutr 25*: 555-558, 1972

7. Davidson, Sir Stanley *et al. Human Nutrition and Dietetics* 6th ed., New York: Churchill Livingstone, 1975, p 112

8. Williams, R. *Nutrition Against Disease*. New York: Bantam Books, 1971, p 299

9. Davidson, S. *op cit*, p 112

10. Pfeiffer, C. *Mental and Elemental Nutrients*. New Canaan, Ct: Keats Publ, 1975, p 272

11. Rodale, J. *The Complete Book of Minerals for Health*. Emmaus, Pa: Rodale Books, 1972, pp 661-662

12. Davidson, S. *op cit*, pp 115-116

13. Macy, I *Nutrition and Chemical Growth in Childhood I*. Springfield, Il: Charles C. Thomas, 1942, p 13

14. Williams, R. *Biochemical Individuality*. Austin, Tx: Univ Texas Press, 1955, p 137

15. Davidson, S. *op cit*, p 116

16. Cheraskin, E., Ringsdorf, Wm, with Brecher, A. *Psychodietetics*. New York: Bantam Books, 1974, pp 87-88

17. Crosby, Wm. Lead-Contaminated Health Food. *JAMA 237*: 2627-2629, 1977

18. Schroeder, H. *The Poisons Around Us*. Bloomington, In: University Press, 1974, p 51

19.   *Ibid*, p 56
20.   *Ibid*, p 56
21.   Lin-Fu, J. Undue absorption of lead among children—a new look at an old problem. *New J Eng Med 186*: 702-710, 1972
22.   Schroeder, H. *op cit*, p 43
23.   *Ibid*, p 55
24.   Ashmead, H. Ecology, chelation, and animal experimentation. *J App Nutr 24*: 11, 1972
25.   Schroeder, H. *op cit*, p 41
26.   Chattopadhyay, A. and Jervis, R. Hair as an indicator of multi-element exposure of population groups. in *Trace Substances in Environmental Health VII*. Edited by Hemphill, D. Columbia, Mo: Univ of Missouri, 1974, p 36
27.   Underwood, E. *op cit*, p 413
28.   Holmes, H. *et al*. Effects of vitamin C on lead poisoning. *J Lab Clin Med 24*: 1126, 1939
29.   Clarke, N. Atherosclerosis, occlusive vascular disease and EDTA. *Am J Card 6*: 233-235, 1960
30.   Hambidge, K. Chromium nutrition in man. *Am J Clin Nutr 27*: 505-514, 1974
31.   Schroeder, H. *The Trace Elements and Man*. Old Greenwich, Ct: Devin-Adair, 1973, p 72
32.   Schroeder, H. *The Poisons Around Us*. p 126
33.   *Ibid*
34.   Underwood, E. *op cit*, p 267
35.   Hambidge, K. *op cit*, 504-514
36.   Schroeder, H. *The Trace Elements and Man*. p 63
37.   Hambidge, K. *op cit*, pp 505-514
38.   Shrader, R. *et al*. Pancreatic pathology in manganese deficient guinea pigs. *J Nutr 94*: 269-281, 1968
39.   Rubenstein, A. *et al*, Manganese-induced hypoglycaemia. *Lancet*, Dec 1962, pp 1348-1351
40.   Randall, G., Schulte, R., and Corey, R. Correlation of plant manganese with extractable soil manganese and soil factors. *Soil Sci Soc Am J 40*: 282-287
41.   Sauchelli, V. *Trace Elements in Agriculture*. New York: Van Nostrand Reinhold, 1969, p 226
42.   Underwood, E. *op cit*, pp 177-178
43.   *Ibid*, p 180
44.   *Ibid*, p 190
45.   Kunin, R., Manganese and niacin in the treatment of drug-induced dyskinesias in *Literature Survey of Selected Articles on Hair Analysis. Vol II*, Hayward, Ca: Mineralab, 1976
46.   Pfeiffer, C. *op cit*, p 255
47.   Pfeiffer, C. Iliev, V., and Goldstein, L. Blood histamine, basophil counts, and trace elements in the schizophrenias in *Orthomolecular Psychiatry*. Edited by Hawkins, D. and Pauling, L., San Francisco: W. H. Freeman, 1973, p 504

48.   *Ibid*
49.   Leeser, O. and Boyd, L. *Textbook of Homeopathic Materia Medica.* Philadelphia, Pa: Boericke and Tafel, 1935, pp 796-699
50.   Boericke, Wm. *Pocket Manual of Homeopathic Materia Medica.* New York: Boericke and Runyon, 1927   pp 683-684
51.   Pfeiffer, C. in *Orthomolecular Psychiatry*, p 499
52.   Pinto, O., and Huggin, H. Mercury poisoning in America. *J Intern Acad Prev Med 3*: 42-58, 1976
53.   Peterson, R. *et al*, Interrelationship of dietary silver with copper in the chick. *Poultry Sci 54*: 771-774, 1975
54.   Leeser, O. and Boyd, L. *op cit*, p 800
55.   Pfeiffer, C. *Mental and Elemental Nutrients.* pp 167-398
56.   Pfeiffer, C. in *Orthomolecular Psychiatry* p 489
57.   O'Dell, B. *et al*, Connective tissue defect in the chick resulting from copper deficiency. *Proc Soc Exp Biol Med 108*: 402-405, 1961
58.   Kelly, W., Kesterson, J. and Carlton, N. Myocardial lesions in the offspring of female rats fed a copper deficient diet. *Exp Molec Patho 20*: 40-56, 1974
59.   Isaacs, J. *et al*, Trace metals, vitamins and hormones in ten-year treatment of coronary atherosclerotic heart disease. Paper delivered at Texas Heart Instit Symp. on Coronary Artery Med and Surg., Houston, Tx, Feb 1974, p 3
60.   Underwood, E. *op cit*, p 71
61.   *Ibid* p. 219
62.   Michaelsson, G. *et al*, Effects of oral zinc and vitamin A in acne. *JAMA 237*: 401, 1977
63.   Underwood, E. *op cit*, p 232
64.   *Ibid*, p 218
65.   Pfeiffer, C., *Mental and Elemental Nutrients* p 231
66.   Underwood, E. *op cit*, p 213
67.   Prasad, A. Zinc deficiency in man. *Am J Dis Child 130*: 359-361, 1976
68.   Pfeiffer, C. *Mental and Elemental Nutrients.* pp 238-241
69.   Underwood, E. *op cit*, p 197
70.   Sauchelli, V. *op cit*, p 120
71.   Keefer, R. and Singh, R. Influence of soil characteristics and fertilizer treatments on trace element composition of sweet corn grain. Morgantown, WV: West Virginia Univ, Agr. Exp. State. Scientific Paper, no. 1117, 1977
72.   Underwood, E., *op cit*, p 229
73.   Hambidge, K. *et al*, Low levels of zinc in hair, anorexia, poor growth, and hypogenesis children. *Pediat Res 6*: 868, 1972
74.   Underwood, E. *op cit*, p 217
75.   Battistone, G. The effect of zinc injected as salt or chelate on bone healing in guinea pigs in *Trace Substances in Environmental Health IV*, Proc Univ No 4th Ann Conf on Trace Subst in Environ Hlth., Edited by Hemphill, D. Columbia, Mo: Univ of Mo, 1971, p 266
76.   Reinhold, J. Phytate destruction by yeast fermentation in whole

wheat meals. *J Am Diet Assn 66*: 38, 1975

77.   *Ibid*
78.   Buell, G. Some biological aspects of cadmium toxicology. *J Occup Med 17*: 193, 1975
79.   Schroeder, H. *op cit*, p 62
80.   Perry, H. Jr., and Erlanger, M. Metal-induced hypertension following chronic feeding of low doses of cadmium and mercury. *J Lab Clin Med*, April 1974, pp 541-457
81.   Schroeder, H. *et al*, Action of a chelate of zinc on trace metals in hypertensive rats. *Am J Phys 214*: 796-800, 1968
82.   Schroeder, H. Cadmium as a factor in hypertension. *J Chronic Dis 18*: 647-656, 1965
83.   Carroll, R. The relationship of cadmium in the air to cardiovascular disease death rates, *JAMA 198*: 267-269, 1966
84.   Schroeder, H. Relation between mortality from cardiovascular disease and treated water supplies. *JAMA 172*: 1902-1908, 1960
85.   Underwood, E. *op cit*, p 248
86.   Buell, G. *op cit*, pp 189-195
87.   Morgan, J. 'Normal' lead and cadmium content of the human kidney. *Arch Environ Hlth 24*: 364-368, 1972
88.   Syversen, T., *et al*, Cadmium and zinc in human liver and kidney. *Scand J Clin Lab Invest 36*: 251, 1976
89.   Buell, G. *op cit*, pp 189-195
90.   Underwood, E. *op cit*, p 251
91.   Buell, G. *op cit*, p 192
92.   *Ibid*, pp 189-195
93.   Der. R., *et al*, Environmental interaction of lead and cadmium on reproduction and metabolism of male rats. in *Trace substances in Environmental Health X*. Edited by Hemphill, D., Columbia, Mo: Univ of Mo, 1976, pp 505-517
94.   Shakman, R. Nutritional influences on the toxicity of environmental pollutants. *Arch Environ Hlth 28*: 105-113, 1974
95.   Underwood, E. *op cit*, p 250
96.   *Ibid*, p 251
97.   Hadjimarkos, D. The role of selenium in dental caries. in *Trace Substances in Environmental Health IV*, 1971, p 301
98.   Kilness, A., and Hochberg, F. Amyotrophic lateral sclerosis in a high selenium environment. *JAMA 237*: 2843-2844, 1977
99.   Sauchelli, V. *op cit*, p 45
100. Underwood, E. *op cit*, p 37
101. *Ibid*, pp 25-26
102. *Ibid*, p 26
103. *Ibid*, p 25
104. Ashmead, D., The need for chelated trace minerals, in *Vet Med*, April 1974, pp 467-468
105. Pfeiffer, C. *Mental and Elemental Nutrients.* pp 250-251
106. Underwood, E. *op cit*, p 46
107. Kempner, W. Treatment of hypertensive vascular disease with rice

diet. *Am J Med 4*: 545-577, 1948
108. Mitchell, H. *Nutrition and Climatic Stress.* Springfield, Il: Charles C. Thomas, 1951, p 92-93
109. Davidson, S. *op cit*, p 98
110. More proof of salt-hypertension link. *JAMA 237*:1305,1307-08, 1977
111. Dahl, L. Salt and hypertension. *Am J Clin Nutr 25*: 231-244, 1972
112. More proof of salt-hypertension link. *JAMA 237*: 1305, 1397-1308, 1977
113. Boles, R. Rice, D, *et al*, Conservative management of Meniere's disease: Furstenberg regimen revisited. *Ann Otol Rhino Laryn 84*: 513-517, 1975
114. Rodale, J. *The Complete Book of Minerals for Health.* Emmaus, Pa: Rodale Books, 1976, p 143
115. Meneely, G. *Qualitas Plantarum—Plant Foods for Human Nutrition 23*: 3-31, 1973
116. Meneely, G., and Battarbee, H. *Present Knowledge in Nutrition.* New York: The Nutrition Foundation, 1976, p 259-279
117. Hutner, S., Inorganic nutrition. *Ann Rev Microbiol 26*: 132, 313-338, 1972
118. Gerson, M. *A Cancer Therapy—Result of 50 Cases.* Del Mar, Ca: Totality Books, 1975
119. Rodale, J. *op cit*, p 124
120. Sauer, H. *et al*, Associations between drinking water and death rates. in *Trace Substances in Environmental Health IV*, 1971, p 318
121. Cameron, W. Trace element toxicity associated with a public water supply. in *Trace Substances in Environmental Health X.* 1976, p 25
122. Costain, Wm. The action of fluorides. *Canad Med Assn J 181*: 954, 1959
123. Schroeder, H. *The Trace Elements in Man.* p 15
124. Yiamouyiannis J. and Burk, D. Fluoridation and cancer: Age-dependence of cancer mortality related to artificial fluoridation. *Fluoride 10*: 102-123, 1977
125. Leeser, O. *Textbook of Homeopathic Materia Medica.* Philadelphia, Pa: Boericke & Tafel, 1935, p 724
126. Shakman, R. Nutritional influences on the toxicity of environmental pollutants. *Arch Environ Hlth 28*: 105-113, 1974
127. Ershoff, B. Antitoxic effects of plant fiber. *Am J Clin Nutr 27*: 1395-1398, 1974
128. Warren, H. *et al*, Variations in the copper, zinc, lead and molybdenum content of some British Columbia vegetables. in *Trace Substances in Environmental Health IV, 1971, pp 94-104*
129. Underwood, E. *op cit*, p 465
130. Warren, H. Medical geology and geography. *Science 23*: 536, 1965
131. Keefer, R., and Singh, R. Influence of soil characteristics and fertilizer treatments on trace element composition of sweet corn grain. WV: Univ Agr Exp Stat, Scientific paper no. 1117, pp 20-28
132. Hutner, S., Inorganic nutrition. *Ann Rev Microbiol 26*: 317, 1972
133. Underwood, E. *op cit*, p 207

CHAPTER 9

1. Katz, L. *et al, Nutrition and Atherosclerosis.* Philadelphia, Pa: Lea and Febiger, 1958, pp 16-20
2. Davis, Adelle, *Let's Eat Right to Keep Fit.* New York: New American Library, 1954, pp 273-303
3. *Nutrition Almanac,* New York: McGraw Hill, 1973
4. Davidson, Sir Stanley, *et al, Human Nutrition and Dietetics.* New York: Churchill Livingstone, 1975
5. Davis, A. *op cit,* p 275
6. Watt, B. and Merrill, A. *Composition of Foods.* USDA Agricultural Handbook no 8, New York: Dover, 1975, p 421

CHAPTER 10

1. Ganong, W. *Review of Medical Physiology.* 7th ed., Los Altos, Ca: Lange, 1975, p 356
2. Osborn, N., Noriskin, J., and Staz, J. A comparison of crude and refined sugar and cereals in their ability to produce in vitro decalcification of teeth. *J Dent Res 16:* 165-171, 1937
3. *Dental,* U.S. Dept. HEW, Publ, no. (HSM) 72-8132, Vol III, p 89
4. Adams, R., and Murray, F., *Minerals: Kill or Cure?* New York: Larchmont, 1974, pp 27-28
5. Newbold, H. *Mega-Nutrients for Your Nerves.* New York: Peter H. Wyden, 1975, p 201
6. Pavlov, I., *The Work of the Digestive Glands.* Transl by Thompson, W., 2nd ed., London: Charles Griffin & Co, 1910
7. Davidson, Sir Stanley, *et al, Human Nutrition and Dietetics.* 6th ed., New York: Churchill Livingstone, 1975, p 629
8. Davenport, H. *Physiology of the Digestive Tract.* 4th ed., Chicago, Il: Year Book Medical Publ, 1977, p 225
9. Williams R. *Biochemical Individuality.* Austin Tx: Univ of Texas, 1956, pp 60-61
10. Felber, J, *et al,* Modulation by food, of hormonal system regulating rat pancreatic secretion. *Lancet,* July 1974, p 185-187
11. Pavlov, I, *op cit*
12. Hepner, G. Altered bile acid metabolism in vegetarians. *Dig Dis 20:* 398, 1975
13. Mott, G. *et al,* Lovering of serum cholesterol by intestinal bacteria in cholesterol-fed piglets. *Lipids 8:* 478-481, 1973

CHAPTER 11

1. Davenport, H. *Physiology of the Digestive Tract.* 4th ed., 1977, Chicago, Il: Year Book Medical Publ, 1961
2. Coates, M. The influence of the gut microflora on the nutrition of its host. *Biblthca Nutr Dieta 22:* 101–108, 1974

3. Clarke, J. *et al*, Bacteriology of the gut and its clinical implications. *West J Med 121*: 390-403, 1974
4. Coates, M. *op cit*, p 101
5. Hill, M. and Drasar, B. The normal colonic bacterial flora. *Gut 16*: 318-323, 1975
6. *Ibid*, p 319
7. Moore, W., and Holdeman, L. Discussion of current bacteriological investigations of the relationships between intestinal flora, diet, and color cancer. *Cancer Res 35*: 3418-3420, 1975
8. Coates, M. *op cit*, p 101
9. Luckey, R. Bicentennial overview of intestinal microecology. *Am J Clin Nutr 30*: 1753-1761, 1977
10. Cummings, J. The colon: absorptive, secretory and metabolic functions. *Digestion 13*: 232-240, 1975
11. Cummings, J. Absorption and secretion by the colon. *Gut 16*: 323-329, 1975
12. Cummings, J. *Digestion 13*: 232-240, 1975
13. Onderdonk, A. *et al*, The role of the intestinal microflora in experimental colitis. *Am J Clin Nutr 30*: 1819-1825, 1977
14. Davenport, H. *op cit*, p 255
15. Cummings, J., *Digestion 13*: 232-249, 1975
16. Davenport, H. *op cit*, p 253
17. Levitt, M. *et al*, Hydrogen catabolism in the colon of the rat. *J Lab Clin Med 184*: 163-167, 1974
18. Coates, M. *op cit*, pp 101-108
19. Neale, G. *et al*, The metabolic and nutritional consequences of bacterial overgrowth in the small intestine. *Am J Clin Nutr 25*: 1409-1417, 1972
20. Clarke, J. *op cit*, pp 390-403
21. Haenel, H. Human normal and abnormal gastrointestinal flora. *Am J Clin Nutr 23*: 1433-1439, 1970
22. Clarke, J. *op cit*, pp 390-403
23. Neale, G. *op cit*, pp 1409-1417
24. *Ibid*
25. Luckey, T. Bicentiennial overview of intestinal microecology. *Am J Clin Nutr 30*: 1753-1761, 1977
26. Coates, M. *op cit*, pp 101-108
27. Clarke, J. *op cit*, pp 390-403
28. Levitt, M. Production and excretion of hydrogen gas in man. *New Eng J Med 281*: 122-127, 1969
29. Abrams, G. Microbial effects on mucosal structure and function. *Am J Clin Nutr 30*: 1880-1886, 1977
30. Hill, M. and Drasar, B. The normal colonic bacterial flora. *Gut 16*: 318-323, 1975
31. Moore, W., and Holdeman, L. Discussion of current bacteriological investigations of the relationships between intestinal flora, diet and colon cancer. *Cancer Res 35*: 3418-3420, 1975
32. Hill, M. *op cit*, pp 318-323

33. Moore, W., and Holdeman, L. *op cit*, pp 3418-3420
34. *Ibid*
35. Dubos, R., and Schaedler, R., Some biological effects of the digestive flora. *Am J Med Sci 244*: 265-271, 1962
36. Speck, M. Interactions among lactobacilli and man. *J Dairy Sci 59*: 338-343, 1976
37. Haenel, H. *op cit*, p 1433-1439
38. Dubos, R., Russell, W., Schaedler, R., Costello, R. and Hoet, P. Indigenous, normal and autochthonous flora of the gastrointestinal tract. *J Exp Med 122*: 67-75, 1965
39. A funny thing happened on the way to get some yogurt.(editorial) *JAMA 182*: 1329-1330, 1962
40. Williams, R. *Nutrition Against Disease*. New York: Bantam Books, 1971, pp 299-300
41. Clarke, J. *op cit*, pp 390-403
42. Moore, W., and Holdeman, L. *op cit*, pp 3418-3420
43. Jones, I. Effects of processing by fermentation on nutrients. in *Nutritional Evaluation of Food Processing*. 2nd ed., Edited by Harris, R., and Karmas, E., Westport, Ct: AVI Publ, 1975, p 343
44. Aleksandrowicz, J. The potential role of mycotoxins and of trace elements in prophylaxis of leukemia. in *Trace Substances in Environmental Health X*. Edited by Hemphill, D., Columbus, Mo: Univ of Missouri, 1976, pp 133-135
45. Clarke, J. *op cit*, pp 390-403
46. Seneca, H., Henderson, E., and Collins, A. Bactericidal properties of yogurt. *Am Pract Digest Treatm 1*: 1252-1259, 1950
47. Wang, H., Ruttle, D., and Hesseltine, C. Antibacterial compound from a soybean product fermented by rhizopus oligosporus. *Proc Soc Exp Bio Med 131*: 579-583, 1969
48. Mott, G., Moore, R., Redmond H., Reiser, R. Lowering of serum cholesterol by intestinal bacteria in cholesterol-fed piglets. *Lipids 8*: 428-431, 1973
49. Forbes, M., Park, J., and Lev, M. Role of the intestinal flora in the growth response of chicks to dietary penicillin. *Ann NY Acad Sci 78*: 321-327, 1959
50. Van der Waaij, D., *et al*. Reconventionalization following antibiotic decontamination in man and animals. *Am J Clin Nutr 30*: 1887-1895, 1977
51. Hill, M., and Drasar, B. *op cit*, pp 318-323
52. Davenport, H., *op cit*, p 255
53. Ershoff, B. Antitoxic effects of plant fiber. *Am J Clin Nutr 27*: 1395-1398, 1974
54. Clarke, J. *op cit*, pp 390-403
55. Mendeloff, A. A critique of fiber deficiency. *Digest Dis 21*: 109-112, 1976
56. Symposium on Nutrition in the Causation of Cancer. *Cancer Res 35*: Nov 1975
57. Reddy, B., and Weisburger, J. Effects of high risk and low risk diets

for colon carcinogenesis on fecal microflora and steroids in man. *J Nutr 105*: 878-884, 1975

58. Vijayagopalan, P., and Kurup, P. Effect of dietary starches on the serum, aorta and hepatic lipid levels in cholesterol-fed rats. *Atherosclero 11*: 257-264, 1970

59. Williams, R. *Nutrition Against Disease.*New York: Bantam Books, 1971, p 260

60. Jenkins, D. *et al*, Effect of pectin, guar, gum and wheat fiber on serum-cholesterol. *Lancet*, May 1975, pp 1116-1117

61. Vijayagopalan, P., *et al*, Fiber content of different dietary starches and their effect on lipid levels in high fat-high cholesterol diet fed rats. *Artheroscler 17*: 156-160, 1973

62. Davenport. H. *op cit*, p 255

63. Ershoff, B. *op cit*, pp 1395-1398

64. Ornstein, R. *The Psychology of Consciousness*. New York: Penguin Books, 1972

65. Swami Rama, *et al. Yoga and Psychotherapy*. Glenview, Il: Himalayan Institute, 1976

CHAPTER 12

1. *The Essene Gospel of Peace.*. Transl by Szekely, E.B., San Diego, Ca: Academy of Creative Living, 1971, p 20

2. Null, G., and Staff, S. *The Complete Question and Answer Book of General Nutrition.* New York: Dell, 1972

3. Luckey, T. Bicentennial overview of institutional microecology. *Am J. Clin Nutr 30*: 1753-1761, 1977

4. Savage, D. Interactions between the host and its microbes. in *Microbiology of the Gut.* Edited by Clarke, R., and Bauchop, T., New York: Academic Press, 1977, pp 277-310

5. Luckey, T. *op cit*, pp 1753-1761

6. Crohn, B., and Drosd, R. Halitosis. *JAMA 117*: 2242-2245, 1941

7. Davenport, H. *Physiology of the Digestive Tract.* 4th ed., Chicago, Il: Year Book Medical Publ, 1977, p 253

8. Abrams, G. Microbial effects of mucosal structure and function. *Am J Clin Nutr 30*: 1880-1886, 1977

CHAPTER 13

1. Fassett, D. Oxalates. in *Toxicants Occurring Naturally in Foods. Washington, D.C.: National Academy* of Sciences, 1973, p 359

2. Davidson, Sir Stanley, *et al, Human Nutrition and Dietetics.* 6th ed., New York: Churchill Livingstone, 1975, p 215

3. Van Veen, A. Toxic properties of certain unusual foods. in *Toxicants Occurring Naturally in Foods, pp 495-502*

4. Davidson, S. *op cit*, p 274

5. Aykroyd, W., and Doughty, J. *Legumes in Human Nutrition*. Rome: FAO of the U.N., 1964

6. Liener, I. Protease inhibitors and hemagglutinins of legumes. in *Evaluation of Proteins for Humans.* Edited by Bodwell, C., Westport, Ct: AVI Publ, 1977, pp 296-297

7. *Ibid*, p 300

8. Aykroyd, W. *op cit* p 65-66

9. Lee, F. *Basic Food Chemistry.* Westport, Ct: AVI Publ, 1975, pp 307-308

10. Singleton, V., and Kratzer, F. Plant phenolics. in *Toxicants Occurring Naturally in Foods.* pp 309-345

11. Williams, R. *Biochemical Individuality.* Austin, Tx: Univ. of Texas Press, 1956, p 108

12. *Ibid*

13. Coon, J. Natural food toxicants—a perspective. in *Present Knowledge in Nutrition.* 4th ed., New York: The Nutrition Foundation, 1976, p 530

14. Bordia, A., *et al*, Effect of the essential oils of garlic and onion on alimentary hyperlipemia. *Atheroscler 21*: 15-19, 1975

15. Lee, F. *op cit*, p 334

16. Ritchie, J. Central nervous system stimulants, II The xanthines. in *Pharmacological Basis of Therapeutics.* 4th ed., Edited by Goodman, L., and Gilman, A., London: Macmillan, 1970, p 359

17. Grieve, M. *A Modern Herbal.* Vol II, New York: Dover, pp 597-598

18. Meyer, C. *American Folk Medicine.* New York: The New American Library, 1973, p 261

19. *Ibid*, p 300

20. Bodel, P., Cotran, R. and Kass, E., Cranberry juice and the antibacterial action of hippuric acid. *J Lab Clin Med 54*: 881-888, 1959

21. Townsend, J., and Luckey, T. Hormoligosis in pharmacology. *JAMA 173*: 128-132, 1960

22. Luckey, T. Hormology as the scientific basis of Homeopathy. *J Am Inst of Homeop 69*: 220-237

23. Albrecht, Wm. Mycorrhiza VII: Proteins, amino acids and benzene rings. *Let's Live*, Sept-Oct 1964, pp 42-43

24. Luckey, T. Insecticide hormoligosis. *J Econ Entomol 61*: 7-12, 1968

25. Zwerdling, D. The pesticide treadmill. *Nat Pks and Conserv Mag*, Sept 1977, p 17

26. Coon, J. *op cit*, p 536

27. Garard, I. *The Story of Food.* Westport, Ct: AVI Publ, 1974 pp 69-70

28. *Ibid*, p 73

29. Sinclair, Upton *The Jungle.* New York: Doubleday & Co., 1906, p 131

30. Garard, I. *op cit*, p 100

31. *Ibid*, pp 68-106

32. Corbett, T. *Cancer and Chemicals.* Chicago, Il: Nerson-Hall, Sept 1977, p 65

33. BHT: Weighing the Benefits and Risks. *Nutrition Action.* Sept 1977, pp 6-7

34. Feingold, B. *Why Your Child is Hyperactive.* New York: Random House, 1974
35. Report to the Nutrition Foundation. Nat Adv Comm on Hyperkinesis and Food Additives, New York: Nutrition Foundation, 1975
36. Food additives and hyperactivity. *Science 199:* 516, 1978
37. Selander, P. Carrot soup in the treatment of infantile diarrhea. *J Pediat 30:* 742, 1950
38. Coon, J. *op cit,* pp 530-531

CHAPTER 14

1. Tobe, J. *How to Conquer Arthritis.* St. Catherine's Ont: Provoker Press, 1976
2. Douglass, J. and Rasgon, I. Diet and diabetes. *Lancet,* Dec 1976, p 1306 (letter)
3. Davidson, Sir Stanley, *et al Human Nutrition and Dietetics.* 6th ed., New York: Churchill Livingstone, 1975, p 255
4. Vaughan, D. Processing effects in *Evaluation of Proteins for Humans.* Edited by Bodwell, C., Westport, Ct: AVI Publ, 1977, p 255
5. *Ibid,* pp 255-269
6. Jensen, L. *Man's Foods.* Champaign, Il: The Garrard Press, 1953, p 7
7. *Ibid,* pp 7-8
8. *Ibid,* p 8
9. Wrench, G. *The Wheel of Health,* New York: Schocken Books, 1972, p 139
10. Haagen-Smit, A.J. Smell and taste. *Sci Am 186:* 28-32, 1952

CHAPTER 15

1. *Charaka Samhita.* Jamnagar, India: Shree Gulabkunverba Ayurvedic Soc, 1949
2. *Sushruta Samhita,* Translated by Dhishagratna, K. Benares, India: Chowkhamba Sanskrit Studies, 1963
3. Steggerda, F. Richards, E., and Rackis, J. Effects of various soybean products on flatulence in the adult man. *Proc Soc Exp Biol Med 121:* 1235-1239, 1966

CHAPTER 16

1. Davidson, Sir Stanley, *et al Human Nutrition and Dietetics.* New York: Churchill Livingston, 1975, p 240
2. Latham, M. *Planning and Evaluation of Applied Nutrition Programmes.* Rome: FAO of the U.N., 1972, p 58
3. Jones, I. Effects of processing by fermentation on nutrients. in *Nutritional Evaluation of Food Processing.* 2nd ed., Edited by Harris, R., and Karmas, E., Westport, Ct: AVI Publ, 1975, p 339
4. *Ibid*
5. Possible effects of aflatoxin consumption by man in *Food Cosmet*

Toxicol 14: 151-152, 1976

6. Lee, F. *Basic Food Chemistry.* Westport, Ct: AVI Publ, 1975, p 104
7. Some kitchen experiments with aluminum. *Lancet,* Jan 1913, pp 54-55
8. Underwood, E. *Trace Elements in Human and Animal Nutrition,* New York: Academic Press, 1977, p 432
9. Some kitchen experiments with aluminum. *Lancet,* Jan 1913, pp 54-55
10. Lewis, S. The assimilation of aluminum by the human system. *Biochem J 25*: 2162-2167, 1931
11. Mayer, J. *A Diet for Living.* New York: David McKay Co, 1972, p 208
12. Diamant, Wm. and Gamertoglio, J. Aluminum intoxication. *New Eng J Med 294*: 1129-1131, 1976 (letter)
13. Lee, R. The effect of aluminum compounds in foods. Milwaukee, Wi: Lee Found for Nutr Res, Oct 1946, pp 62-69
14. Diamant, Wm., and Gamertoglio, J. *op cit*, pp 1129-1131
15. Ulmer, D. Toxicity from aluminum antacids. *New Eng J Med 294*: 219, 1976
16. Sherrard, D. The myth of aluminum toxicity. *New Eng J Med 290*: 750, 1974 (letter)
17. Alfrey, A. *et al*, The dialysis encephalopathy syndrome. *New Eng J Med 294*: 184-188, 1976
18. Berlyne, G., *et al*. Aluminum toxicity in rats. *Lancet 1*: 564-567, 1972
19. Alfrey, A. and Kaehhy, W. *New Eng J Med 294*: 1131, 1976 (letter)
20. James, C. Medical report on aluminum poisoning, *Brit Med J.* April 1932, p 686
21. Tchijevsky, A. and Tchijevskaya, J. Aluminum as a factor contributing to the rise and progress of different pathologic processes in the organism. *Acta Medica Scand 83*: 501-505, 1934
22. Karel, M., and Heidelbaugh, N. Effects of packaging on nutrients. in *Nutritional Evaluation of Food Processing,* p 430
23. Davidson, S. *op cit*, p 256
24. Lachance, P. Effects of preparation and service of food on nutrients. in *Nutritional Evaluation of Food Processing,* p 499
25. Aykroyd, W., and Doughty, J. *Wheat in Human Nutrition.* Rome: FAO of the U.N., 1970, p 35
26. *Charaka Samhita.* Jamnagar, India, 1949, Vol II, Shree Gulabkunverba Ayurvedic Society, Sutrashana 25: 39, p 407
27. Williams, R. *Nutrition Against Disease.* New York: Bantam Books, 1971, p 298-299
28. Davidson, S. *op cit*, p 243
29. Grieve, M. *A Modern Herbal.* Vol 1, New York: Dover, 1971, p 253
30. Mathur, K., Khan, M., and Sharma, R. Hypocholesterolaemic effect of Bengal gram: a long-term study in man. *Brit Med J 1*: 30-31, 1968
31. Luyken, R. *et al*, The influence of legumes on the serum cholesterol level. *Voeding 23*: 447, 1962
32. Kervran, L. *Biological Transmutations.* Binghamton, NY: Swan

House, 1972, p 104-105

33.   Davidson, S. *op cit*, p 256

CHAPTER 17

1.   Newbold, H. *Mega-Nutrients for Your Nerves*. New York: Peter H. Wyden, 1975, p 70
2.   Crapo, P. Reaven, G. and Olefsky, J. Plasma glucose and insulin responses to orally administered simple and complex carbohydrates. *Diabetes 25*: 741-747, 1976
3.   Palm, J. *Diet Away Your Stress, Tension, and Anxiety*. New York: Pocket Books, 1977, pp 222-234
4.   Cahill, G. and Soeldner, J. A non-editorial on non-hypoglycemia. *New Eng J Med 291*: 905-906, 1974
5.   Orthomolecular Psychiatry. Edited by Hawkins, D. and Pauling, L. San Francisco, Ca: W. H. Freeman 1973, p 449
6.   Ogden, E. The abused liver. *Brit Homeop J 63*: 130-134, 1974
7.   Davenport, H. *Physiology of the Digestive Tract*. Chicago, Il: Year Book Medical Publ, 1977, p 184
8.   Cleave, T. *The Saccharine Disease*. New Canaan, Ct: Keats Publ, 1975, p 147
9.   Davenport, H. *op cit*, p 184
10.   *Ibid*, p 82
11.   Swami Rama *et al Yoga and Psychotherapy*. Glenview, Il: Himalayan Institute, 1976, pp 226-232
12.   Freedman, M., Rosenman, R., and Carroll, V. Changes in the serum cholesterol of blood clotting times in men subjected to cyclic variations of occupational stress. *Circ 18*: 852-861, 1958 quoted in Mind as Slayer, Mind as Healer. Pelletier, K. New York: Delta, 1977, p 90
13.   Liquid protein warning issued. *Am Med News*, Nov 4, 1977, p 11
14.   FDA Drug Bulletin 8: 2-4, 1978
15.   Hackler, R., In vitro indices: relationships to estimating protein value for the human. in *Evaluation of Proteins for Humans*. Edited by Bodwell, C., Westport, Ct: AVI Publ, 1977, p 61
16.   Stunkard, A. Obesity and the denial of hunger. *Psychosom Med 21*: p 281-289, 1959
17.   Stunkard, A. and Koch, C. The interpretation of gastric motility. *Arch Gen Psychiat 11*: 74-81, 1964
18.   Schachter, S. Obesity and eating. *Science 161*: 751-756, 1968,
19.   *Ibid*
20.   Thorpe, T. Effects of hatha yoga and meditation on anxiety and body image. in *Meditational Therapy*. Edited by Swami Ajaya, Glenview, Il: Himalayan Institute, 1977
21.   Johnson, M., Burke, B., and Mayer, J. Relative importance of inactivity and overeating in the energy balance of obese high school girls. *Am J Clin Nutr 4*: 37, 1956
22.   Williams, R. *Nutrition Against Disease*. New York: Bantam Books, 1971, p 106
23.   *Ibid*.

24.   Gerrard, D. *One Bowl.* New York: Random House, 1974

CHAPTER 18

1.   Cleckley, H. *et al.* Nicotinic acid in the treatment of atypical psy-
      chotic states. *JAMA 112*: 2107-2110, 1939
2.   *Ibid*
3   Hoffer, A. Mechanism of action of nicotinic acid and nicotinamide
      in the treatment of schizophrenia. in *Orthomolecular Psychiatry.*
      Edited by Hawkins, D., and Pauling, L. San Francisco, Ca: W. H.
      Freeman pp 202-278, 1973
4.   Spies. T. *et al.* The mental symptoms of pellagra. Their relief with
      nototinic acid. *Am J Med Sci 169*: 461-475, 1938
5.   Hoffer, A., *et al.* Treatment of schizophrenia with nicotinic acid and
      nicotinamide *J Clin Exp Psychopath* and   *Quart Rev Psychiat Nevr*
      18: 131-159, 1977
6.   Williams, R. *Biochemical Individuality.* Austin Tx: Univ of Texas,
      1956, p 153
7.   Pauling, L. Orthomolecular psychiatry. *Science 160*: 265-271, 1968
8.   Hoffer, A (Personal Communication) Jan, 1977
9.   Hoffer, A., in *Orthomolecular Psychiatry.* pp 202-203
10.   *Megavitamin and Orthomolecular Therapy in Psychiatry.* Report of
      the Am Psychiatr. Assn. task force on vitamin therapy in psychiatry.
      Washington, D.C.: Am. Psychiat. Assn., 1973
11.   *Ibid*
12.   Hoffer, A., and Osmond, H. *Megavitamin Therapy.* Reply to Am
      Psychiat. Assn. task force report on megavitamin and orthomolecular
      therapy in psychiatry. Regina, Saskatchewan: Canadian Schizophrenia
      Foundation, 1976
13.   Pauling, L. *et al.* Results of a loading test of ascorbic acid, niacinamide
      and pyridoxine in schizophrenic subjects and controls. in *Ortho-
      molecular Psychiatry,* pp 18-34
14.   Hoffer, J. Megavitamin treatment of schizophrenia. *Canad Psychiat
      Assn J 20*: 492-494, 1975
15.   Wittenborn, J. A search for responders to niacin supplementation.
      Arch Gen Psychiat 31: 547, 1974
16.   Pfeiffer, C. *Mental and Elemental Nutrients.* New Canaan, Ct: Keats
      Publ, 1975, p 112
17.   Stein, S. Some observations on pyridoxine and L-tryptophan in a
      neuropsychiatric medical regimen. *Ann NY Acad Sci 166*: 210, 1969
18.   Pfeiffer, C. *op cit*
19.   Williams, R. *op cit*, p 13-14
20.   Davenport, H. *Physiology of the Digestive Tract.* Chicago, Il: Year
      Book Medical Publ, 1977, pp 183-184
21.   Ellis, F., and Nasser, S. A pilot study of vitamin B_{12} in the treatment
      of tiredness. *Brit J Nutr 30*: 277-283, 1973
22.   Lucksch F. Vitamin C and schizophrenia. *Wien Klin Wochenschr 53*:
      1009, 1940, quoted in *Nutrition Against Disease*, Williams, R., New

York: Bantam Books, 1971, p 332

23. Herjanic, M. Ascorbic acid and schizophrenia. in *Orthomolecular Psychiatry.* pp 303-315
24. Pauling, L. *et al, op cit,* p 18
25. Herjanic, M. *op cit* pp 303-315
26. *Ibid*
27. Davidson, S. *et al, Human Nutrition and Dietetics.* New York: Churchill, Livingston, 1975, p 159
28. Vander Kamp, H. A biochemical abnormality in schizophrenia involving ascorbic acid. *Int J Neuro Psychiat 2*: 204-205, 1966
29. Herjanic, M. *op cit,* p 311
30. Roddis, L. *James Lind, Founder of Nautical Medicine.* New York, Ny: Henry Schuman, 1950, p 64
31. Davis, Adelle, *Let's Eat Right to Keep Fit.* New York: New Amer Lib 1954, p 68
32. Tenbergen, N. Ethology and stress diseases. *Science 185*: p 20-27, 1974
33. Klotz, S. Allergy screening consultation service to an inpatient psychiatric service. in *Clinical Ecology.* Edited by Dickey, L, Springfield, Il: Charles C. Thomas, 1976, p 715
34. Coca, A. *The Pulse Test.* New York: Lyle Stuart, 1956
35. Newbold, H., *Meganutrients for Your Nerves.* New York, Ny: Peter H. Wyden, 1975, p 47
36. Philpott, Wm. Allergy and ecology in orthomolecular psychiatry. in *Clinical Ecology*, p 735
37. Klotz, S. *op cit,* p 709
38. *Ibid*, pp 708-718
39. Randolph, T.G. Historical development of clinical ecology. in *Clinical Ecology.* pp 9-17
40. Stein, M., *et al,* Influence of brain and behavior on the immune systum. *Science 166*: 435-440, 1969
41. *Ibid*
42. Pelletier, K. *Mind as Healer, Mind as Slayer.* New York: Delta, 1977, p 65
43. Davidson, S. *op cit,* p 525
44. Rajalakshmi, R., Deodhar, A., and Ramakrishnan, C. *Acta Paediat 54*: 375-382, 1965
45. Rajalakshmi, R., Subbulakshmi, G., Ramakrishnan, C., Joshi, S. and Bhatt, R. Biosynthesis of ascorbic acid in human placenta. *Curr Sci 36*: 45-46, 1967

CHAPTER 19

1. *Charaka Samhita.* Jamnagar, India: Shree Gulabkunverba Ayurvedic Soc., 1949. Sutrasthana 5:3, Vol II, p 68
2. *Charaka*, Sutrasthana 27: 345, Vol II p 557
3. *Charaka*, Sutrasthana 7:36-37, Vol II pp 114-115
4. Alther, L. *Organic Farming on Trial. Nat Hist 81*: 23, 1972

5. Gerrard, D. *One Bowl.* New York: Random House, 1974
6. Williams, R. *Physician's Handbook of Nutritional Science.* Springfield, Il: Charles C. Thomas, 1975, pp 95-96

CHAPTER 20

1. Barnard, G. and Stevenson, J. Fresh evidence for a biophysical field in *Main Currents Mod Thought 24*: 115-122, 1968
2. Kervran, L. *Biological Transmutations.* Binghamton, NY: Swan House Publ, 1972
3. Kervran, L. *Transmutations A Faible Energie.* Paris: Librairie Maloine 1964
4. *Ibid*, p 16
5. *Ibid*
6. *Ibid*, p 18
7. Moyse.Respiration et Metabolisme Azote (de la Feuille), Edited by Hermann, 1950. Cited in *Biological Transmutations.* p 82
8. Kervran. L., *Biological Transmutations*, pp 27-28
9. *Ibid*, p 156
10. Foucault, M. *Les Mots et Les Choses.* Paris: Gallimard, 1966, p 7
11. Kervran, L. *Biological Transmutations*, p 52
12. Kervran. L. *Transmutations A Faible Energie*, p 68

Index

BOOKS PUBLISHED BY THE HIMALAYAN INSTITUTE

Living with the Himalayan Masters Spiritual Experiences of Swami Rama	Swami Ajaya (ed)
Yoga and Psychotherapy	Swami Rama, R. Ballentine, M.D., Swami Ajaya
Emotion to Enlightenment	Swami Rama, Swami Ajaya
Freedom from the Bondage of Karma	Swami Rama
Book of Wisdom,—Ishopanishad	Swami Rama
Lectures on Yoga	Swami Rama
Life Here and Hereafter	Swami Rama
Marriage, Parenthood and Enlightenment	Swami Rama
Meditation in Christianity	Swami Rama, et al.
Superconscious Meditation	Pandit U. Arya, Ph.D.
Philosophy of Hatha Yoga	Pandit U. Arya, Ph.D.
Yoga Psychology	Swami Ajaya
Psychology East and West	Swami Ajaya (ed)
Foundations, Eastern & Western Psychology	Swami Ajaya (ed)
Meditational Therapy	Swami Ajaya (ed)
Diet and Nutrition	R. M. Ballentine, M.D.
Theory and Practice of Meditation	R. M. Ballentine, M.D.(ed)
Science of Breath	R. M. Ballentine, M.D. (ed)
Joints and Glands Exercises	R. M. Ballentine, M.D. (ed)
Yoga and Christianity	Justin O'Brien, Ph.D.
Faces of Meditation	S.N. Agnihotri, Justin O'Brien (ed)
Art and Science of Meditation	L. K. Misra, Ph.D. (ed)
Swami Rama of the Himalayas	L. K. Misra, Ph.D. (ed)
Science Studies Yoga	James Funderburk, Ph.D.
Homeopathic Remedies	D. Anderson, M.D., D. Buegel, M.D., D. Chernin, M.D.
Hatha Yoga Manual I	Samskrti and Veda
The Swami and Sam	Brandt Dayton
Himalayan Mountain Cookery	Mrs. R. Ballentine, Sr.
Chants from Eternity	
Thought for the Day	
Spiritual Diary	
The Yoga Way Cookbook	